CRITICAL CARE INTERDISCIPLINARY OUTCOME PATHWAYS

Kimberley A. Rutherford Basham, ARNP, MSN, CS, CCRN

President
Healing Matters
Louisville, Kentucky

Vickie A. Samuels Miracle, EdD, RN, CCRN

Senior Clinical Coordinator
Jewish Hospital Heart and Lung Institute
Louisville, Kentucky

W.B. SAUNDERS COMPANY

A Division of Harcourt Brace & Company
Philadelphia   London   Toronto   Montreal   Sydney   Tokyo

W. B. SAUNDERS COMPANY

A Division of Harcourt Brace & Company

The Curtis Center
Independence Square West
Philadelphia, Pennsylvania 19106

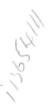

Library of Congress Cataloging-in-Publication Data

RT 120.I5   C735   1988
    Critical care interdisciplinary outcome pathways / Kimberley A.
Rutherford Basham, Vickie Ann Samuels Miracle. — 1st ed.
      p. cm.
    ISBN 0-7216-7373-2
    1. Intensive care nursing—Decision making. 2. Critical path analysis.
I. Miracle, Vickie Ann Samuels. II Title.
    [DNLM: 1. Critical pathways—organization & administration. 2. Critical
Care—organization & administration. 3. Treatment Outcome.
WX 162 B299c 1998]
610.73'61—DC21
DNLM/DLC
                                    98-5490

CRITICAL CARE INTERDISCIPLINARY OUTCOME PATHWAYS   ISBN 0-7216-7373-2

Printed in the United States of America

Last digit is the print number: 9   8   7   6   5   4   3   2   1

CRITICAL CARE INTERDISCIPLINARY OUTCOME PATHWAYS

This book is dedicated to my special family. To Morris, my husband—Thank you for believing in me! I could not have done this without your constant love and support. To my precious children—Erin and Greg—Thanks for all of your patience when Mom was glued to the computer! I love you both very much.

K.A.R.B.

To my wonderful and supportive husband, David, and our daughter, Jennifer. I could not have taken on a project of this magnitude without your love, support, and patience. Thank you.

V.A.S.M.

Reviewers

Terry Chambliss, MHS, PT
Assistant Professor of Physical Therapy
University of Evansville
Evansville, Indiana

Diane G. Jusekelis, MS, RD, LD, CNSD
Mercy Hospital Medical Center
Des Moines, Iowa

Patricia A. Kelly, RN, CS-FNP, CCRN, CEN
Brookville, Ohio

Reita S. Keyes, PhD
Mississippi College School of Nursing
Clinton, Mississippi

Jackie B. Lewis, RN
Methodist Alliance Home Care
Memphis, Tennessee

Carole Thompson, PhD, RN, CCRN, CS
College of Nursing
University of Tennessee, Memphis
Memphis, Tennessee

Laura L. Wood, MSN, CNA
McFaul & Lyons, Inc.
Trenton, New Jersey

Contributors

Kimberley A. Rutherford Basham, ARNP, MSN, CS, CCRN
President
Healing Matters
Louisville, Kentucky

"Congestive Heart Failure" / "Myocardial Infarction" / "Acute Respiratory Failure" / "Chronic Obstructive Pulmonary Disease" / "Chronic Ventilator-Dependent Patients" / "Pneumonia" / "Pulmonary Embolism" / "Gastrointestinal Bleeding" / "Acute Head Injury" / "Acute Renal Failure" / "Endstage Renal Disease/Kidney Transplantation" / "Adrenal Crisis" / "Disseminated Intravascular Coagulation" / "Sepsis/Systemic Inflammatory Response Syndrome" / "Coronary Artery Bypass Grafting" (Patient Education Outcome Pathway) / "Pneumonia" (Patient Education Outcome Pathway)

Therese Beatty, RN, BSN
Clinical Nurse Specialist
St. Jude Medical, Pacesetter Division
Louisville, Kentucky

"Pacemakers" (Patient Education Outcome Pathway)

Mary S. Carroll, RN, BSN
Clinical Coordinator
University Cardiothoracic Surgical Associates
University of Louisville
Louisville, Kentucky

"Minimally Invasive Cardiac Surgery"

Liza S. Cowart, RN, BSN, CCRN
Coronary Care Unit Staff Nurse
Kidney Transplant Recipient's Spouse
Baptist Hospital East
Louisville, Kentucky

"Kidney Transplant" (Patient Education Outcome Pathway)

Carolyn A. Pyrch Cunningham, MS, RN, CS
Manager, Pulmonary Rehabilitation
Frazier Rehab Center
Jewish Hospital
Louisville, Kentucky

"Lung Volume Reduction Surgery"

Emma Harris, RN, CCRN
Charge Nurse, Intensive Care Unit
Baptist Hospital East
Louisville, KY

"Subarachnoid Hemorrhage"

Patricia C. Mader, RN, CEN
Staff RN
Baptist Hospital East
Louisville, Kentucky

"Thrombolytic Therapy"

Donna R. Meador, MSN, RN, CEN
Clinical Nurse Specialist
Jewish Hospital
Louisville, Kentucky

"Acute Ischemic Stroke"

Vickie A. Samuels Miracle, EdD, RN, CCRN
Senior Clinical Coordinator
Jewish Hospital Heart and Lung
  Institute
Louisville, Kentucky

"Coronary Artery Bypass Surgery" / "Heart Transplantation" / "Interventional Cardiology" / "Peripheral Vascular Disease" / "Valve Replacement" / "Vascular Emergencies" / "Asthma" / "Cirrhosis and Portal Hypertension" / "Guillain-Barré Syndrome" / "Diabetic Ketoacidosis" / "Burns" / "Obstetric Crises" / "Asthma" (Patient Education Outcome Pathway) / "Cardiac Catheterization" (Patient Education Outcome Pathway) / "Interventional Cardiology" (Patient Education Outcome Pathway) / "Valve Replacement" (Patient Education Outcome Pathway)

Patricia G. Rogers, RN, RVT
Vascular Nurse Specialist
Surgical Care Associates
Louisville, Kentucky

"Carotid Endarterectomy"

Joyce Ann Schepers, BSN, CCRN
ICU Staff Nurse
Baptist Hospital East
Louisville, Kentucky

"Pancreatitis"

Peggy S. Schmidt, RN, BSN
Staff Nurse, Intensive Care Unit
Baptist Hospital East
Louisville, Kentucky

"Transsphenoidal Hypophysectomy"

Suzette L. Sewell, RN, BSN, CCRN
Critical Care Connections, Inc.
Louisville, Kentucky

"HIV"

Anita J. Stiles, RN, MSN
Critical Care Clinical Nurse Specialist
Department of Veterans Affairs
Medical Center
Louisville, Kentucky

"Acute Pain Management" / "Chronic Pain Management" / "Lung Cancer" / "Trauma"

Carolyn Voelker, MSN, RN, CS
Clinical Nurse Specialist
Jewish Hospital
Louisville, Kentucky

"Thoracic Surgery" / "Thoracic Surgery" (Patient Education Outcome Pathway)

Marlot A. Wiggington, RN, MN, CCRN
Program Coordinator
Heart, Spine and Neuroscience Centers
Norton Hospital
Louisville, Kentucky

"Abdominal Aortic Aneurysm"

Christy Yates, CCRN, MSN, ARNP
Family Nurse Practitioner
FernCreek Medical Center
Louisville, Kentucky

"Dysrhythmias" / "Dysrhythmias" (Patient Education Outcome Pathway)

Foreword

This book is an important reference for clinicians who practice in the critical care environment and are struggling to achieve patient outcomes with increasing limitations on resources and time. This excellent text provides guidelines on how to care for critically ill patients using an integrated model. This model is based on using interdisciplinary collaboration to achieve short- and long-term patient outcomes.

As critical care practice has evolved over the last four decades, significant advances have been made in diagnostic techniques, care approaches, treatments, and monitoring. In many ways, today's world of critical care is unrecognizable when compared with the formative days of this specialty. Each discipline involved in the care of the critically ill has also made significant progress in the knowledge and expertise needed to care for these complex patients. With these changes, there has been an increasing need to collaborate across disciplines in order to achieve optimal patient outcomes. However, progress in this area has been slow. Discipline practice is still very independent in the care of critically ill patients. Achieving integration and interdependence among the critical care disciplines is still a desirable but not often attained goal.

Today's critical care environment faces escalating costs, limitations on resources, and very limited lengths of stay by patients. Critical care clinicians are challenged to accomplish numerous patient outcomes in a very short time period, while simultaneously completing the planning that is needed to ensure continued care in other settings. Because of these limitations and challenges, integrated care across disciplines is no longer an option. Care can no longer be disjointed across disciplines or compartmentalized as patients move to different care settings. Fully integrated care across disciplines is the only way to achieve patient outcomes and ensure that care is fluid across settings and targeted toward *shared* outcomes. For these reasons, this integrated interdisciplinary approach to care is now being mandated by our patients, our respective disciplines, our organizations, and our payers.

Considering these environmental constraints, one easily recognizes the importance of achieving *interdisciplinary* care in order to deliver clinically effective and cost-efficient care to critically ill patients. However, until now, there has been a lack of tools and guidelines to facilitate this type of integration.

Basham and Miracle have created an excellent tool to facilitate the integration of disciplines in the care of the critically ill and help us meet these challenges. They have taken 43 critical care diagnoses and developed interdisciplinary pathways, each of which addresses all aspects of the critically ill patient. These pathways provide an overview of the patient's care from admission to critical care through recovery at home or at a rehabilitation facility. The pathways are tools the interdisciplinary team can use as a basis for care. They are holistic guidelines, addressing needs of patients that go beyond their medical needs. In addition, the pathways are designed so that it is easy to incorporate additional components to individualize care for a given patient and family.

Various disciplines worked together to create these pathways. Therefore, they speak authentically to the integration of the roles and talents in the disciplines that are accountable for outcomes of critically ill patients.

In the current environment, the only way to meet optimal patient outcomes is to have maximum integration of everyone who provides care to the critically ill patient. Using the *Critical Care Interdisciplinary Pathways* text, all disciplines working with the patient are driven by the same plan, a plan that (1) identifies outcomes that flow from one care setting to another; (2) addresses all the needs of the patient and family, including their education needs; (3) keeps the team focused on the future goals of the patients, even if they are to be achieved in another setting. For all these reasons, this text is a *timely* and an *essential* resource for all clinicians who are searching for a way to meet patient needs in this challenging environment.

Christine Breu, RN, MN, CNAA, FAAN
Director of Operations
Hospice of Louisville
Louisville, Kentucky

Preface

The vision of the American Association of Critical Care Nurses (AACN) is "a healthcare system driven by the needs of patients and families where critical care nurses make their optimal contribution."[1] This means the provision of critical care occurs in any environment, not just an intensive care or coronary care unit. Due to the changing health care climate, critical care is provided in many settings including, but not limited to, intensive care units, coronary care units, transitional care units, telemetry units, cardiac catheterization labs, post-anesthesia units, and in the home. Patients who are now in critical care units probably would not have survived several years ago. Patients currently on medical/surgical units were in critical care units just a few years ago. Thus, critical care is now provided in a variety of settings.

Because of this, it is important for health care providers in any environment caring for critically ill patients to become more familiar with the care of these patients. Since patients move in and out of critical care at an ever increasing pace, practitioners must be familiar with all aspects of care and not just the few days the patient may actually spend in the critical care unit. Practitioners planning the care of the critically ill patient must begin with the end in mind. The buzzword today for these ends is "outcome." As Stephen Covey related in his book *The Seven Habits of Highly Effective People,* start with the end in mind.[2] Health care providers must do the same. We can no longer be concerned with only the care provided in our particular units. We must plan care with the end or outcome in mind from the time the patient enters our unit.

Hospital administrators, unit managers, quality assurance staff, third-party reimbursers, and consumers are interested in looking at clinical outcomes. Almost all evaluations of care now look at clinical outcomes. How is this patient doing compared to the majority of patients following coronary artery bypass grafting or an exacerbation of chronic obstructive pulmonary disease? These outcomes, like objectives, must be measurable so evaluation can occur. Critical care now and in the future will be evaluated by how well our patients meet these out-

[1] American Association of Critical Care Nurses. (1997). Communication at National Teaching Institute, Orlando, Florida, May 18–22.
[2] Covey, S.R. (1989). *The seven habits of highly effective people.* New York: Simon and Schuster.

comes—and not just the outcomes in the hospital, as we will also need to supply data on how our patients are doing long after discharge.

The purpose of this book is to provide health care practitioners at the bedside—wherever that "bed" may be in *any* setting—with established outcome criteria, pathways, and interventions needed to reach the desired outcomes. In addition, these pathways incorporate a interdisciplinary approach since collaboration among the entire health care team is essential to improving patient outcomes. One of the limitations of the current health care system has been each discipline working with the patient with little or no communication among the team members. This practice is no longer acceptable or relevant for future health care practice. Care must be based on holistic, caring principles, focusing not only on physical needs but also on emotional, psychological, and spiritual needs. These pathways stress the importance of an interdisciplinary approach when planning, providing, and evaluating care of the critically ill during hospitalization and after discharge. This interdisciplinary approach will promote the necessary collaboration and communication among the various health care providers so optimal outcomes may be met.

We excluded specific reference to which discipline performs an intervention since this may vary among institutions. For instance, in some hospitals, a registered dietitian may be responsible for teaching dietary restrictions to cardiac patients. In other hospitals, it may be a nurse educator or cardiac rehabilitation nurse who does the teaching. In some hospitals, an occupational therapist is responsible for teaching energy-conservation techniques to COPD (chronic obstructive pulmonary disease) patients. In other hospitals, pulmonary rehabilitation nurses do this teaching. Our main purpose is to include all appropriate interventions so that each institution can then determine which discipline will actually provide them. The term "advanced practice nurse" is used to describe a licensed RN who is either a clinical nurse specialist, an advanced registered nurse practitioner, a nurse midwife, or a nurse anesthetist.

This book began as a result of the second edition of *Critical Care Nursing,* which included 17 pathways.[3] These pathways were included in the second edition to stress the importance of collaboration among the disciplines and to provide the highest quality care to critically ill patients. For this book, these 17 pathways have been updated. In addition, 26 new pathways have been added. We have also added 10 pathways that focus on patient education in terms of outcomes. We have included throughout the most common diagnoses critical care nurses encounter in any setting.

The reader should feel free to use the pathways as a resource and to individualize them to meet the needs of a particular patient population and/or organization. The contributors of these pathways are experts in their clinical field with extensive experience at the bedside and in various practice roles. The pathways have been reviewed by clinical nurse experts as well as members of other disciplines, such as physical therapists, dietitians, and occupational therapists, to strengthen the interdisciplinary approach.

Some of the information is consistent among pathways. There is a core of nursing science that is applicable to all patients regardless of the diagnosis or setting. The result is repetition in each pathway in some areas. For example, in every pathway you will see the outcome: "The patient will be protected from harm." We as health care providers take appropriate measures, which are standard among disorders, to protect our patients from harm.

The clinical pathways have been divided into three phases: Diagnosis/Stabi-

---

[3] Clochesy, J.M., Breu, C., Cardin, S., Whittaker, A.A, Rudy, E. (1996). *Critical care nursing,* 2nd ed. Philadelphia: W.B. Saunders.

lization, Acute Management, and Recovery. We did not include any specific time frames since the length of time in any one stage will vary from patient to patient and institution to institution. For example, the majority of patients undergoing open heart surgery, either coronary artery bypass grafting or valve replacement, will be in the "Diagnosis/Stabilization Phase" for only a few hours before moving into the "Acute Management Phase." However, the occasional open heart surgical patient may be in this phase for a longer period of time. The pathways are written so that specific outcomes must be met before the patient can progress to the next phase. The "Acute Management Phase" can occur while the patient remains in the critical care unit or after the patient has transferred to a stepdown unit. Again, the phases are meant to be flexible based on the unique needs and progress of each individual patient. The last phase, "Recovery," can occur before the patient is discharged and will continue after discharge. Remember, the majority of a patient's recovery occurs outside the hospital setting. However, the patient's care can still be planned and evaluated even after the patient leaves the hospital environment and enters either the home environment or long-term care. In fact, in many acute care facilities, patients are routinely called at 30 days to determine whether optimal outcomes have been met. The follow-up period may be even longer in some settings. The pathways, therefore, stress the importance of discharge planning from the time of admission until after discharge.

In each pathway the reader will find ten areas of concern to critical care nurses and health care providers. These are (1) Coordination of Care; (2) Diagnostics; (3) Fluid Balance; (4) Nutrition; (5) Mobility; (6) Oxygenation/Ventilation; (7) Comfort; (8) Skin Integrity; (9) Protection and Safety; and (10) Psychosocial/Self-Determination. For example, if you are interested in the nutritional needs of the burn patient, simply turn to the "Burns" pathway and go to the "Nutrition" section. All of the patient care pathways are presented in the same manner.

One particularly important aspect of this book is that these pathways stress an active role of the patient and family in all aspects of care, from diagnosis and stabilization to acute management and recovery. We have stressed this because of the increasing need for the patient and family to be actively involved in all aspects of care, including coordination of care, fluid balance, nutrition, mobility, oxygenation/ventilation, comfort, skin integrity, protection/safety, psychosocial/self-determination, and diagnostics.

The last ten pathways provide patient and family education for a variety of conditions or procedures. Again, these pathways are meant to serve as a resource for health care providers of all disciplines, and they can be adapted to meet the needs of many patients in a multitude of settings. Each of these patient education pathways is divided into areas specific to that topic. For example, cardiac catheterization patient education pathway is divided into three sections: before, during, and after the procedure, including post-discharge care. Each patient education pathway may be slightly different to meet the needs of that particular patient population. The patient education pathways have been written so they are adaptable as patient handouts.

The first chapter deals with the creation of a healing, caring, and humane environment. Various methodologies can be used to care for the patient and family, beyond the more traditional forms of health care. This chapter provides the reader with alternative techniques that can be used to promote healing and comfort in the patient and family. Environment plays an important role in the care and recovery of patients, as Florence Nightingale first theorized.[4] Techniques in these pathways include imagery, massage, humor, and music therapy. This chap-

---

[4] Nightingale, F. (1992). *Notes on nursing.* Philadelphia: J.B. Lippincott. (First published in 1859.)

ter challenges the reader to incorporate these emerging therapies into daily practice to create a more complete healing environment for patients and their families.

On the inside cover of this book is a list of the abbreviations used in this text. We have also included a list of normal laboratory values, hemodynamic parameters, weaning parameters, and arterial blood gases referred to in the pathways. For instance, we state in many of the pathways under the Fluid Balance Section, "Monitor and treat hemodynamic parameters." We list the parameters to monitor and treat in the pathways. Then the normal values to these parameters are listed in the appendix.

The future of critical care is constantly changing and ever challenging for health care professionals in all settings. As more care moves out of the hospital setting and into the home or extended care facilities, these pathways will continue to provide guidelines to meet these ever-changing health care needs. This book is meant to serve as a resource for critical care professionals wherever care is provided. Flexibility will be one of the criteria for success in the future as we endeavor to build "a health care system driven by the needs of patients and families where critical care nurses make their optimal contribution."[5]

---

[5] American Association of Critical Care Nurses. (1997). Communication at National Teaching Institute, Orlando, Florida, May 18–22.

Acknowledgments

We would like to acknowledge the following people who helped, encouraged, motivated, and inspired us on this project:

- The editors of *Critical Care Nursing,* 2nd ed., W.B. Saunders, 1994:
  John M. Clochesy, PhD, RN, CS, FAAN, FCCM
  Christine Breu, RN, MN, CNAA, FAAN
  Suzette Cardin, RN, DNSc, CNAA
  Alice A. Whittaker, RN, MS
  Ellen B. Rudy, RN, PhD, FAAN

- The contributors to *Critical Care Nursing,* 2nd ed., W.B. Saunders, 1994

- Barbara Nelson Cullen
  Senior Editor, Nursing Books
  W.B. Saunders

- The contributors to this book

- All the critical care nurses we have worked with during our careers. We have learned so much from you.

- Our families who put up with us during this project.

Contents

PATIENT EDUCATION OUTCOME PATHWAYS

Creating a Healing Environment

Critical care practitioners have enormous potential to create or destroy healing environments. The environment that surrounds a patient can definitely influence the outcome. Nurses and other critical care professionals are not always aware just how significantly their own behaviors, attitudes, and comments can impact on the patient. Both extremes of creating or destroying healing environments for patients can be witnessed in the critical care setting. Consider the following examples.

One day in a busy intensive care unit, it was unusually hectic. Tension was paramount. One of the nurses was already complaining about her tough day. Then her patient, Mrs. M., needed to be taken to the x-ray department for a CT scan. Mrs. M. was nervous and anxious. She had a tracheostomy tube and was on a ventilator so could not readily verbalize her feelings, although her worried expression communicated her fear. The nurse left the room to get a portable monitor to use for transportation to and from the x-ray department. When she returned, she was very angry and exploded, "I'm so tired of the incompetence around here! This thing is going to be dead by the time we get downstairs!" Someone had forgotten to plug in the portable monitor, which recharges the battery. The nurse was afraid the battery of the portable monitor might not last through the entire trip to and from x-ray. One look at Mrs. M. and it was obvious the patient thought the nurse meant that *she* would probably die before the procedure was finished. Mrs. M. became restless and anxious, began thrashing about in bed, and attempted to get up and call for her family. Her respiratory rate, heart rate, and blood pressure all increased. The nurse was not even aware that the patient was reacting to her comment! Words, tone, and actions do impact the environments we create around our patients even if we are not directly communicating with them. How many times have you had a bad day or were tired and didn't want to be at work? Was your negative energy unknowingly projected onto a patient you might have interacted with? It's quite possible.

Here's a different example. Maggie is a critical care nurse who works in the coronary care unit. Each morning as she enters her patients' rooms she says, "Hi, I'm Maggie—I'll be taking care of you today." Then she always finds something positive to say about the patient—their heart rate is not as fast, their blood pressure has improved, they have better color or more life in their eyes. Then she'll add, "We're going to have a good day today." Invariably Maggie's patients do well. Not only that, but in many cases they require less pain medication or antianxiolytics than they did during the previous shift.

These two examples illustrate just how powerful a role critical care nurses play in creating or destroying healing environments. Patients in critical care units are very vulnerable because of their critical illnesses. If they are intubated or sedated, they may not be able to verbalize what they are feeling, which may further increase their stress and negative emotions. The field of psychoneuroimmunology has supported the interactive nature of psychophysiologic variables. Conclusive evidence indicates that thoughts and emotions affect the neurologic, endocrine, and immune systems.[1] Our thoughts, images, attitudes, and feelings are generated in the frontal cortex. The frontal cortex connects with the limbic system, which in turn communicates with the hypothalamus, which controls the pituitary gland. Chemical messengers literally connect the entire mind-body via neurotransmitters, hormones, immunomodulators, and neuropeptides. Our mind and body are connected at every cell. Nothing happens to us physically that doesn't affect us psychologically, and nothing happens to us psychologically that doesn't affect us physically. This is the whole premise of psychoneuroimmunology. Imagine just how much stress and negative energy could be experienced by a patient in a critical care area. They may be frightened of all the equipment, alarms, and noise that constantly surround them. They may not be able to sleep comfortably. They may also be fearful about the outcome of their critical illness. All health care workers must be cognizant of the patients' and families' potential stress/anxiety and attempt to surround them with supportive, loving, healing environments.

Norman Cousins was one of the first to realize that if stress, anxiety, and constant pressure can make us ill, then couldn't positive emotions contribute to our health and well-being? He was diagnosed with ankylosing spondolitis, a collagen vascular disorder with a grim prognosis. He knew that stress had contributed significantly to his illness. Research has since demonstrated that stress causes the release of cortisol, epinephrine, and norepinephrine, which over time can negatively affect the body. Cousins had a lot of influential friends, among them Allen Funk (host of the television program *Candid Camera*). He began to watch clip after clip that always ended with the line, "Smile, you're on *Candid Camera*." He found that ten minutes of belly-slapping laughter provided two hours of pain-free rest, which he had been unable to achieve with traditional pain medications. His initial hypothesis was correct: positive emotions can impact our physical state just as the negative emotions do. Cousins was able to help cure himself of a serious disease.[2] His experience has incredible significance for us as critical care professionals.

Healing environments can be enhanced in many ways. First, become aware of how you approach patients each day. Learn to create a real sense of presence

---

[1] B. Dossey, The psychophysiology of bodymind healing. In B. Dossey et al. (Eds.), *Holistic nursing, a handbook for practice* (2nd ed.) (Gaithersburg, Md.: Aspen, 1995), pp. 87–111.

[2] N. Cousins, *Anatomy of an illness as perceived by the patient* (New York: Bantam Books, 1979).

by consciously connecting with what the patient is experiencing. Use direct eye contact, introduce yourself, and call the patient by name. Approach all interventions in a calm, competent manner, fully aware of how each one is impacting your patient or his or her family.

Many complementary therapies can significantly enhance healing environments. Music therapy may be very effective in helping a patient to relax. If the patient is less stressed, less oxygen will be consumed. More of the patient's energy can be used for healing instead of the stress response. Cathie Guzzetta has studied the impact of music therapy on critically ill patients for many years, including patients in various clinical settings such as coronary care units, cardiac catheterization laboratories, oncology units, and AIDS units.

Guzzetta's results have given us tremendous insight into using music therapy effectively. For instance, when using music therapy it's important to first go through a general relaxation exercise. The four significant elements of relaxation are comfortable position, quiet environment, passive attitude, and focused concentration.[3] Choose music that appeals to the patient. No one music will be right for everyone. The music should be slow, soothing, and relaxing, without words. A new type of music called nontraditional (or meditative music) typically has wide appeal. It has no central rhythm, beat, or harmonic progression. Usually people haven't heard it before so no associations with memories or emotions are triggered. Be cautious. Not all the music labeled nontraditional is slow and soothing. Experiment with different types of music and ideally allow the patient to indicate his or her preference.[4]

Mrs. R. was an elderly obese woman with chronic obstructive pulmonary disease. She was on a ventilator and unable to be weaned with standard protocols. She had been a professor of music at the local university in her earlier years and still had a great appreciation for classical music. Her husband carefully chose just the right blend of classical music that would help her relax. The tape was played daily through her weaning trials. As she listened to the tapes, her heart rate decreased, her respiratory rate decreased, and her tidal volumes increased. She was able to eventually wean off the ventilator.

Touch therapy can be very relaxing for patients. Patients expect nurses to touch them. Even patients who are not typically comfortable with touch usually do respond to a nurse's touch in the face of their vulnerability within a critical care setting. So many times it is necessary to touch patients while performing interventions that are unpleasant—turning them when they are in pain, suctioning them, or getting them up to a chair—that it is crucial to balance the negative touch with some positive touch. Hold the patient's hand or give patients a back rub to help them relax and feel better. Many types of interventional touch such as healing touch and therapeutic touch are becoming more commonplace. Other therapies that direct or impact energy flow, such as Amma therapy, Reike, acupressure, acupuncture, Jin Shin Do, and reflexology, are being used in conjunction with traditional medical practice.

Guided imagery has also been utilized to help maximize one's healing potential. Barbara Dossey, who has done extensive work in this area, emphasizes that imagery is more than just visualization. Imagery incorporates all the senses and can be viewed as an interface between the body, mind, and spirit. It can be an extremely potent healing resource.[5] I once observed a nurse use imagery very effectively with her patient who was having a triple lumen catheter inserted. The

[3] C. Guzzetta, *The art of caring: music therapy: hearing the melody of the soul* (Audiotape Series, Sounds True Audio, 1996).

[4] Ibid.

[5] B. Dossey, *The art of caring: imagery: awakening the inner healer* (Audiotape Series, Sounds True Audio, 1996).

physician had difficulty inserting the catheter and had to stick the patient several times. After the second or third stick, I heard the nurse say to the patient, "OK, let's take a trip. Want to go to Florida? Imagine you are lying on a raft in the ocean. The sun is beating down on you. Every once in a while a wave gently rocks you to sleep." Not only did the patient relax, but so did the physician. He was able to get the catheter in on the next attempt.

Guided imagery has been used to help enhance traditional treatment. For instance, cancer patients who are receiving chemotherapy often visualize the chemotherapy as little "Pac men" chomping away at the cancer cells. They also imagine their own natural killer cells becoming enhanced and able to conquer and destroy the cancer or tumor cells.

Families can be a vital factor in creating a healing environment. The love and support from family members, significant others, or close friends can greatly improve a patient's well-being and enhance the healing process. In each of the outcome pathways, we have included families as part of the patient's routine care. Despite the positive research regarding families and a patient's healing process, some critical care units continue to restrict family visitation. Some nurses are uncomfortable caring for a patient in front of family members. Nurses have also verbalized that the family takes up too much time with questions, which takes away from their time to care for the patient. The nurse's discomfort and need for control becomes the basis for wanting restricted visitation. Yet whose needs are actually being met—the patient's or the nurse's? Some nurses find it difficult to deal with families' anxieties without becoming defensive and negative. It's crucial to view the families' negative reactions as a call for help. Perhaps the family needs additional reassurance, counseling, or information regarding the patient's illness. Perhaps they need help with stress management. Remember, many times the families' love and support can be just as therapeutic for the patient as Versed or morphine. Encourage the family to be involved in the patient's care, to ask questions or give suggestions freely. They know the patient better than anyone else.

Our modern-age treatment has come full circle to the Hippocratic ideal that the treatment of disease is a dual process. One part is the systematic medical treatment. The other part is full activation of a patient's own healing system. The patient is not just a passive vessel into which we pour our interventions, but a sovereign human being capable of generating powerful responses to disease.[6] We've done a great job in advancing the science of medicine. We've not done so well in helping to activate a person's own healing system. Creating healing environments for patients will enhance the activation of a patient's own healing potential!

---

[6] N. Cousins, Finding the healer within. In R. Smolan, P. Moffitt, and M. Naythons (Eds.), *The power to heal: ancient arts and modern medicine* (New York: Prentice Hall Press, 1990), pp. 143–145.

CRITICAL CARE INTERDISCIPLINARY OUTCOME PATHWAYS

CHAPTER 1

Cardiovascular Pathways

Abdominal Aortic Aneurysm
Interdisciplinary Outcome Pathway

COORDINATION OF CARE

Diagnosis/Stabilization Phase		Acute Management Phase		Recovery Phase	
Outcome	Interventions	Outcome	Interventions	Outcome	Interventions
All appropriate team members and disciplines will be involved in the plan of care.	Develop the plan of care with the patient/family, primary care physician, vascular surgeon, cardiologist, radiologist, nephrologist, general surgeon, RN, advanced practice nurse, RCP, pastoral care, social worker, and discharge planners.	All appropriate team members and disciplines will be involved in the plan of care.	Initiate planning for anticipated discharge and call home health as indicated. Begin teaching patient/family about care at home. Initiate vascular rehabilitation program if available. Update the plan of care with all team members. Assess social support system.	Patient will understand how to maintain optimal health at home.	Consult home health as necessary. Provide guidelines concerning care at home and any follow-up visits. Provide patient/family with phone numbers of resources available to answer questions.

DIAGNOSTICS

Diagnosis/Stabilization Phase		Acute Management Phase		Recovery Phase	
Outcome	Interventions	Outcome	Interventions	Outcome	Interventions
Patient/family will understand any tests or procedures that need to be completed (i.e., VS, I & O, hemodynamic monitoring, x-rays, Doppler ultrasound, MRI, CT scan).	Explain all procedures and tests to patient/family. Be sensitive to individualized needs of patient/family for information. Establish effective communication technique with patient while intubated.	Patient will understand any tests or procedures that need to be completed (removal of indwelling lines, hemodynamic monitoring, cardiac monitoring, coughing and deep breathing, IS, EKG).	Explain procedures and tests needed to assess recovery from surgery. Be sensitive to individualized needs of patient/family for information. Anticipate need for further diagnostic tests such as ultrasound or angiography and any intervention that may result. Provide appropriate patient/family education. Initiate referrals to dietitian, home health, social services, PT, as indicated.	Patient will understand meaning of diagnostic tests in relation to continued health (lab tests, exercise program).	Review with patient/family before discharge the results of lab and diagnostic tests. Discuss any abnormal values and appropriate measures patient can take to help return those values to normal. Provide instruction on care at home after discharge: • when to call the doctor • care of incision • activity progression/limitations • medications • diet • signs of decreased orientation, such as confusion Follow up referrals to dietary, home health, social services, PT, as indicated.

FLUID BALANCE

Diagnosis/Stabilization Phase		Acute Management Phase		Recovery Phase	
Outcome	Interventions	Outcome	Interventions	Outcome	Interventions
Patient will achieve optimal hemodynamic status as evidenced by: • MAP > 70 mmHg • hemodynamic parameters WNL • UO > 0.5 mL/kg/hr • absence of dysrhythmias • adequate LOC • clear lung sounds • absence of JVD Patient demonstrates optimum peripheral tissue perfusion as evidenced by: • warm, pink pain-free extremities with palpable pulses • UO > 0.5 mL/kg/hr • normal LOC • normal liver enzymes Patient demonstrates optimum renal tissue perfusion as evidenced by: • UO > 0.5 mL/kg/hr • SCR ≤ 1.0 • BUN ≤ 20 Patient demonstrates optimum cardiac output as evidenced by: • SvO$_2$ 60–75 • normal BP • normal HR	Monitor and treat cardiovascular parameters: • dysrhythmias • BP • PA pressures • PCWP • CO/CI • SVR/PVR • SV • SvO$_2$ • I & O • LOC • evidence of tissue perfusion Monitor lab values: electrolytes, Mg^{++}, Hgb, Hct, PT, PTT, ACT if available, platelets, CK, CK-MB. Observe for signs of bleeding and administer blood products as needed; assess response. Blood products may include packed red cells, fresh frozen plasma, platelets, and/or cryoprecipitate. Monitor for signs of complications: hypovolemic shock, embolism, thrombus formation, GI complications, stroke, acute renal failure, colon ischemia, spinal cord ischemia, MI, infection, hypertension. Keep systolic blood pressure < 120 mmHg. Administer and titrate vasopressor agents as needed. Assess lung sounds q4h and PRN. Assess impact of related factors influencing renal perfusion—cardiac function, medications. Assess peripheral pulses, color, movement/sensation of lower extremities q1–2h and PRN.	Patient will maintain optimal hemodynamic status. Patient will remain free of bleeding. Patient demonstrates optimum peripheral tissue perfusion. Patient demonstrates optimum renal tissue perfusion. Patient demonstrates optimum cardiac output.	Monitor/report patient's response to therapeutic regimen. Assess neurologic status q2–4h and PRN. Continue to assess for complications of abdominal aortic aneurysm, as listed earlier. Monitor and treat cardiovascular parameters. Monitor renal status closely. Keep UO > 0.5 mL/kg/hr. Weigh daily. I & O q1–2h and PRN. Assess need for diuretics and potassium replacement. Monitor patient's response to treatment. Assess lung sounds q4h and PRN. Monitor laboratory data related to coagulation—PT/PTT, platelets, fibrinogen, bleeding time. Monitor vasoactive drips to optimize hemodynamic status as ordered.	Patient will maintain optimal hemodynamic status.	Continue as in Acute Management Phase. Instruct patient/family in signs of fluid imbalance and when to seek medical attention such as increasing SOB, dyspnea on exertion, weight gain of > 3 lbs. in one week, JVD, 2–3 pillow orthopnea, or peripheral edema.

Abdominal Aortic Aneurysm Interdisciplinary Outcome Pathway (continued)

FLUID BALANCE (continued)

Diagnosis/Stabilization Phase		Acute Management Phase		Recovery Phase	
Outcome	Interventions	Outcome	Interventions	Outcome	Interventions
	Assess impact of related factors influencing tissue perfusion (i.e., risk factors, BP, medications, PVD). Assess for risk factors influencing cardiac output—cardiac disease, fluid status.				

NUTRITION

Diagnosis/Stabilization Phase		Acute Management Phase		Recovery Phase	
Outcome	Interventions	Outcome	Interventions	Outcome	Interventions
Patient will be adequately nourished as evidenced by: • stable weight • weight not >10% below or >20% above IBW • albumin >3.5 g/dL • total protein 6–8 g/dL • prealbumin >15 • total lymphocyte count 1,000–3,000	NPO until extubation. If extubation is delayed greater than 24h, assess need for alternative nutritional therapy such as enteral feedings. Consult dietitian or nutritional support team to determine and direct nutritional support. Assess bowel sounds, abdominal distension, abdominal pain and tenderness q4h and PRN. Initiate clear liquids and monitor response. Monitor serum protein, albumin, and prealbumin levels. Assess pattern of N & V, as indicated. Monitor appetite, food/fluid intake. Assess stools for frequency, consistency, character.	Patient will be adequately nourished. Patient demonstrates optimum GI tissue perfusion.	Monitor/report patient's response to treatment. Assess bowel sounds, abdominal distension, abdominal pain and tenderness q4h and PRN. Advance to DAT and monitor response. Continue enteral feedings until patient consuming at least three-quarters caloric need. Monitor serum protein and albumin lab values. Assess patient for risk of hypercholesterolemia and hyperlipidemia and begin assessment of patient's usual diet. NG tube to low intermittent suction until bowel sounds are present. Administer antiemetics, H$_2$ blockers, and/or antacids as needed. Monitor gastric pH (normal value 3–5). Weigh daily. I & O.	Patient will be adequately nourished. Patient demonstrates knowledge/skill in activities designed to restore/promote/maintain optimum GI tissue perfusion.	Consider calorie count to assure patient consuming three-quarters caloric need. Teach patient/family about heart healthy diet: • total fat <30% of daily intake • total saturated fat <10% of daily intake • total daily cholesterol intake <300 mg • caloric reduction if indicated • sodium restriction if indicated Teach patients about dietary supplements (antioxidants, oat bran, fiber, vitamins and minerals).

MOBILITY

Diagnosis/Stabilization Phase		Acute Management Phase		Recovery Phase	
Outcome	Interventions	Outcome	Interventions	Outcome	Interventions
Patient will maintain normal ROM and muscle strength.	Turn at least q2h, if hemodynamically stable, and monitor response. Begin passive/active-assist ROM exercises. Bed rest until extubated, unless extubation delayed >24h.	Patient will achieve optimal mobility.	PT consult to assess ambulation mobility, muscle flexibility, strength, and tone. OT consult to determine functional ability for ADLs. PT/OT to help determine and direct activity goals. Progress exercise as tolerated: dangle, OOB TID to QID, and walking 50 feet. Provide physical assistance or assistive devices as necessary. Monitor response to increased activity. Decrease if adverse events occur: tachycardia, chest discomfort, bleeding, ectopy. Begin teaching patient/family principles of a progressive exercise program.	Patient will achieve optimal mobility.	Continue to progress exercise as tolerated and monitor response. Walk at least 200–300 feet TID to QID. Assess ability to negotiate stairs if part of home environment. Teach patient/family about home exercise program. Decrease activity if tachycardia, chest discomfort, hypotension, or dyspnea occurs. Provide patient with home exercise program.

OXYGENATION/VENTILATION

Diagnosis/Stabilization Phase		Acute Management Phase		Recovery Phase	
Outcome	Interventions	Outcome	Interventions	Outcome	Interventions
Patient will have adequate gas exchange as evidenced by: • SaO_2 >90% • SpO_2 >92% • ABGs WNL • clear breath sounds • respiratory rate, depth, and rhythm WNL • CXR normal • absence of dyspnea, cyanosis, and secretions • Hgb and Hct WNL.	Assess for influencing factors (i.e., smoking, lung disease). Monitor ventilator settings and hemodynamic variables before, during, and after weaning. Wean ventilator and monitor response: • wean FIO_2 to keep SpO_2 >92% • monitor effects of anesthesia and wean ventilator accordingly • after extubation, apply supplemental oxygen	Patient will have adequate gas exchange.	Instruct and assist patient in proper deep breathing and coughing. Have patient give return demonstration. Monitor and treat oxygenation/ventilation disturbances, such as decreased pO_2 and increased pCO_2. Wean O_2 therapy and/or mechanical ventilation as tolerated. Provide humidification. Reinforce the use of IS. Use chest splint pillow or abdominal splint pillow if indicated. Have patient demonstrate proper use. Suction PRN.	Patient will have adequate gas exchange.	Continue as in Acute Management Phase. CXR before discharge. Continue IS. Continue discussion on smoking cessation. Refer to Smokers Anonymous or other available support groups.

Abdominal Aortic Aneurysm Interdisciplinary Outcome Pathway (*continued*)

OXYGENATION/VENTILATION (continued)

Diagnosis/Stabilization Phase		Acute Management Phase		Recovery Phase	
Outcome	Interventions	Outcome	Interventions	Outcome	Interventions
	Assess respiratory functioning, including lung sounds, respiratory muscle strength, respiratory rate and depth, coughing ability, and CXR. If not intubated, apply supplemental O_2. Monitor with pulse oximetry. Reinforce use of IS when extubated. Teach patient proper use of IS and have patient give return demonstration.		Observe effect of increased activity on respiratory status. Monitor with pulse oximetry. Observe for complications of vascular emergencies that may impair oxygenation/ventilation: thrombus formation, embolus, shock, bleeding, ARDS. If applicable, begin discussion on smoking cessation. Plan activities to provide rest periods.		

COMFORT

Diagnosis/Stabilization Phase		Acute Management Phase		Recovery Phase	
Outcome	Interventions	Outcome	Interventions	Outcome	Interventions
Patient will be as comfortable and pain free as possible as evidenced by: • no objective indicators of discomfort • no complaints of discomfort	Assess quantity and quality of pain using pain scale or visual analogue tool. Administer narcotics and monitor response. Assess effects of analgesics on ability to wean from ventilator, if applicable. Anticipate need for analgesia and provide as needed. If patient is intubated, establish effective communication technique with which patient can communicate discomfort and need for analgesics. Provide a quiet environment to potentiate analgesia. Provide reassurance in a calm, caring, competent manner.	Patient will be as relaxed and pain free as posssible.	Continue as in Diagnosis/Stabilization Phase. Provide chest or abdominal splint pillow, as indicated, and instruct on proper use. Have patient demonstrate proper use. Provide uninterrupted periods of rest. Teach patient relaxation techniques and have patient give return demonstration. Use touch therapy, humor, music therapy, and imagery to promote relaxation. Involve family in strategies. Provide analgesics as needed before ambulation and any other procedures.	Patient will be as relaxed and pain free as possible.	Progress analgesics to oral medications as needed; assess response. Use sedatives as indicated and assess response. Continue alternative methods to promote relaxation as listed earlier. Teach patient/family alternative methods to promote relaxation at home. Teach self-medication after discharge.

Teach patient proper use of PCA pump, if used.
Use sedatives as indicated.
Observe for complications of abdominal aortic aneurysm that may cause increase in discomfort (ischemic bowel, DVT, pulmonary embolus, infection, dehiscence, MI).

SKIN INTEGRITY

Diagnosis/Stabilization Phase		Acute Management Phase		Recovery Phase	
Outcome	Interventions	Outcome	Interventions	Outcome	Interventions
Patient will have intact skin without abrasions or pressure ulcers. Patient will be afebrile and without objective signs of infection.	Preop shower/scrub with antibacterial agent. Temperature q4h and PRN. Rewarm slowly. Suggested methods of rewarming include warm blankets, warm air blankets, warm IV fluids, warmed, humidified O₂. Begin passive/active-assist ROM exercises. Assess all bony prominences at least q4h and treat if needed. Use preventive pressure-reducing devices if patient is at high risk for developing pressure ulcers. Treat pressure ulcers according to hospital protocol.	Patient will have intact skin without abrasions or pressure ulcers. Patient will be afebrile and without objective signs of infection. Patient will have healing wounds.	Same as Diagnosis/Stabilization Phase. Temperature q4h unless elevated, then more frequently as indicated. Continue ROM exercises. Keep surgical site covered for 24h, then open to air unless actively draining. Assess incision sites for signs and symptoms of infection q4h and PRN. Culture if necessary. Wash incisions daily proximally to distally with sterile soap and water. Assess all bony prominences at least q4h and treat if needed. Assess skin adjacent to surgical wounds for symptoms of tape burns, allergies. Initiate referrals to wound/skin advanced practice nurse, as indicated. Monitor integrity of all dressings. Assess skin for presence/absence of turgor q4h and PRN.	Patient will have intact skin without abrasions or pressure ulcers. Patient will be afebrile and without objective signs of infection. Patient will have healing wounds.	Assess all bony prominences at least q4h and treat if needed. Assess and cleanse incisions as described earlier. Teach patient/family proper skin care at home: • care of incision • appropriately fitting shoes and garments • diet • avoidance of tape • signs and symptoms of infection • when to call the physician Assess patient/family understanding of skin care.

Abdominal Aortic Aneurysm Interdisciplinary Outcome Pathway (continued)

PROTECTION/SAFETY

Diagnosis/Stabilization Phase		Acute Management Phase		Recovery Phase	
Outcome	Interventions	Outcome	Interventions	Outcome	Interventions
Patient will be protected from possible harm.	Assess need for wrist restraints if patient is intubated, has a decreased level of consciousness, or is agitated and restless. Explain need for restraints to patient/family. Assess response to restraints, if used, and check q1–2h for skin integrity and impairment to circulation. Follow hospital protocol for use of restraints. Remove restraints as soon as patient is able to follow instructions. Provide sedatives as needed. Secure all drains.	Patient will be protected from possible harm.	If need still exists for restraints, check q1–2h for skin integrity. Provide support when dangling, getting OOB, and ambulating; monitor response. Use gait belt as indicated for ambulation. PT consult as indicated. Determine appropriate pressure prevention: sheepskin, sequential pump stockings, special mattress, foot cradle. Institute as appropriate.	Patient will be protected from possible harm.	Teach patient/family about any physical limitations in activity after discharge. Provide patient with a written list of these limitations/restrictions. Assess understanding and reinforce as necessary. Provide support with ambulation and climbing stairs.

PSYCHOSOCIAL/SELF-DETERMINATION

Diagnosis/Stabilization Phase		Acute Management Phase		Recovery Phase	
Outcome	Interventions	Outcome	Interventions	Outcome	Interventions
Patient will achieve psychophysiologic stability. Patient will demonstrate a decrease in anxiety as evidenced by: • vital signs WNL • subjective report of decreased anxiety • objective signs of decreased anxiety	Assess patient's/family's past and present coping mechanisms. Provide patient/family opportunities for verbalization of feelings. Assess physiologic effects of critical care environment on patient (hemodynamic variables, psychological status, signs of increased sympathetic response). Provide sedatives as indicated. Take measures to reduce sensory overload, such as providing uninterrupted rest periods.	Patient will achieve psychophysiologic stability. Patient will demonstrate a decrease in anxiety.	Continue as in Diagnosis/Stabilization Phase. Provide adequate rest periods. Continue to include patient/family in all aspects of care. Continue to assess coping ability of patient/family and take measures as indicated. Maintain quiet environment. Instruct patient in relaxation techniques, imagery, soft music, humor. Assess patient's understanding of techniques.	Patient will achieve psychophysiologic stability. Patient will demonstrate a decrease in anxiety.	Provide instruction on coping mechanisms after discharge. Refer to outside services or agencies as appropriate (chaplain, social services, psychiatry, home health). Continue to assess coping ability of patient and family. Include patient/family in decisions regarding care. Address concerns patient may have about impact on daily life: ADLs, recreation, sexual functioning, return to work, and driving.

If patient is intubated, develop effective interventions to communicate with patient such as magic slate, pen and pencil, alphabet board.

Use calm, caring, reassuring manner.

Answer all patient/family questions honestly and thoroughly.

Allow flexible visitation to meet patient and family needs.

Carotid Endarterectomy
Interdisciplinary Outcome Pathway

COORDINATION OF CARE

Diagnosis/Stabilization Phase		Acute Management Phase		Recovery Phase	
Outcome	Interventions	Outcome	Interventions	Outcome	Interventions
All appropriate team members and disciplines will be involved in the plan of care.	Develop the plan of care with the patient, family, primary physician, vascular surgeon, cardiologist, RN, advanced practice nurse, RCP (if needed), chaplain, and social worker.	All appropriate team members and disciplines will be involved in the plan of care.	Initiate planning for anticipated discharge with family and with social services if indicated. Begin teaching patient and family about home care. Initiate plans for subacute short stay if needed. Update the plan of care with appropriate team members.	Patient and family will understand how to maintain optimal health at home.	Provide guidelines concerning home care and date of follow-up visit with surgeon and primary care physician. Provide family with phone number of resource person available to answer questions.

DIAGNOSTICS

Diagnosis/Stabilization Phase		Acute Management Phase		Recovery Phase	
Outcome	Interventions	Outcome	Interventions	Outcome	Interventions
Patient will understand any tests or procedures that need to be completed (angiogram, duplex scan carotids, lab studies, EKG, CXR, hemodynamic monitoring, vital signs, I & O, MRI, or thallium stress as indicated).	Establish effective communication with patient and family. Explain all procedures and tests to patient and family and give them educational booklets to review prior o surgery. Be sensitive to individual needs of patient and family.	Patient will understand any procedures or tests ordered (removal of lines, incentive spirometer, pulse oximetry, lab work, metered dose inhaler, coughing and deep breathing, increase in activity).	Explain procedures and tests needed to assess recovery from surgery. Be sensitive to individual needs of patient and family and their need for understanding the procedures. Anticipate need for further diagnostic tests such as duplex scan carotids, and any intervention that may result.	Patient will understand the need for continuation of some procedures and tests in relation to achieving optimum health (lab tests, incentive spirometry; increased activity; coughing and deep breathing; cessation from smoking, follow-up carotid duplex scans; anticoagulants if indicated).	Review results of all tests with patient and family before discharge and explain the need to continue specific measures. Discuss any abnormal results and explain to patient the appropriate measures to return these to normal. Give patient and family discharge instruction sheet for home care and follow-up visits with surgeon. Discuss this with patient and family in detail.

FLUID BALANCE

Diagnosis/Stabilization Phase		Acute Management Phase		Recovery Phase	
Outcome	Interventions	Outcome	Interventions	Outcome	Interventions
Patient will achieve/maintain optimal hemodynamic status as evidenced by: • normal LOC for patient • clear lung sounds • hemodynamic parameters WNL	Initiate IV fluids as ordered. Monitor for dysrhythmias. Monitor BP. Initiate access to monitor hemodynamic parameters as ordered. Arterial line for BP. Pulmonary artery catheter for CO, PAP, PCWP, and CVP. Maintain NPO status. Monitor lab values: electrolytes, Hgb, Hct, PT, PTT, platelets, BUN, creatinine. Monitor for complications: • bleeding • neurologic events • hypertension • tracheal shift	Patient will maintain optimal hemodynamic status.	Monitor for dysrhythmias. Monitor BP. Monitor I & O. Administer IV fluids as ordered. Ice chips; advance to clear liquids when fully awake. Monitor lab values: SMA7, Hgb/Hct. Monitor neurovascular checks q1h. Monitor and treat cardiac variables.	Patient will maintain optimal hemodynamic status.	Advance diet to low fat, low cholesterol foods. Discontinue IV fluids. Monitor I & O. Discuss need for heart healthy diet with patient and family. Neurovascular checks q4h until discharge.

NUTRITION

Diagnosis/Stabilization Phase		Acute Management Phase		Recovery Phase	
Outcome	Interventions	Outcome	Interventions	Outcome	Interventions
Patient will be adequately nourished as evidenced by: • stable weight • weight not >10% below or >20% above IBW • albumin >3.5 g/dL • prealbumin >15 • total protein 6–8 g/dL • total lymphocyte count 1,000–3,000	NPO; initiate IV fluids.	Patient will be adequately nourished.	NPO until fully awake. Continue IV fluids until tolerating solid food. When awake: ice chips to clear liquids to low fat, low cholesterol diet. I & O. Monitor response to intake.	Patient will be adequately nourished.	Low fat, low cholesterol diet. Involve dietitian if diet counseling indicated. Teach patient and family the necessity of heart healthy diet. Give patient heart healthy grocery list of low fat, low cholesterol foods. Teach patients about supplements (i.e., antioxidants, oat bran, fiber, vitamins and minerals).

Carotid Endarterectomy Interdisciplinary Outcome Pathway (continued)

MOBILITY

Diagnosis/Stabilization Phase		Acute Management Phase		Recovery Phase	
Outcome	Interventions	Outcome	Interventions	Outcome	Interventions
Patient will maintain optimal mobility.	Bed rest through preop phase and immediate postop phase. Passive/active-assist ROM exercises.	Patient will return to preop mobility status.	Turn and position q2h until fully awake. Increase activity as tolerated by monitoring response to the activity: • BP • HR • neurologic response. Decrease if adverse events occur. Begin with dangle at bedside to sitting in recliner QID to walking around nursing station QID. Neurovascular checks q1h.	Patient will achieve optimal mobility.	Up as desired with help. Neurovascular check q4h until discharge. BP q4h until discharge. Send instructions home with patient concerning allowed activities (climbing stairs, driving car, exercise activity). Discuss these activities with the patient and family. Teach patient and family about home exercise program.

OXYGENATION/VENTILATION

Diagnosis/Stabilization Phase		Acute Management Phase		Recovery Phase	
Outcome	Interventions	Outcome	Interventions	Outcome	Interventions
Patient will have adequate gas exchange as evidenced by: • clear breath sounds • respiratory rate, depth, and rhythm WNL • ABGs WNL • normal CXR • SpO_2 > 96% or WNL for patient	Pulmonary consult if history of pulmonary disease. Assess respiratory function including lung sounds, respiratory rate and depth. Review CXR. ABGs, pulmonary function studies if history of COPD. Teach use of incentive spirometer.	Patient will have adequate gas exchange as evidenced by SpO_2 > 96% or WNL for patient.	Incentive spirometer at bedside. Encourage use q2h while awake. May increase frequency if patient has a history of smoking. Turn, cough, and deep breathe q2h. O_2 N.C. at 2L/minute, if SpO_2 <96%. Metered dose inhaler if previous pulmonary history or smoker. Neurovascular checks q1h. Observe for possible complications: • bleeding • stroke • tracheal shift. Continuous pulse oximetry.	Patient will have adequate gas exchange.	Increase ambulation. Teach patient and family the importance of incentive spirometer. Include smoking counseling if patient is a smoker. Neurovascular checks q4h until discharge. VS q4h until discharge. DC pulse oximetry.

COMFORT

Diagnosis/Stabilization Phase		Acute Management Phase		Recovery Phase	
Outcome	Interventions	Outcome	Interventions	Outcome	Interventions
Patient will be comfortable, with reduced anxiety.	Review preop and postop procedure with patient and family. Administer preop medication as ordered per anesthesia. Provide reassurance. Anticipate need for analgesia and provide as needed. Assess response.	Patient will be as pain free and relaxed as possible.	Anticipate need for, administer pain medication and monitor response. Use visual analogue scale to objectively assess pain. Provide comfort measures, including position in bed, dressing placement, and elevation of head. Provide reassurance in a calm, caring manner. Answer questions. Observe for complications (tracheal shift, bleeding, neurologic deficit). Use sedative if significantly anxious/restless. Assist patient with relaxation techniques.	Patient will be relaxed and pain free.	Progress to oral pain medications as needed and assess response. Instruct patient and family about use of analgesics and sedatives after discharge. Discuss wound care with patient and family as means of pain control. May resume all aspects of personal hygiene including showering and shampooing hair. Continue alternative methods to promote relaxation such as meditation, music therapy, humor therapy, or guided imagery.

SKIN INTEGRITY

Diagnosis/Stabilization Phase		Acute Management Phase		Recovery Phase	
Outcome	Interventions	Outcome	Interventions	Outcome	Interventions
Patient will be without objective signs of infection. Skin will be intact without abrasion or pressure ulcers.	Temperature q4h. Assess all bony prominences at least q4h and treat if needed.	Patient will have intact skin without abrasions, pressure ulcers, or wound infection.	Turn q1h with back care. Temperature q4h unless elevated; then as indicated. Sterile dressing to neck incision for 24h. Replace if drainage. Check dressing and/or incision q1h and PRN. Ambulate evening of surgery if possible.	Patient will be afebrile without objective sign of infection. Skin will be intact without pressure areas.	Teach patient and family proper care of incision: • wash with warm water and soap daily • apply lotion (e.g., vitamin E) to neck up to incision line • avoid high neck clothing that could irritate skin. Teach signs of wound infection: • redness • swelling • hot to touch

Carotid Endarterectomy Interdisciplinary Outcome Pathway (continued)

PROTECTION/SAFETY

Diagnosis/Stabilization Phase		Acute Management Phase		Recovery Phase	
Outcome	Interventions	Outcome	Interventions	Outcome	Interventions
Patient will be protected from possible harm.	Bed rest following medications such as sedative or analgesics.	Patient will be protected from possible harm.	Complete bed rest until fully awake. Assistance with getting OOB and ambulating; monitor response. Teach patient the need for assistance with ambulation.	Patient will be protected from possible harm.	Teach patient and family allowances and limitations of activity following discharge: • may go up and down stairs • may ride in car; no driving until after first follow-up visit • may take short walks • no heavy lifting (<10 pounds) for 4 weeks • may perform light housework. Give patient and family discharge instruction sheet.

PSYCHOSOCIAL/SELF-DETERMINATION

Diagnosis/Stabilization Phase		Acute Management Phase		Recovery Phase	
Outcome	Interventions	Outcome	Interventions	Outcome	Interventions
Patient will achieve psychophysiologic stability. Patient will demonstrate a decrease in anxiety as evidenced by: • vital signs WNL • subjective report of decreased anxiety.	Assess physiologic effects of hospitalization and surgery on patient and family (e.g., psychological and emotional status and hemodynamic variables). Provide education as needed. Provide preop sedation to patient as indicated. Notify social services if indicated to begin preparing for discharge needs (e.g., meals, extended care facility). Allow flexible visiting to meet needs of patient and family.	Patient will achieve psychophysiologic stability. Patient will demonstrate a decrease in anxiety.	Assess physiologic effects of critical care environment on patient and family (e.g., psychological and emotional status and hemodynamic variables). Continue to educate patient and family. Provide adequate rest periods. Give emotional support and encouragement to patient and family. Continue to include family in all aspects of care. Maintain a secure, quiet, and caring environment.	Patient will achieve psychophysiologic stability. Patient will demonstrate a decrease in anxiety.	Provide patient with discharge instructions with specifics of activities and office follow-up. Provide patient and family with phone number of resource person to answer questions. Refer patient to outside service or agency (e.g., Meals on Wheels or social services as indicated on admission). Continue to assess coping ability of patient and family. Address concerns patient may have about impact on daily life: ADLs, recreation, sexual functioning, and return to work.

Congestive Heart Failure
Interdisciplinary Outcome Pathway

COORDINATION OF CARE

	Diagnosis/Stabilization Phase		Acute Management Phase		Recovery Phase	
	Outcome	Interventions	Outcome	Interventions	Outcome	Interventions
	All appropriate team members and disciplines will be involved in the plan of care.	Develop the plan of care with the cardiologist, primary physician(s), cardiovascular surgeon, RN, advanced practice nurse, PT, RCP, pharmacist, chaplain, and outcome manager.	All appropriate team members and disciplines will be involved in the plan of care.	Update the plan of care with the patient/family, other team members, social services, dietitian, cardiac rehabilitation, OT, and discharge planner. Include pharmacist in decisions concerning pharmacologic treatment in an effort to decrease costs.	All appropriate team members and disciplines will be involved in the plan of care.	Involve the CHF clinic coordinator, if available, and/or home health for follow-up if needed. Prepare patient for possible home inotrope therapy. Stress need for team approach in managing CHF and need for compliance with medical regimen. Evaluate patient for possible surgical intervention (transplant, ventricular remodeling, cardiomyoplasty).

DIAGNOSTICS

	Diagnosis/Stabilization Phase		Acute Management Phase		Recovery Phase	
	Outcome	Interventions	Outcome	Interventions	Outcome	Interventions
	Patient will understand any tests or procedures that must be completed such as hemodynamic assessments, ABGs, echocardiogram, CXR, EKG, and lab work.	Explain all procedures and tests to patient. Be sensitive to patient's and family's individualized needs for information.	Patient will understand any tests or procedures that must be completed.	Explain procedures and tests that must be completed (cardiac enzymes, endomyocardial biopsy, nuclear scans, cardiac angiography, diagnostic workup for heart transplantation, cardiomyoplasty, ventricular remodeling, and investigational treatments).	Patient will understand the meaning of diagnostic tests in relation to continuing health.	Review with patient before discharge results of EKG, any abnormal lab values, and appropriate measures patient can take to help return to normal. Provide patient with guidelines concerning follow-up care. Explain any additional procedures that may be done such as metabolic testing and exercise stress testing. Cardiac teaching; • signs and symptoms of CHF, dysrhythmias, angina, MI • medications • diet • activity • when to call physician • risk factor modification • energy-saving techniques

Congestive Heart Failure Interdisciplinary Outcome Pathway (continued)

FLUID BALANCE

Diagnosis/Stabilization Phase		Acute Management Phase		Recovery Phase	
Outcome	Interventions	Outcome	Interventions	Outcome	Interventions
Patient will achieve optimal hemodynamic status as evidenced by: • MAP >70 mmHg • VS WNL • optimal hemodynamic function • UO >0.5 mL/kg/hr • free from abnormal EKG changes and/or dysrhythmias • normal heart sounds • PCWP <15 mmHg • SVR <1,200 dynes/second/cm² • SvO₂ 60–75%	Monitor and treat cardiac parameters: • BP • PA pressures • PCWP • CO/CI • SV/SI • SvO₂ • SVR/PVR • left and right ventricular stroke work index • dysrhythmias • LOC • evidence of tissue perfusion Monitor effects of medications closely; if patient is on ACE inhibitors, MAP may be as low as 50 mmHg as long as patient is asymptomatic (SvO₂ 60–75%). Anticipate need for vasopressor agents. Assess VS, heart sounds, and hemodynamics before and after any vasoactive, diuretic, and/or cardiac medication is given or dosage change. Anticipate need for pharmacologic interventions for dysrhythmias. Monitor and treat lab values: electrolytes, Mg⁺⁺, phosphorus, and cardiac enzymes. Monitor for signs of complications that can occur with CHF: • pulmonary edema • cardiogenic shock • dysrhythmias • renal insufficiency or failure • hepatic insufficiency or failure • systemic emboli	Patient will maintain optimal hemodynamic status.	Monitor hemodynamic parameters and treat patient as needed. Convert vasoactive medications to oral derivatives. Monitor effect on hemodynamics closely. Monitor lab values and treat patient as needed. Evaluate patient for further therapeutic options such as transplant, cardiomyoplasty, or ventricular remodeling. Explain risks and benefits clearly to patient/family. Support patient/family physically and psychologically if further therapeutic options are exercised. Monitor for PND and orthopnea. Monitor response to medications (i.e., ACE inhibitors and diuretics). Note: Digitalis is no longer a mainstay of therapy for the CHF patient. It is primarily used in the CHF patient to help control HR and rhythm.	Patient will maintain optimal hemodynamics.	Monitor hemodynamic values and treat patient as needed. Teach patient/family: • medication regimen • signs and symptoms of CHF (dyspnea on exertion, shortness of breath, 2–3 pillow orthopnea, weight gain of 3 or more pounds, JVD, peripheral edema) • importance of reporting symptoms to physician • how to adjust diuretic therapy based on daily weight • if on digitalis, daily pulse taking and signs of digitalis toxicity Teach patients who are severely hyponatremic and unresponsive to diuretics and ACE inhibitors to restrict fluid intake.

Monitor for conditions that can increase the symptomatology of CHF:
- mitral stenosis
- mitral regurgitation
- aortic stenosis
- aortic regurgitation
- papillary muscle dysfunction
- ventricular septal defect
- dysrhythmias
- MI

NUTRITION

Diagnosis/Stabilization Phase		Acute Management Phase		Recovery Phase	
Outcome	Interventions	Outcome	Interventions	Outcome	Interventions
Patient will be adequately nourished as evidenced by: • stable weight • weight not >10% below or >20% above IBW • albumin >3.5 g/dL • prealbumin >15 • total protein 6–8 g/dL • total lymphocyte count 1,000–3,000 • cholesterol <200 mg/dL	Assess nutritional status. Monitor for albumin, prealbumin, total protein, cholesterol, triglycerides, and sodium. Assess need for fluid restriction.	Patient will be adequately nourished.	Monitor response to low sodium/heart healthy diet. Weigh daily. Involve dietitian. Teach patient/family: • total fat <30% of daily intake • total saturated fat <10% of daily intake • total daily cholesterol intake <300 mg/day • total daily sodium intake <2–3 g depending on severity of CHF • caloric reduction if needed • potassium supplements if on chronic diuretic therapy • diet supplements for cachectic patients • for patients with alcoholic cardiomyopathy, complete restriction from alcohol; for all other patients, limit alcohol intake to one drink per day Assess signs and symptoms of GI distress and take appropriate measures: anorexia, N & V, abdominal distension, hepatomegaly.	Patient will be adequately nourished.	Continue diet teaching. Assess understanding. Reinforce as needed. Continue fluid restriction if indicated.

Congestive Heart Failure Interdisciplinary Outcome Pathway (continued)

NUTRITION (continued)

Diagnosis/Stabilization Phase		Acute Management Phase		Recovery Phase	
Outcome	Interventions	Outcome	Interventions	Outcome	Interventions
			Fluid restriction if indicated. Patient may need smaller portions at more frequent intervals.		

MOBILITY

Diagnosis/Stabilization Phase		Acute Management Phase		Recovery Phase	
Outcome	Interventions	Outcome	Interventions	Outcome	Interventions
Patient will achieve optimal mobility and participate in spaced activities. Patient will receive optimal rest.	PT consult when indicated to assess ambulation mobility, muscle flexibility, strength, and tone. OT consult to determine functional ability for ADLs. PT/OT to help determine activity goals. Allow frequent rest periods between activities. Allow flexible visitation if it promotes rest of patient. If IABP or VAD in place, limit activities as needed.	Patient will achieve optimal mobility.	Progress exercise as tolerated. Monitor response to exercise and increased activity. Decrease activity if adverse events occur (tachycardia, dyspnea, ectopy, syncope, hypotension, chest discomfort, crackles after activity). Monitor exercise with pulse oximetry and cardiac monitor. Teach patient pursed-lip breathing technique and how to coordinate breathing with activity for energy conservation. Have patient give return demonstration. Use an exertion scale for the patient to rate level of work with activity.	Patient will achieve optimal mobility.	Continue as in Acute Management Phase. Assist patient and family in developing home exercise program. Teach patient/family energy-saving techniques. Refer to CHF clinic or cardiac rehabilitation program if applicable. Improving exercise tolerance is essential in this group of patients.

OXYGENATION/VENTILATION

Diagnosis/Stabilization Phase		Acute Management Phase		Recovery Phase	
Outcome	Interventions	Outcome	Interventions	Outcome	Interventions
Patient will have adequate gas exchange as evidenced by: • SaO_2 > 90% • SpO_2 > 92% • ABGs WNL • clear breath sounds • normal heart sounds • respiratory rate, depth, and rhythm WNL • CXR WNL Patient will have adequate tissue oxygenation as evidenced by: • alertness and orientation to time, place, and person • normal LOC • UO > 0.5 mL/kg/hr	Monitor and treat oxygenation status per ABGs and/or SpO_2. Monitor and treat ventilatory status per chest assessment, ABGs, adventitious breath sounds, and CXR. Support patient with O_2 therapy and/or mechanical ventilation. Monitor for signs of fluid overload: • I & O • daily weight • JVD • crackles • S3 • S4 • altered LOC • evidence of tissue perfusion to all major organs • abdominal distension Restrict fluid when indicated. Monitor IABP and VAD as necessary. Monitor for signs and symptoms of impaired circulation and infection. Keep HOB elevated.	Patient will have adequate gas exchange. Patient will maintain adequate tissue perfusion.	Continue as in Diagnosis/Stabilization Phase. Monitor and treat oxygenation/ventilation disturbances. Wean oxygen therapy and/or mechanical ventilation as tolerated. Observe for complications that may impair oxygenation/ventilation: • exacerbation of CHF • mitral stenosis • mitral regurgitation • pulmonary embolus • cardiogenic shock Be prepared to administer medications, such as beta-blockers and ACE inhibitors. Beta-blockers help reduce the activity of the sympathetic nervous system. However, monitor closely for adverse pulmonary effects.	Patient will have adequate gas exchange. Patient will maintain optimal tissue perfusion.	Continue as in Acute Management Phase. Teach patient pulmonary signs and symptoms of CHF. Involve home health agency and respiratory care if home oxygen is indicated. Teach patient hazards of smoking, secondhand smoke, and environmental factors that can contribute toward development of atherosclerotic heart disease.

COMFORT

Diagnosis/Stabilization Phase		Acute Management Phase		Recovery Phase	
Outcome	Interventions	Outcome	Interventions	Outcome	Interventions
Patient will be as comfortable as possible as evidenced by: • no objective indicators of discomfort	Provide adequate rest periods between activities. Keep HOB elevated to enhance breathing comfort. Maintain quiet supportive environment to minimize catecholamine levels.	Patient will be as comfortable as possible.	Provide uninterrupted periods of rest. Teach patient relaxation techniques. Have patient give return demonstration.	Patient will be as comfortable as possible. Patient will have decreased dyspnea with rest and exertion.	Teach patient/family relaxation and complementary therapy techniques. Teach pursed-lip breathing and have patient give return demonstration.

Congestive Heart Failure Interdisciplinary Outcome Pathway (continued)

COMFORT (continued)

Diagnosis/Stabilization Phase		Acute Management Phase		Recovery Phase	
Outcome	Interventions	Outcome	Interventions	Outcome	Interventions
• no complaints of discomfort	Assess quantity and quality of discomfort. Use visual analogue scale. Administer narcotics and/or nitroglycerin for chest discomfort and monitor response. Provide reassurance in a calm, caring, competent manner.		Use complementary therapies such as touch therapy, humor, music therapy, and imagery to promote relaxation. Involve family in strategies.		

SKIN INTEGRITY

Diagnosis/Stabilization Phase		Acute Management Phase		Recovery Phase	
Outcome	Interventions	Outcome	Interventions	Outcome	Interventions
Patient will have intact skin without abrasions or pressure ulcers.	Assess skin integrity and all bony prominences q4h and PRN. Use preventive pressure-reducing devices if patient is at high risk for pressure ulcer development. Treat pressure ulcers according to hospital protocol. If IABP or VAD in place, monitor condition of skin at entry site q2h and PRN.	Patient will have intact skin without abrasions or pressure ulcers.	Continue as in Diagnosis/Stabilization Phase.	Patient will have intact skin without abrasions or pressure ulcers.	Teach patient/family proper skin care.

PROTECTION/SAFETY

Diagnosis/Stabilization Phase		Acute Management Phase		Recovery Phase	
Outcome	Interventions	Outcome	Interventions	Outcome	Interventions
Patient will be protected from possible harm.	Assess need for wrist restraints if patient is intubated, has a decreased LOC, or is unable to follow commands. If restrained, follow hospital protocol for use of restraints. Explain need for restraints to patient and family. If IABP is in place, you may need to restrain the appropriate lower extremity.	Patient will be protected from possible harm.	Provide physical assistance when dangling or beginning progressive exercise program. Assess mental status and take appropriate measures as indicated.	Patient will be protected from possible harm.	Provide physical assistance or assistive devices with ambulation and progressive exercise. Teach patient/family about physical limitations the patient may have. Reinforce energy conservation techniques

PSYCHOSOCIAL/SELF-DETERMINATION

Diagnosis/Stabilization Phase		Acute Management Phase		Recovery Phase	
Outcome	Interventions	Outcome	Interventions	Outcome	Interventions
Patient will achieve psychophysiologic stability. Patient will demonstrate a decreased level of anxiety as evidenced by: • VS WNL • mental status WNL • patient reports feeling less anxious • objective signs of decreased anxiety Patient will begin acceptance process of CHF.	Assess physiologic effect of critical care environment on patient (i.e., physical signs of sympathoadrenal stress response). Assess patient for appropriate level of stress. Assess personal responses (affective and/or feelings) of patient regarding critical illness. Observe patient's patterns of thinking and communication. Use calm, competent, reassuring approach to interventions. Arrange for flexible visitation to meet needs of patient and family. Assess and observe factors that make patient/family fearful or anxious.	Patient will achieve psychophysiologic stability. Patient will demonstrate a decrease in anxiety. Patient will continue acceptance of CHF.	Continue as in Diagnosis/Stabilization Phase. Determine coping ability of patient/family and take appropriate measures to meet their needs (i.e., explain condition, equipment, and medications; provide frequent condition reports; use easy to understand terminology; repeat information as needed; allow family to visit; and answer all questions).	Patient will achieve psychophysiologic stability. Patient will demonstrate a decrease in anxiety. Patient will continue acceptance of CHF.	Continue to assess patient for psychophysiologic stability. Include patient/family in decisions regarding care. Discuss end-of-life decisions if appropriate. Provide emotional support and instructions on coping mechanisms for a chronic illness. Inform patient/family of local support groups. Refer to outpatient counseling if needed after discharge. Discuss high readmission rate and ways to decrease (i.e., early recognition and treatment of recurrent CHF). Teach patient/family about other risk factors for heart disease and how to modify. Continue and reinforce teaching as started in Acute Management Phase.

Congestive Heart Failure Interdisciplinary Outcome Pathway *(continued)*

PSYCHOSOCIAL/SELF-DETERMINATION (continued)

	Diagnosis/Stabilization Phase	Acute Management Phase		Recovery Phase
Outcome	Interventions	Outcome	Interventions	Outcome	Interventions
	Take measures to reduce patient's and family's anxiety, fear, and/or sensory overload: • initiate family conferences • utilize consistent caregivers • support services • flexible visitation Use sedatives and antianxiety agents as appropriate, and monitor response.				Address concerns patient may have about impact on daily life: ADLs, recreation, sexual functioning, return to work, and driving.

Coronary Artery Bypass Surgery Interdisciplinary Outcome Pathway

COORDINATION OF CARE

Diagnosis/Stabilization Phase		Acute Management Phase		Recovery Phase	
Outcome	Interventions	Outcome	Interventions	Outcome	Interventions
All appropriate team members and disciplines will be involved in the plan of care.	Develop plan of care with patient/family, primary physician, cardiovascular surgeon, cardiologist, pulmonologist, hematologist, anesthesiologist, RN, advanced practice nurse, perfusionist, RCP, and chaplain.	All appropriate team members and disciplines will be involved in the plan of care.	Update the plan of care with patient/family, other team members, PT, cardiac rehabilitation, discharge planner, dietitian, and social services. Assess social support systems. Initiate planning for discharge and call home health as indicated. Begin teaching patient/family about care at home. Assess ability to manage at home versus extended care.	Patient will understand how to maintain optimal health at home.	Provide guidelines concerning care at home and any follow-up visits. Arrange first postop visit for patient prior to discharge. Assist with travel arrangements if necessary. Provide patient/family with phone number of resources available to answer questions. Refer to outpatient cardiac rehabilitation program.

DIAGNOSTICS

Diagnosis/Stabilization Phase		Acute Management Phase		Recovery Phase	
Outcome	Interventions	Outcome	Interventions	Outcome	Interventions
Patient will understand any tests or procedures that must be completed (VS, I & O, CO, hemodynamic monitoring, hyperthermia unit, CXR, lab work, chest tubes, invasive devices, EKG, suctioning, VAD, IABP).	Explain all procedures and tests to patient/family. Be sensitive to individualized needs of patient/family for information. Establish effective communication technique with intubated patient.	Patient will understand any tests or procedures that must be completed (removal of indwelling lines and chest tubes, lab work, CXR, IS, coughing and deep breathing, antithrombotic hose).	Explain procedures and tests needed to assess recovery. Be sensitive to individualized needs of patient/family for information. Be prepared to repeat information frequently.	Patient will understand meaning of diagnostic tests in relation to continued health (lab tests, increase in activity, coughing and breathing, IS).	Review with patient before discharge the results of lab tests, CXR, and surgery. Discuss abnormal values and measures patient can take to help return to normal. Provide guidelines concerning follow-up care. Provide instruction on care at home: • when to call physician • care of incision(s) • activity limitations • medications • diet • graft patency • return of symptoms • late complications (pericarditis, CHF) • cardiac rehabilitation

Coronary Artery Bypass Surgery Interdisciplinary Outcome Pathway (continued)

FLUID BALANCE

Diagnosis/Stabilization Phase		Acute Management Phase		Recovery Phase	
Outcome	Interventions	Outcome	Interventions	Outcome	Interventions
Patient will achieve optimal hemodynamic status as evidenced by: • MAP >70 mmHg • hemodynamic parameters WNL • UO >0.5 mL/kg/hr • return to normothermic state • free from abnormal EKG changes • free of dysrhythmias Patient will remain free from bleeding.	Monitor and treat cardiac parameters: • HR • BP • PA pressures • PCWP • CO/CI • SV/SI • SvO$_2$ • SVR/PVR • ST segment • I & O • LOC • peripheral pulses • evidence of tissue perfusion • dysrhythmias Rewarm slowly and monitor temperature and signs of shivering. Methods of rewarming include head covering, radiant light, warming blankets, and/or vasodilators. Anticipate need for epicardial pacing and/or pharmacologic agents. Monitor for complications and treat as appropriate: • hypotension • bleeding • hypertension • dysrhythmias • MI • respiratory failure • renal failure • electrolyte imbalance • DIC Monitor for cardiac tamponade: decreased CO, increased CVP, pulsus paradoxus, widening cardiac silhouette, distant heart sounds. Notify physician immediately.	Patient will maintain optimal hemodynamic status. Patient will remain free from dysrhythmias.	Monitor and treat cardiac parameters as appropriate. Assist with chest tube and indwelling line removal and monitor patient afterward. In some facilities, nurses may remove chest tubes and indwelling lines. Follow hospital protocol. Monitor and treat symptomatic dysrhythmias: supraventricular, ventricular, and bradycardia. Consider need for dysrhythmia prophylaxis. Monitor for potential complications of CABS: CVA, MI, bleeding. Begin patient/family teaching on cardiovascular system, current treatment, and expected clinical course. Monitor lab values: Hgb, Hct, platelets, SMA-6. Weigh daily. I & O. Assess need for diuretics and/or potassium repletion.	Patient will maintain optimal hemodynamic status.	Monitor and treat cardiac parameters as appropriate. Continue to monitor for complications. Continue cardiac teaching. Discuss fluid management as appropriate with patient (i.e., fluid or sodium restriction, daily weight, observation for edema). Assess for understanding. Reinforce as needed. Assist with pacing wire removal and monitor patient after pacing wires removed.

Maintain VAD or IABP if used.

Monitor for complications associated with use of VAD or IABP and notify physician should they occur: bleeding, decreased peripheral circulation, dissection of the aorta, thrombus formation, septicemia, infection, hemolysis, air embolus.

Monitor lab values: Mg^{++}, Hgb, Hct, PT, PTT, ACT if available, platelets, K^+, CK-MB, cardiac troponin, glucose, BUN, and creatinine.

Assess for sudden increase or decrease in chest tube drainage, equalization of filling pressures, widening mediastinum, decrease in blood pressure, and pulsus paradoxus.

NUTRITION

Diagnosis/Stabilization Phase		Acute Management Phase		Recovery Phase	
Outcome	Interventions	Outcome	Interventions	Outcome	Interventions
Patient will be adequately nourished as evidenced by: • stable weight • weight not >10% below or >20% above IBW • albumin >3.5 g/dL • prealbumin >15 g/dL • total protein 6–8 g/dL • total lymphocyte count 1,000–3,000 • cholesterol <200 mg/dL	Keep patient NPO until extubation. If extubation is delayed >24h, assess need for alternative nutritional therapy. Monitor response to clear liquids. Remove NG tube (if utilized) once extubated. Monitor protein and albumin lab values. Administer antiemetics, H_2 blockers, and/or antacids as needed.	Patient will be adequately nourished. Patient will remain free from nausea. Patient will demonstrate return of appetite.	Advance to heart healthy diet (low fat, low cholesterol) as tolerated. Monitor response to diet. Involve dietitian: • if eating less than half of food on tray • for unanticipated weight loss • for albumin <3 • for education on heart healthy diet Weigh daily. Assess bowel sounds. Administer laxatives/stool softeners as needed.	Patient will be adequately nourished.	Teach patient/family about heart healthy diet: • total fat <30% of daily intake • total saturated fat <10% of daily intake • total daily cholesterol intake <300 mg • calorie restriction if indicated • sodium restriction if indicated Continue laxatives/stool softeners if needed. Teach patient about dietary supplements (i.e., antioxidants, oat bran, fiber, vitamins and minerals).

Coronary Artery Bypass Surgery Interdisciplinary Outcome Pathway (continued)

MOBILITY

Diagnosis/Stabilization Phase		Acute Management Phase		Recovery Phase	
Outcome	Interventions	Outcome	Interventions	Outcome	Interventions
Patient will maintain normal ROM and muscle strength.	Bed rest until extubated unless extubation delayed > 24h. If extubation is delayed, consult PT for appropriate exercises. When patient is hemodynamically stable, may be up in chair. Begin passive/active-assist ROM exercises. Dangle after extubation.	Patient will achieve optimal mobility.	Progress exercise as tolerated: dangle, bathroom privileges, OOB for meals, and walking 50 feet. Monitor response to increased activity. Decrease if adverse events occur (tachycardia, chest discomfort, dyspnea, ectopy, bleeding). Provide physical assistance or assistive devices as necessary. Assess symptoms that may occur in lower extremities in patients with SVGs: pain, paresthesia, numbness. Begin patient/family teaching on principles of a gradual exercise program. Initiate cardiac rehabilitation.	Patient will achieve optimal mobility.	Walk at least 200 to 300 feet TID to QID. Walk up and down one flight of stairs, particularly if stairs at home. Teach patient/family about home exercise program. Refer to outpatient cardiac rehabilitation.

OXYGENATION/VENTILATION

Diagnosis/Stabilization Phase		Acute Management Phase		Recovery Phase	
Outcome	Interventions	Outcome	Interventions	Outcome	Interventions
Patient will have adequate gas exchange as evidenced by: • SaO_2 >90% • SpO_2 >92% • ABGs WNL • clear breath sounds • respiratory rate, depth, and rhythm WNL • CXR WNL	Monitor ventilator settings and wakefulness and determine readiness to wean. Determine if patient meets early extubation criteria. Monitor hemodynamic variables before, during, and after weaning. Wean ventilator and monitor patient response: • wean FIO_2 to keep SpO_2 >92% • monitor effects of anesthesia and wean ventilator accordingly • after extubation, apply supplemental oxygen	Patient will have adequate gas exchange.	Monitor and treat oxygenation/ventilation status per ABGs, SpO_2, chest assessment, and CXR. Monitor closely for hypoxemia or dyspnea related to atelectasis and/or pleural effusion. Evaluate need for thoracentesis. Assess chest tubes for drainage/presence of air leaks. Support patient with oxygen therapy as indicated to keep SpO_2 > 92%. Reinforce use of IS.	Patient will have adequate gas exchange.	Obtain CXR before discharge. Reinforce teaching about IS and use of chest splint pillow at home.

	Diagnosis/Stabilization Phase		Acute Management Phase		Recovery Phase	
	Outcome	Interventions	Outcome	Interventions	Outcome	Interventions
		Assess respiratory functioning, including lung sounds, respiratory muscle strength, respiratory rate and depth, coughing ability, and CXR. Monitor pulse oximetry to keep SpO$_2$ > 92%. Reinforce use of IS (with inspiratory hold) when extubated.		Monitor for complications that may impair oxygenation/ventilation: pneumonia, atelectasis, pulmonary embolus, and CHF. Provide chest splint pillow and instruct on proper use. Have patient give return demonstration.		

COMFORT

	Diagnosis/Stabilization Phase		Acute Management Phase		Recovery Phase	
	Outcome	Interventions	Outcome	Interventions	Outcome	Interventions
	Patient will be as comfortable and pain free as possible as evidenced by: • no objective indicators of discomfort • no complaints of discomfort • normal VS	Anticipate need for analgesia and provide as needed. Use a pain scale or visual analogue tool. Assess response to all analgesics and effects on ability to wean from ventilator when indicated. Use newer NSAIDs with fewer sedative effects. Establish effective communication technique with intubated patient with which he or she can communicate discomfort and need for analgesics.	Patient will be as relaxed and comfortable as possible.	Anticipate need for analgesics and provide as needed. Assess response. Remember, descriptors of discomfort will change from sharp pain to dull ache as recovery progresses. Teach patient proper use of PCA pump. Provide chest splint pillow and instruct on proper use. Have patient give return demonstration. Provide uninterrupted periods of rest. Assist patient with relaxation techniques. Use touch therapy, humor, music therapy, and imagery to promote relaxation. Provide analgesics as needed before chest tube removal, ambulation, and any other uncomfortable procedures.	Patient will be as relaxed and comfortable as possible.	Progress analgesics to oral medications as needed and monitor response. Teach patient/family regarding analgesic administration and potential side effects for after discharge. Continue alternative methods to promote relaxation. Teach patient/family alternative methods to promote relaxation at home. Have patient/family give return demonstration. Provide uninterrupted periods of rest. Inform patient to report any discomfort to physician.

Coronary Artery Bypass Surgery Interdisciplinary Outcome Pathway (continued)

SKIN INTEGRITY

Diagnosis/Stabilization Phase		Acute Management Phase		Recovery Phase	
Outcome	Interventions	Outcome	Interventions	Outcome	Interventions
Patient will have intact skin without abrasions or pressure ulcers. Patient will return to normothermia. Patient will have healing wounds.	Rewarm slowly; monitor temperature and signs of shivering. Use radiant lights, warm IV fluids, and warm blankets. In some institutions, patients are not kept as hypothermic as before. Adapt rewarming techniques according to temperature of patient after surgery. Assess all bony prominences at least q4h and treat if needed. Maintain integrity of all dressings. Consider mattress overlay.	Patient will have intact skin without abrasions, pressure ulcers, or wound infections. Patient will have healing wounds.	Assess all bony prominences at least q4h and treat if needed. Use preventive pressure-reducing devices if patient is at high risk for developing pressure ulcers. Treat pressure ulcers according to hospital protocol. Use antithrombotic hose and elevate legs to minimize edema. Ambulate patient on postop Day 2 if possible. Assess sternotomy incision and leg incisions for drainage, erythema, and induration. Use sterile technique when changing bandages. Teach patient/family proper skin care at home: • incision care • antithrombotic hose • signs and symptoms of infection • how to minimize edema • when to call physician	Patient will have intact skin without abrasions, pressure ulcers, or infections. Patient will have healing wounds.	Assess all wounds/incisions for signs and symptoms of infection. Culture if necessary. Reinforce importance of proper hygiene and wound care postop. Continue patient/family teaching on skin care at home. Assess understanding and reinforce as needed.

PROTECTION/SAFETY

Diagnosis/Stabilization Phase		Acute Management Phase		Recovery Phase	
Outcome	Interventions	Outcome	Interventions	Outcome	Interventions
Patient will be protected from possible harm.	Assess need for wrist restraints while patient is intubated, has a decreased LOC, or is agitated and restless. Explain need for restraints to patient/family. Assess response to restraints and check q1–2h for skin integrity and impairment to circulation.	Patient will be protected from possible harm.	Provide support when dangling or getting OOB; monitor response. Isolate pacing wires. Assess symptoms in lower extremities in patients with SVGs: numbness, pain, paresthesia.	Patient will be protected from possible harm.	Provide support with ambulation and climbing stairs. Teach patient/family about physical limitations such as no lifting/pulling objects over 10–15 pounds for 2–3 months after surgery, no driving until approved by surgeon, when sexual activity may resume, and when patient may return to work.

Remove restraints as soon as patient is awake from anesthesia and able to follow instructions.
Follow hospital protocol regarding use of restraints.
Provide sedatives/antianxiety agents as needed.
Isolate pacing wires.

Review signs and symptoms of infection and when to call physician.
Isolate pacing wires until removed.

PSYCHOSOCIAL/SELF-DETERMINATION

Diagnosis/Stabilization Phase		Acute Management Phase		Recovery Phase	
Outcome	Interventions	Outcome	Interventions	Outcome	Interventions
Patient will achieve psychophysiologic stability. Patient will demonstrate a decrease in anxiety as evidenced by: • VS WNL • LOC WNL • subjective reports	Assess physiologic effects of critical care and/or open heart recovery environment on patient (hemodynamic variables, psychological status, signs of increased sympathetic response). Provide sedatives as indicated. Take measures to reduce sensory overload. Develop effective interventions to communicate with patient while intubated. Use calm, caring, competent, and reassuring approach with patient and family. Allow flexible visitation to meet patient and family needs. Determine emotional impact and coping ability of patient and take appropriate measures to meet needs (provide frequent condition reports, repeat information, use easy to understand terminology, answer questions, allow to verbalize feelings). Conduct a family needs assessment and employ measures to meet identified concerns.	Patient will achieve psychophysiologic stability. Patient will demonstrate a decrease in anxiety.	Take measures to decrease sensory overload. Provide adequate rest periods. Provide sedatives as needed. Continue to include family in aspects of care. Continue to assess coping ability of patient/family and take measures as indicated. Involve patient/family in health care decisions.	Patient will achieve psychophysiologic stability. Patient will demonstrate a decrease in anxiety. Patient will understand that full recovery may take 2–6 months.	Provide adequate rest periods. Continue to assess coping ability of patient and family. Provide information on coping mechanisms for use after discharge. Refer to outside services or agencies as appropriate (chaplain, social services, support group, home health, cardiac rehabilitation). Include patient/family in decisions concerning care. Address concerns patient may have about impact on daily life: ADLs, recreation, sexual functioning, return to work, and driving.

Dysrhythmias
Interdisciplinary Outcome Pathway

COORDINATION OF CARE

Diagnosis/Stabilization Phase		Acute Management Phase		Recovery Phase	
Outcome	Interventions	Outcome	Interventions	Outcome	Interventions
All appropriate team members and disciplines will be involved in plan of care.	Develop the plan of care with the patient/family, primary physician, emergency department physician (if applicable), cardiologist, RN, advanced practice nurse, and RCP.	All appropriate team members and disciplines will be involved in the plan of care.	Update the plan of care with the patient/family, other team members, pharmacist, dietitian, and discharge planner. Assess social support systems. Assess learning needs regarding patient's dysrhythmia and treatment. Begin teaching patient/family about care at home. Initiate discharge planning.	Patient will understand how to maintain optimal health at home.	Discuss with patient and family home care instructions and need for follow-up visits. Provide guidelines regarding discharge instructions. Provide educational material on dysrhythmias and their management. Provide phone numbers of resources available to answer questions.

DIAGNOSTICS

Diagnosis/Stabilization Phase		Acute Management Phase		Recovery Phase	
Outcome	Interventions	Outcome	Interventions	Outcome	Interventions
Patient will verbalize understanding of tests or procedures regarding current hospitalization (VS, cardiac monitoring, EKG, Holter monitoring, EP study, IV line, lab work).	Assess patient's readiness to learn. Explain tests and procedures to patient/family. Explain what a cardiac cath lab is like and what the patient will experience during an EP study and final ICD testing. Explain what an operating room is like and what the patient will experience during an implantable cardioverter defibrillator (ICD) insertion. Ask for questions after explanations given, and provide answers. Be sensitive to individualized needs of patient/family for information.	Patient will verbalize understanding of tests or procedures regarding current hospitalization.	Assess patient's learning needs. Explain procedures and tests to patient/family, answering any questions they may have. Provide any literature/videotapes/audiovisual aids available regarding procedures, tests, and the hospital. Encourage patient to discuss fears and concerns.	Patient will verbalize understanding of tests/procedures related to continued health.	Review with patient before discharge results of diagnostic tests. Provide patient with guidelines concerning follow-up care. Provide instructions on care at home after discharge (as applicable): • medications • follow-up visits • pacemaker phone transmission • activity limitations • actions to take should dysrhythmia occur again or worsen • actions to take should chest discomfort, shortness of breath occur • diet • when to call physician/come to the ER

FLUID BALANCE

Diagnosis/Stabilization Phase		Acute Management Phase		Recovery Phase	
Outcome	Interventions	Outcome	Interventions	Outcome	Interventions
Patient will achieve and/or maintain optimal hemodynamic status as evidenced by: • MAP > 70 mmHg • UO > 0.5 mL/kg/hr • skin turgor with good resiliency • capillary refill < 2 seconds • hemodynamic parameters WNL • normal respiratory exam • normal EKG • normal heart sounds	Monitor cardiac parameters and treat as needed: • HR • heart rhythm • BP • respiratory rate and rhythm • CO/CI • SV/SI • SpO₂ • PR interval • QRS • T wave • ST segment • QT interval • I & O Maintain patient IV line. Patient will be NPO at least 6 hours prior to an EP study or an ICD insertion. Deliver IV fluids at a rate in accordance with cardiac parameters. Monitor lab values: SMA-18, CBC, PT, PTT, cardiac enzymes, ABGs. Assess capillary refill, peripheral pulses, LOC, skin temperature, and presence of peripheral edema. Auscultate lung sounds q4h and PRN.	Patient will maintain optimal hemodynamic status and a stable rhythm.	Continue as in Diagnostic/Stabilization Phase Obtain a 12/15/18 lead EKG. Monitor HR and rhythm using an EKG lead most likely to show changes in the rhythm (i.e., Lead II for atrial rhythms, MCL1 for ventricular ectopy/rhythm). Monitor as many different leads simultaneously as possible (i.e., Lead II and MCL1). Assess signs and symptoms related to dysrhythmias. If patient symptomatic (decreased tissue perfusion, hypotension, chest pain, altered LOC, SOB, pulmonary congestion, decreased oxygen saturation), treat according to ACLS protocol and hospital policy. Monitor cardiac heart sounds (S3 with impending CHF, S4 with heart failure, murmur with high outflow states or valvular disease). Administer oxygen according to SpO₂. Monitor with pulse oximetry. Maintain SpO₂ > 92%. Monitor lab values: • SMA: especially K⁺, cardiac enzymes, BUN/creatinine, LFT if on medications metabolized in the liver • CBC (anemia could be a contributing factor) • myoglobin/troponin levels (if suspect AMI) • drug levels • thyroid studies (if suspect hyper/hypothyroid)	Patient will maintain optimal hemodynamic status.	Continue as in Acute Management Phase. Perform routine postop care after ICD insertion including incisional care. Continue cardiac teaching regarding care of catheter insertion site after an EP study. Monitor maintenance medications and drug levels. Continue patient education regarding: • current rhythm • actions to take if dysrhythmia occurs again • medications including dosage, benefits, side effects, and interactions • follow-up information • care of incision site, if applicable • any future interventions

Dysrhythmias Interdisciplinary Outcome Pathway (*continued*)

FLUID BALANCE (continued)

Diagnosis/Stabilization Phase		Acute Management Phase		Recovery Phase	
Outcome	Interventions	Outcome	Interventions	Outcome	Interventions
			• PT, PTT (if on anticoagulants or anticipate initiation of them as with atrial fibrillation)		
			• INR		
			Observe for cardiac complications:		
			• angina		
			• acute MI		
			• CHF		
			• pulmonary edema		
			• cardiogenic shock		
			• change in LOC		
			• syncope		
			• N & V		
			Provide age-appropiate education regarding dysrhythmia and its management.		
			Monitor catheter insertion site for an EP study. If bleeding is noted, apply pressure immediately and notify physician. Instruct patient to apply pressure when he or she sneezes or coughs and call nurse if feels sensation of warmth or wetness.		
			Monitor patient during and after ICD insertion. If ventricular fibrillation occurs, follow ACLS protocols. Check patient's chart for ICD program, pacemaker program information, and number of therapies.		
			Management of dysrhythmias (per ACLS protocol).		

Management of unstable brady-cardias:

- atropine 0.5–1 mg IV (repeat dose every 3–5 minutes up to a total of 0.03 mg/kg). Transcutaneous pacing is preferred over atropine in AV block at the His-Purkinje level (Type II AVB and CHB with wide QRS).
- transcutaneous pacing (verify patient tolerance and mechanical capture. Use analgesic and sedation PRN).
- dopamine 5–20 mcg/kg/minute
- epinephrine 2–10 mcg/kg/minute
- Never treat bradycardias with ventricular escape beats with lidocaine

Management of stable bradycardias:

- continue to observe (unless second-degree Type II AVB and CHB in which a permanent pacemaker may be indicated)
- have transcutaneous pacemaker close to patient

Management of unstable tachycardias:

- may give brief trial of medications
- immediate synchronized cardioversion, especially if HR > 150; sedate if patient can tolerate it
- verify defibrillator is in sychronized mode and run strip
- charge to appropriate joules (start at 50–100 joules)
- look and call "all clear"; then cardiovert
- observe rhythm for change; repeat cardioversion as needed

Dysrhythmias Interdisciplinary Outcome Pathway (continued)

DIET AND FLUIDS (continued)

	Diagnosis/Stabilization Phase		Acute Management Phase		Recovery Phase	
Outcome	Interventions	Outcome	Interventions	Outcome	Interventions	Outcome
			• monitor patient response during and after treatment; if patient too sedated, may need temporary airway assistance • if cardioversion unsuccessful, administer medications as in "Management of Stable Tachycardias" **Management of stable tachycardias:** • **Atrial fibrillation or atrial flutter:** diltiazem (usually first choice), beta-blockers, verapamil (caution: beta-blockers combined with IV verapamil may cause severe hypotension), digoxin, procainamide, quinidine • **Paroxysmal SVT (PSVT):** (1) vagal maneuvers (cough, Valsalva maneuver); (2) adenosine 6 mg IV over 1–3 seconds; (3) adenosine 12 mg IV over 1–3 seconds (in 1–2 minutes if first dose unsuccessful); (4) repeat adenosine 12 mg over 1–3 seconds (1–2 minutes later if still needed). • **Further treatment if QRS narrow:** (1) verapamil 2.5–5 mg IV; (2) verapamil 5–10 mg IV (in 15–30 minutes if first dose unsuccessful); (3) consider digoxin, beta-blockers, or diltiazem.		

- **Further treatment if QRS wide:** (1) lidocaine 1–1.5 mg/kg IV; (2) procainamide 20–30 mg/minute if lidocaine unsuccessful (maximum 17 mg/kg).

If patient remains tachycardic despite medications, proceed to synchronized cardioversion.

- **Wide complex tachycardia of uncertain type:** (1) lidocaine 1–1.5 mg IV; may repeat every 5–10 minutes at 0.5–0.75 mg/kg IV to maximum of 3 mg/kg; (2) adenosine 6 mg IV over 1–3 seconds; (3) adenosine 12 mg IV over 1–3 seconds (in 1–2 minutes if first adenosine dose unsuccessful); (4) may repeat adenosine 12 mg IV over 1–3 seconds if second dose unsuccessful; (5) procainamide 20–30 mg/minimum (maximum 17 mg/kg); (6) bretylium 5–10 mg/kg over 8–10 minutes (maximum 30 mg/kg over 24h).

If patient remains tachycardic, proceed to synchronized cardioversion.

- **Ventricular tachycardia:** (1) lidocaine 1–1.5 mg/kg; may repeat every 5–10 minutes at 0.5–0.75 mg/kg IV to maximum of 3 mg/kg; (2) procainamide 20–30 mg/minute (maximum 17 mg/kg); (3) bretylium 5–10 mg/kg over 8–10 minutes (maximum 30 mg/kg over 24h).

If patient remains tachycardic, proceed to synchronized cardioversion.

Dysrhythmias Interdisciplinary Outcome Pathway (continued)

NUTRITION

Diagnosis/Stabilization Phase		Acute Management Phase		Recovery Phase	
Outcome	Interventions	Outcome	Interventions	Outcome	Interventions
Patient will maintain a diet appropriate to his or her condition. Patient will be NPO for at least 6h prior to an EP study and ICD insertion.	Patient will begin on clear liquids and advance to heart healthy diet. Monitor response to diet. Patient will be NPO for at least 6h prior to an EP study or ICD insertion.	Patient will remain NPO during procedures. Patient will advance diet as tolerated.	Patient will be NPO during cardiac procedures. Patient may restart fluids immediately after procedures. Patient will advance diet as tolerated after the procedures and response assessed. Consult dietitian to help determine and direct nutritional support.	Patient will be adequately nourished.	Continue monitoring response to diet. Teach patient/family about heart healthy diet: • total fat <30% of daily intake • total saturated fat <10% of daily intake • total cholesterol <300 mg/day • caloric reduction if indicated • sodium reduction if indicated

MOBILITY

Diagnosis/Stabilization Phase		Acute Management Phase		Recovery Phase	
Outcome	Interventions	Outcome	Interventions	Outcome	Interventions
Patient will be mobile as appropriate to his or her hemodynamic stability.	Patient will remain on bed rest until complete assessment and evaluation is made regarding appropriate activity level. Monitor patient's response to slow progressive activity. Patient will be on bed rest for several hours after an EP study. Patient's activity level post ICD insertion will vary according to patient's condition.	Patient will be mobile as appropriate to his or her hemodynamic stability. Patient will lie still during diagnostic tests and procedures.	Continue as in Diagnostic/Stabilization Phase. HOB may be elevated to maximize lung expansion and decrease SOB if present. Instruct patient to lie still during diagnostic tests and an EP study. Administer analgesics and sedatives as necessary during the procedures. After an EP study: (1) patient will remain on bed rest for several hours (according to hospital policy); (2) patient must keep involved extremity (usually a leg) still with pressure bandage in place;	Patient will achieve optimal mobility.	Continue to advance activity according to patient's tolerance. Teach patient/family about warning signs indicating patient should decrease activity: • SOB • chest discomfort • dizziness/syncope • fatigue • palpitations Instruct patient on home activity limitations after an EP study: • no lifting > 10 pounds for at least a week. • stairs may be taken slowly

Instruct patient on home activity limitations after an ICD insertion:
- no lifting > 5 pounds for 4 weeks
- avoid above the shoulder arm movements for 4 weeks
- ask physician when patient can drive, return to work, resume sexual functioning, and resume full ADLs.

Refer to cardiac rehabilitation program if applicable.

(3) HOB may be increased 30 degrees approximately 3h after the procedure or according to hospital protocol.

After an ICD insertion: (1) patient will remain on bed rest according to hospital policy; (2) advance activity as tolerated; (3) the arm may be immobile up to 24h; (4) an ice bag may be placed over the insertion site to decrease swelling.

Slowly progress activity level according to patient's tolerance. Ambulate with assistance the first time patient gets up. Monitor response to activity. Consult OT/PT as needed.

Monitor response to increased activity. Decrease activity if adverse events occur (tachycardia, chest discomfort, bleeding, dyspnea, ectopy, and hypotension).

Initiate cardiac rehabilitation if applicable.

OXYGENATION/VENTILATION

Diagnosis/Stabilization Phase		Acute Management Phase		Recovery Phase	
Outcome	Interventions	Outcome	Interventions	Outcome	Interventions
Patient will have adequate gas exchange as evidenced by: • $SaO_2 > 90\%$ • $SpO_2 > 92\%$ • ABGs WNL • respiratory rate, depth, and rhythm normal • CXR normal	Monitor respiratory rate and effort. Monitor shortness of breath/dyspnea. Monitor and treat any adventitious breath sounds, especially any change from baseline, such as increased crackles. Monitor pulse oximeter/ABGs. Apply supplemental oxygen to maintain $SpO_2 > 92\%$. Involve RCP as needed. Elevate HOB to ease ventilation.	Patient will have adequate gas exchange.	Continue as in Diagnosis/Stabilization Phase. While patient on bed rest, elevate HOB 30 degrees and encourage coughing and deep breathing at least q2h. During an EP study, patient may be asked to take a deep breath, hold his or her breath, or cough. Utilize pulse oximetry during an EP study.	Patient will have adequate gas exchange.	Instruct patient/family to report any dyspnea that may occur after discharge.

Dysrhythmias Interdisciplinary Outcome Pathway (*continued*)

COMFORT

Diagnosis/Stabilization Phase		Acute Management Phase		Recovery Phase	
Outcome	Interventions	Outcome	Interventions	Outcome	Interventions
Patient will be free of discomfort as evidenced by: • no objective indication of discomfort • no complaints of discomfort Patient will be as comfortable as possible during the cardiac procedures.	Have patient remain on bed rest until condition stable. Elevate HOB at least 30 degrees. Maintain a quiet, calm atmosphere. Anticipate need for nitrates, analgesics, and/or sedatives, and provide as needed. Assess response. Obtain 12 lead EKG immediately if chest discomfort/pain should occur with dysrhythmia and report to physician. Encourage patient to report any discomfort before and during an EP study. Instruct patient that numbing of EP study entry site will burn for a few seconds.	Patient will be free of discomfort. Patient will be as comfortable as possible during cardiac procedures.	Instruct patient to communicate any discomfort to staff. Teach patient about the dysrythmia and associated signs and symptoms indicating need for medical attention. Administer sedation before an EP study or ICD insertion. Administer analgesics and sedation as needed during an EP study and assess response. After an EP study, continue to monitor for chest discomfort. Should it occur, obtain a 12 lead EKG immediately. Apply supplemental oxygen and notify physician. Provide reassurance. Instruct patient on antidysrhythmic medications, including dosage, side effects, and interactions. Promote relaxation techniques and stress management resources: • deep breathing • pursed-lip breathing • imagery • music therapy After an ICD insertion: • monitor HR and rhythm • monitor for any dysrhythmia and assess functioning of ICD • administer medications as ordered or per hospital/ACLS protocol • adminster analgesics as needed and assess response • provide supplemental oxygen according to SpO_2	Patient will be free from discomfort.	Determine cause of discomfort. Monitor catheter insertion site post EP study. Monitor incision site post implantable defibrillator insertion. Administer analgesics as needed and assess response. Teach patient/family about stress management and relaxation techniques. Teach patient/family what measures to take should discomfort or dysrhythmia recur.

SKIN INTEGRITY

Diagnosis/Stabilization Phase		Acute Management Phase		Recovery Phase	
Outcome	Interventions	Outcome	Interventions	Outcome	Interventions
Patient will have intact skin without redness or abrasions.	Obtain baseline assessment of patient's skin, especially over bony prominences and other pressure-prone areas. Treat any abrasions according to hospital protocol. Assess tissue perfusion (pulse, pain, color, temperature, signs of decreased perfusion such as altered LOC and decreased UO). Position patient for comfort and pressure relief.	Patient will have intact skin without redness or abrasions.	Assess patient's skin q4h and treat if needed. Utilize pressure-relieving mattresses. Aggressively treat redness/skin breakdown due to pressure according to hospital protocol. Assess catheter entry site after an EP study according to hospital policy. Monitor and treat signs of infection or bleeding. Assess incisional site after an ICD is inserted. Observe for signs of infection or bleeding. If noted, take appropriate measures.	Patient will have intact skin and no evidence of redness or abrasions.	Continue as in Acute Management Phase. Teach patient proper skin care for after discharge.

PROTECTION/SAFETY

Diagnosis/Stabilization Phase		Acute Management Phase		Recovery Phase	
Outcome	Interventions	Outcome	Interventions	Outcome	Interventions
Patient will be protected from possible harm.	Perform risk for falls assessment. Provide sedation as needed and monitor response. Instruct patient to remain in bed until heart rhythm, HR, breathing, and BP are controlled.	Patient will be protected from possible harm.	Reassess patient's risk for falls if vital signs or medications change. Instruct patient to remain on bed rest until assessed by nurse. Instruct patient to call nursing staff before getting OOB for the first time or if light-headedness occurs. Provide physical support as needed. Instruct patient to lie still during an EP study. Provide sedatives as needed and monitor response. Instruct patient to keep extremity used for catheter entry still for several hours after an EP study.	Patient will be protected from possible harm.	Provide physical support with ambulation. Teach patient to avoid activities that may precipitate or aggravate a dysrhythmia (caffeine, stimulants, anxiety, lack of sleep, low potassium). Instruct patient to stop activity and rest if chest discomfort, palpitations, SOB, or dizziness occurs. Teach patient to avoid lifting anything over 10 pounds for 1 week after an EP study. Teach patient to avoid lifting anything over 5 pounds for 4 weeks after an ICD is inserted.

Dysrhythmias Interdisciplinary Outcome Pathway (continued)

PSYCHOSOCIAL/SELF-DETERMINATION

Diagnosis/Stabilization Phase		Acute Management Phase		Recovery Phase	
Outcome	Interventions	Outcome	Interventions	Outcome	Interventions
Patient will maintain psychophysiologic stability. Patient will use effective coping strategies to manage anxiety.	Assess patient's response to the stress of the dysrhythmia and hospitalization. Assess patient's coping skills and take appropriate measures to assist patient with coping. Assess patient's support systems. Provide a calm, caring environment for the patient and family. Involve patient/family in health care decisions. Provide explanations appropriate to patient's condition and readiness to learn.	Patient will maintain psychophysiologic stability. Patient will use effective coping strategies to manage anxiety.	Continue to assess patient's stress response to hospitalization and coping skills. Take measures as necessary. Maximize patient's ability to adapt to the stress of the dysrhythmia and its management, including hospitalization (i.e., relaxation techniques, providing time to verbalize feelings, providing a quiet, supportive environment, having significant others at bedside). Continue explanations regarding dysrhythmia and its management. Administer sedatives as indicated and monitor response. Initiate discharge planning. Call for resources to help patient deal with condition (i.e., CNS, pastoral care). Be sensitive to patient/family's individual needs for information	Patient will maintain psychophysiologic stability. Patient will use effective coping strategies to manage anxiety.	Continue to assess patient's stress response and use of coping skills. Provide information on stress management for use after discharge. Provide community resource information. Refer to appropriate agencies (home health, cardiac rehabilitation, pacemaker clinic). Address concerns patient may have about impact on daily life: ADL, recreation, sexual functioning, return to work, driving.

Heart Transplantation Interdisciplinary Outcome Pathway

COORDINATION OF CARE

Diagnosis/Stabilization Phase		Acute Management Phase		Recovery Phase	
Outcome	Interventions	Outcome	Interventions	Outcome	Interventions
All appropriate team members and disciplines will be involved in the plan of care.	Develop plan of care with patient/family, primary physician(s), cardiothoracic surgeon, cardiologist, pulmonologist, anesthesiologist, RN, advanced practice nurse, transplant team, RCP, social services, and psychologist. Instruct patient/family on the transplant process.	All appropriate team members and disciplines will be involved in the plan of care.	Update plan of care with patient/family, other team members, physical therapist, cardiac rehabilitation staff, discharge planner, dietitian, chaplain, and case manager. Assess social support systems. Initiate planning for anticipated discharge and call home health as indicated. Begin teaching patient/family about care at home. Assess ability to manage care at home.	Patient will understand how to maintain optimal health care at home. Patient will understand importance and necessity of follow-up visits for the rest of his or her life.	Provide guidelines concerning care at home and any follow-up visits. Provide patient/family with phone number of resources available to answer questions. Provide patient/family with phone number of transplant coordinator. Assist patient with arrangements for follow-up visits. Provide patient with schedule of follow-up visits and actions needed for each visit. Refer to a transplant support group.

DIAGNOSTICS

Diagnosis/Stabilization Phase		Acute Management Phase		Recovery Phase	
Outcome	Interventions	Outcome	Interventions	Outcome	Interventions
Patient will understand any tests or procedures that must be completed (VS, I & O, CO, hemodynamic monitoring, hyperthermia unit, CXR, lab work, chest tubes, invasive devices, EKG, cardiac monitoring, VAD, suctioning).	Explain all procedures and tests to patient/family. Be sensitive to individual needs of patient and family for information. Establish effective communication technique with intubated patient.	Patient will understand any tests or procedures that must be completed (removal of indwelling lines and chest tubes, IS, lab work, CXR, coughing and deep breathing, increase in activity, isolation measures, aseptic technique, endomyocardial biopsy).	Explain procedures and tests needed to assess recovery from surgery. Be sensitive to individualized needs of patient and family for information.	Patient will understand meaning of diagnostic tests in relation to continued health (lab tests, increase in activity, coughing and deep breathing, IS, endomyocardial biopsy, all necessary follow-up tests including coronary angiography at least once a year).	Review with patient before discharge the results of lab tests, CXR, rejection episodes, and results of all endomyocardial biopsies. Discuss any abnormal findings and appropriate measures patient can take to help return to normal. Provide patient with guidelines concerning follow-up care. Interact with transplant team to plan discharge and follow-up care.

Heart Transplantation Interdisciplinary Outcome Pathway (continued)

DIAGNOSTICS (continued)

	Diagnosis/Stabilization Phase		Acute Management Phase		Recovery Phase
Outcome	Interventions	Outcome	Interventions	Outcome	Interventions
					Provide instructions on care at home after discharge:
					• when to call the physician
					• care of incision
					• activity limitations
					• medications
					• diet
					• follow-up visits
					• first biopsy after discharge
					Refer to transplant support group.
					Stress need for patient to have list of medications with him or her at all times.

FLUID BALANCE

	Diagnosis/Stabilization Phase		Acute Management Phase		Recovery Phase
Outcome	Interventions	Outcome	Interventions	Outcome	Interventions
Patient will achieve optimal hemodynamic status as evidenced by: • MAP > 70 mmHg • hemodynamic parameters WNL • UO > 0.5 mL/kg/hr • return to normal thermic state • free from abnormal EKG changes • free from dysrhythmias Patient will remain free from bleeding.	Monitor and treat cardiac parameters: • HR • BP • PA pressures • PCWP • CO/CI • SV/SI • SvO$_2$ • SVR/PVR • I & O • LOC • peripheral pulses • evidence of tissue perfusion • dysrhythmias	Patient will maintain optimal hemodynamic status. Patient will remain free from dysrhythmias.	Monitor and treat cardiac variables. Assist with chest tube and indwelling line removal and monitor patient afterward. Begin patient/family teaching on cardiovascular system, current treatment, and expected clinical course. Monitor and treat dysrhythmias. Monitor lab values: Hgb, Hct, platelets, SMA-6. Monitor daily weight. Monitor I & O.	Patient will maintain optimal hemodynamic status.	Continue to monitor all cardiac parameters and treat as needed. Continue cardiac teaching: • daily weight • low salt diet • heart healthy diet • actions to take for sudden weight gain (2–3 pounds overnight) • monitor for edema • when to call physician Assess understanding of cardiac teaching and reinforce as needed.

Rewarm slowly and monitor temperature and signs of shivering. Methods of rewarming include head cover, radiant light, warming blankets, and/or vasodilation.

Anticipate need for antidysrhythmics and/or need for cardiac pacing.

Monitor lab values: K^+, Mg^{++}, Hgb, Hct, PT, PTT, ACT, platelets, cardiac enzymes, cardiac troponin, glucose, creatinine, BUN.

Assess for sudden increase or decrease in chest tube drainage, equalization of filling pressure, widening mediastinum, decrease in blood pressure, and pulsus paradoxus.

Maintain ventricular assist system (VAD) if used.

Maintain IABP if used.

Administer vasopressors and positive inotropic agents as necessary. Monitor response.

Administer positive chronotropic support (i.e., isoproterenol) if needed for bradycardia.

Wean from VAD as tolerated. Monitor for complications of VAD system (bleeding, CVA, thromboembolic events, infection, vascular damage, hemolysis).

Wean from IABP as tolerated. Monitor for complications associated with IABP: infection, limb ischemia, thromboembolic events, bleedings, thrombocytopenia, aortic dissection.

Continue to administer vasopressors and positive inotropic agents as needed and monitor response.

Cardiac monitoring: There will be two p waves for every QRS, since the recipient's native SA node may be left in place. However, the impulses from this SA node will not be transmitted across the donor heart's AV node. In addition, a right BBB is not uncommon.

NUTRITION

Diagnosis/Stabilization Phase		Acute Management Phase		Recovery Phase	
Outcome	Interventions	Outcome	Interventions	Outcome	Interventions
Patient will be adequately nourished as evidenced by: • stable weight • weight not >10% below or >20% above IBW • albumin >3.5 g/dL • prealbumin >15 g/dL	Keep NPO until extubation. If extubation is delayed >24h, assess need for alternative nutritional therapy and initiate as needed. Consult dietitian to determine and direct nutritional support. Monitor response to clear liquids. Remove NG tube (if used) once patient is able to take fluids. Monitor protein and albumin lab values.	Patient will be adequately nourished. Patient will remain free from nausea and demonstrate return of appetite.	Advance to heart healthy diet: • total fat <30% of daily intake • total saturated fat <10% of daily intake • total cholesterol intake of <300 mg per day • calorie restriction if needed • sodium restriction if needed Monitor response to diet. Consider calorie count to assure patient consuming at least three-quarters caloric need.	Patient will be adequately nourished. Patient will achieve/maintain appropriate body weight.	Teach patient/family about heart healthy diet as described earlier. Continue laxatives and/or stool softeners as needed. Caution patient about possible weight gain after transplant secondary to medications. The patient should follow a calorie-restricted diet if needed and implement the prescribed exercise program.

Heart Transplantation Interdisciplinary Outcome Pathway (continued)

NUTRITION (continued)

Diagnosis/Stabilization Phase		Acute Management Phase		Recovery Phase	
Outcome	Interventions	Outcome	Interventions	Outcome	Interventions
• total protein 6–8 g/dL • total lymphocyte count 1,000–3,000 • cholesterol <200 mg/dL	Administer antiemetic, H$_2$ blockers, and/or antacids as needed.		Weigh daily. Assess bowel sounds. Administer laxatives and/or stool softeners as needed.		Teach patient about dietary supplements (i.e., antioxidants, oat bran, fiber, vitamins and minerals).

MOBILITY

Diagnosis/Stabilization Phase		Acute Management Phase		Recovery Phase	
Outcome	Interventions	Outcome	Interventions	Outcome	Interventions
Patient will maintain normal ROM and muscle strength.	Bed rest until extubation and hemodynamically stable. If extubation is delayed >24h, initiate passive/active-assist ROM exercises. May need PT consult. Begin passive/active-assist ROM exercises. Dangle after extubation. Monitor for orthostatic hypotension.	Patient will achieve optimal mobility.	PT consult to assess ambulation, mobility; muscle flexibility, strength, and tone. OT to determine functional ability for ADLs and IADLs. PT/OT to help determine and direct activity goals. Progress exercise as tolerated: dangle, bathroom privileges, OOB for meals, walking 50 feet. Monitor closely for orthostatic hypotension. Monitor response to increased activity. Decrease if adverse events occur: tachycardia, chest discomfort, dysrhythmia, ectopy. Remember, HR may be fast due to denervation of transplanted heart. Provide physical assistance or assistive devices as needed. Begin patient/family teaching on principles of a gradual exercise program. Initiate inpatient cardiac rehabilitation.	Patient will achieve optimal mobility.	Walk at least 200–300 feet TID to QID. Walk up and down one flight of stairs before discharge, particularly if stairs in the home. Teach patient/family about home exercise program. Refer to outpatient cardiac rehabilitation.

OXYGENATION/VENTILATION

Diagnosis/Stabilization Phase		Acute Management Phase		Recovery Phase	
Outcome	Interventions	Outcome	Interventions	Outcome	Interventions
Patient will have adequate gas exchange as evidenced by: • SaO_2 > 90% • SpO_2 > 92% • ABGs WNL • clear breath sounds • respiratory rate, depth, and rhythm WNL • CXR WNL	Monitor ventilator settings and wakefulness. Determine readiness to wean. Monitor hemodynamic variables before, during, and after weaning. Wean ventilator and monitor patient response: • wean FIO_2 to keep SpO_2 >92% • monitor effects of anesthesia and wean ventilator accordingly • after extubation, apply supplemental oxygen Assess respiratory functioning, including lung sounds, respiratory muscle strength, respiratory rate and depth, coughing ability, and CXR. Monitor pulse oximetry and use supplemental oxygen as necessary to keep SpO_2 > 92%. Teach use of IS (with inspiratory hold) when extubated.	Patient will have adequate gas exchange.	Monitor and treat oxygenation/ventilation status per ABGs, SpO_2, chest assessment, and CXR. Monitor closely for hypoxemia or dyspnea related to atelectasis and/or pleural effusion. Evaluate need for thoracentesis. Assess chest tubes for drainage and presence of air leak. Support patient with oxygen therapy as indicated. Monitor with pulse oximetry. Reinforce use of IS. Provide chest splint pillow and instruct on proper use. Have patient give return demonstration. Monitor closely for complications that may impair oxygenation/ventilation: pneumonia, atelectasis, pulmonary embolus, infection.	Patient will have adequate gas exchange.	Obtain CXR before discharge. Reinforce use of IS and chest splint pillow at home. Have patient give return demonstration. Teach patient signs and symptoms of respiratory complications and when to call physician.

COMFORT

Diagnosis/Stabilization Phase		Acute Management Phase		Recovery Phase	
Outcome	Interventions	Outcome	Interventions	Outcome	Interventions
Patient will be as comfortable and pain free as possible as evidenced by: • no objective indicators of discomfort • no complaints of discomfort	Anticipate need for analgesics and provide as needed. Use a pain scale or visual analogue tool. Assess response to all analgesics and effects on ability to wean from ventilator when indicated. Use newer NSAIDs with fewer sedative effects.	Patient will be as relaxed and comfortable as possible.	Anticipate need for analgesics and provide as needed. Assess response. Provide chest splint pillow and instruct on proper use. Have patient give return demonstration. Provide uninterrupted periods of rest.	Patient will be as relaxed and comfortable as possible.	Progress analgesics to oral medications as needed and assess response. Teach patient/family about analgesic administration and potential side effects for after discharge. Continue alternative methods to promote relaxation as listed earlier. Have patient give return demonstration of relaxation techniques.

Heart Transplantation Interdisciplinary Outcome Pathway (continued)

COMFORT (continued)

	Diagnosis/Stabilization Phase		Acute Management Phase		Recovery Phase
Outcome	**Interventions**	**Outcome**	**Interventions**	**Outcome**	**Interventions**
	Establish effective communication techniques with intubated patient with which he or she can communicate discomfort and need for analgesics.		Assist patient with relaxation techniques. Use touch therapy, humor, music therapy, and imagery to promote relaxation. Provide analgesics as needed before chest tube removal, ambulation, and any other procedures.		Instruct patient on stress management techniques. Teach patient/family alternative methods to promote relaxation at home. Refer to a transplant support group. Provide uninterrupted periods of rest.

SKIN INTEGRITY

	Diagnosis/Stabilization Phase		Acute Management Phase		Recovery Phase
Outcome	**Interventions**	**Outcome**	**Interventions**	**Outcome**	**Interventions**
Patient will have intact skin without abrasions or pressure ulcers. Patient will return to normothermic state.	Rewarm slowly; monitor temperature and signs of shivering. To warm, use head cover, warm blankets, radiant lighting, hyperthermia unit. Assess all bony prominences at least q4h and treat as needed. Maintain integrity of all dressings. Utilize mattress overlay.	Patient will have intact skin without abrasions, pressure ulcers, or wound infections. Patient will have healing wounds.	Assess all bony prominences at least q4h and treat as needed. Use preventive pressure-reducing devices if patient is at high risk for developing pressure ulcers. Treat pressure ulcers according to hospital protocol. Assess sternotomy incision(s) for drainage, erythema, and induration. Begin teaching patient/family proper skin care at home: incision care, signs and symptoms of infection.	Patient will have intact skin without abrasions, pressure ulcers, and infection. Patient will continue to have healing wounds.	Assess all wounds/incisions for signs and symptoms of infection. Culture if necessary. Reinforce importance of proper hygiene and wound care postop. Continue patient/family teaching on skin care at home. Assess understanding and reinforce as needed.

PROTECTION/SAFETY

Diagnosis/Stabilization Phase		Acute Management Phase		Recovery Phase	
Outcome	Interventions	Outcome	Interventions	Outcome	Interventions
Patient will be protected from possible harm. Patient will be protected from infection. Patient will be free of rejection episodes.	Assess need for wrist restraints while patient is intubated, has a decreased LOC, or is agitated and restless. Explain need for restraints to patient/family. Assess response to restraints and check q1–2h for skin integrity and impairment to circulation. Remove restraints as soon as patient is awake from anesthesia and able to follow instructions. Follow hospital protocol regarding use of restraints. Provide sedatives/antianxiety agents as needed. Monitor meticulously for signs and symptoms of any infection (renal, wound, respiratory, etc.) due to bacteria or viruses (cytomegalovirus, Epstein-Barr virus, herpes simplex, bacterial infection). Remember, immunosuppressive therapy can mask the signs of infection. Monitor for complications of either VAD or IABP if used. Protective isolation is used at some hospitals but is optional. Administer antibiotics as needed. Use meticulous aseptic technique and handwashing with patient. Administer medications to reduce risk of rejection (cyclosporine, prednisone, etc.). Prepare patient for first endomyocardial biopsy.	Patient will be protected from possible harm. Patient will be free of rejection episodes. Patient will be protected from infection.	Provide physical support when dangling or getting OOB. Monitor response. Teach correct movement and appropriate functional skills to prevent joint stress, strain, or injury. Continue protective isolation if used at your facility. Continue using aseptic technique and meticulous handwashing with patient. Continue to monitor for signs and symptoms of infection. Continue to monitor for complications associated with VAD or IABP if used. Continue to administer antirejection medications. Signs and symptoms of rejection may include: • fever • fatigue • malaise • hypotension • decreased ejection fraction • dysrhythmias • CHF	Patient will be protected from possible harm. Patient will be free from rejection episodes. Patient will be protected from infection.	Provide physical assistance or assistive devices with ambulation and climbing stairs. Teach patient/family about physical limitations after discharge. Review signs and symptoms of infection. Report any signs to physician. Teach patient/family ways to avoid infection after discharge. Continue to administer antirejection medications. Instruct patient on proper way to take and any adverse effects. Instruct patient about need for frequent endomyocardial biopsies the first year. The incidence of biopsies should decrease after the first year. Make sure patient knows that cardiac catheterizations will be done at least yearly to assess for accelerated graft atherosclerosis. Instruct patient on signs and symptoms of rejection and actions to take should symptoms occur. Inform patient of other conditions that may result from long-term immunosuppression therapy: • accelerated graft atherosclerosis • malignancies • nephrotoxicity • hypertension • hyperlipidemia • obesity • osteoporosis

Heart Transplantation Interdisciplinary Outcome Pathway (*continued*)

PSYCHOSOCIAL/SELF-DETERMINATION

Diagnosis/Stabilization Phase		Acute Management Phase		Recovery Phase	
Outcome	Interventions	Outcome	Interventions	Outcome	Interventions
Patient will achieve psychophysiologic stability. Patient will demonstrate a decrease in anxiety as evidenced by: • VS WNL • LOC WNL • subjective reports of decreased anxiety Patient will begin acceptance process of transplant.	Assess physiologic effects of critical care and/or open heart recovery environment on patient (hemodynamic variables, psychological status, signs of increased sympathetic activity). Provide sedatives as indicated. Take measures to reduce sensory overload. Develop effective techniques to communicate with patient while intubated. Use calm, caring, competent, and reassuring approach with patient and family. Allow flexible visitation to meet needs of patient and family. Determine emotional impact and coping ability of patient and take appropriate measures to meet needs. Conduct a family needs assessment and employ measures to meet identified concerns. Initiate discussion of transplant as soon as patient is able. Allow patient to verbalize feelings.	Patient will achieve psychophysiologic stability. Patient will demonstrate a decrease in anxiety. Patient will continue acceptance process of transplant.	Take measures to decrease sensory overload. Provide adequate rest periods, at least 2h of uninterrupted rest as often as possible. Provide sedatives as needed. Continue to include family in aspects of care. Continue to assess coping ability of patient and family and take measures as indicated. Involve patient/family in health care decisions. Allow patient/family to verbalize any feelings concerning the transplanted heart. Obtain psychology or psychiatric consult as needed. Schedule social services to meet with family to discuss financial/insurance considerations. Provide support as needed.	Patient will achieve psychophysiologic stability. Patient will demonstrate a decrease in anxiety. Patient will continue acceptance of transplant.	Provide adequate rest periods. Continue to assess coping ability of patient and family. Provide information on coping mechanisms for use after discharge. Refer to outside agencies or services as appropriate (chaplain, psychologist, transplant support group, social services, home health). Include patient/family in decisions concerning care. The transplant team will assist with discharge planning. Encourage patient/family to discuss feelings concerning the transplant. Refer to outpatient cardiac rehabilitation program. Address concerns patient may have about impact on daily life: ADLs, recreation, sexual functioning, return to work, and driving.

Interventional Cardiology
Interdisciplinary Outcome Pathway

Percutaneous Transluminal Coronary Angioplasty
Coronary Atherectomy
Laser Angioplasty
Intracoronary Stent Placement

COORDINATION OF CARE

Diagnosis/Stabilization Phase		Acute Management Phase		Recovery Phase	
Outcome	Interventions	Outcome	Interventions	Outcome	Interventions
All appropriate team members and disciplines will be involved in the plan of care.	Develop the plan of care with patient/family, primary physician(s), cardiologist, interventional cardiologist, cardiovascular surgeon, RN, and advanced practice nurse. Inform cardiac catheterization (cath) lab staff of the plan of care. Keep cardiovascular surgeon and surgical team aware of plans.	All appropriate team members and disciplines will be involved in the plan of care.	Update plan of care with patient/family, other team members, dietitian, case manager, and cardiac rehabilitation (rehab) staff. Assess social support systems. Initiate planning for discharge. Begin teaching patient/family about care at home.	Patient will understand how to maintain optimal health care at home.	Provide patient/family with: • guidelines concerning care at home and follow-up visits • guidelines concerning any future interventions such as repeat procedures • phone number of resources available to answer questions • medications • activity limitations • diet • referral to outpatient cardiac rehabilitation program

DIAGNOSTICS

Diagnosis/Stabilization Phase		Acute Management Phase		Recovery Phase	
Outcome	Interventions	Outcome	Interventions	Outcome	Interventions
Patient will understand any tests or procedures that must be completed (VS, hemodynamic monitoring, CXR, lab work, history and physical, IV lines, EKG, and cardiac monitoring).	Explain all procedures and tests to patient/family. Explain what patient will see and hear in the cardiac cath lab during the procedure. For example, during a laser angioplasty, all cath lab staff and the patient will wear goggles to protect their eyes from the laser.	Patient will understand any tests and procedures that must be completed during and after the cardiac intervention (EKG, cardiac monitoring, IV lines, indwelling urinary catheter if needed, femoral sheaths, lab tests).	Explain procedures and tests needed to assess response during the cardiac procedure and afterward. Be sensitive to individualized needs of patient/family for information.	Patient will understand meaning of diagnostic tests relative to continued health (results of cardiac interventions, lab tests).	Review with patient before discharge the results of the procedure. Provide pictures if possible. Stress that restenosis occurs in 20–50% of all patients. Discuss any abnormal lab values and appropriate measures patient can take to help return to normal.

Interventional Cardiology Interdisciplinary Outcome Pathway (continued)

DIAGNOSTICS (continued)

	Diagnosis/Stabilization Phase		Acute Management Phase		Recovery Phase	
Outcome	Interventions	Outcome	Interventions	Outcome	Interventions	
	Be sensitive to individualized needs of patient/family for information.				Provide patient with guidelines concerning follow-up care. Provide instruction on care at home after discharge: • care of entry site • diet • when to call physician • actions to take should chest discomfort occur • actions to take should bleeding occur • risk factor modification • activity limitations • medications • follow-up visit	

FLUID BALANCE

	Diagnosis/Stabilization Phase		Acute Management Phase		Recovery Phase	
Outcome	Interventions	Outcome	Interventions	Outcome	Interventions	
Patient will achieve or maintain optimal hemodynamic status as evidenced by: • MAP >70 mmHg • hemodynamic parameters WNL • UO >0.5 mL/kg/hr • free from abnormal EKG changes • free from dysrhythmias Patient will remain free from bleeding.	Monitor and treat cardiac parameters: • HR • BP • CO/CI • SV/SI • SvO_2 • ST segment • I & O • LOC • peripheral pulses • evidence of tissue perfusion • dysrhythmias Patient will be NPO after midnight the night before the cardiac intervention. If the procedure is scheduled for late afternoon, the patient may	Patient will maintain optimal hemodynamic status and remain free from dysrhythmias.	Monitor and treat cardiac parameters. Monitor closely for ST segment changes during the procedure. Time when they occur (i.e., with balloon inflation or after an inflation) and inform physician. Also monitor for ST segment changes after the procedure. Consider the use of continuous ST segment monitoring equipment. Monitor and treat potentially life-threatening dysrhythmias according to hospital protocol. Consider need for dysrhythmia prophylaxis.	Patient will maintain optimal hemodynamic status.	Continue to monitor for signs of bleeding. Continue cardiac teaching: • care of entry site • when to call physician • follow-up visits • any planned future interventions • risk factor modification • increased fluid intake for at least 1 week	

receive a light breakfast. Monitor for signs of dehydration and be prepared to administer IV fluids as necessary.

Monitor lab values: CBC, renal-electrolyte profile, PT, PTT, ACT, cardiac enzymes, cardiac troponin.

Maintain at least two IV lines.

Anticoagulants and/or platelet inhibitors may be ordered prior to the procedure. Administer as ordered and monitor response. Initiate bleeding precautions. Aspirin may be given before the procedure.

If ticlodipine (platelet inhibitor) is ordered, monitor WBC.

Monitor lab values: CBC, platelets, SMA-6, clotting studies, cardiac enzymes, cardiac troponin.

Monitor I & O.

Monitor peripheral pulses distal to entry site. If quality of pulses decreases, notify the physician immediately.

Monitor entry site (usually groin) for bleeding. If bleeding noted, apply pressure immediately and notify physician.

Instruct patient to call nurse if bleeding noted—feeling of warmth and/or stickiness at entry site.

Instruct patient to apply pressure to bandage when he or she sneezes, coughs, or laughs.

Remove femoral sheaths according to hospital protocol. Observe for bleeding, hematoma, loss of peripheral pulses. After sheaths are removed, apply bandage according to hospital protocol. With sheath removal, be prepared to administer atropine in case of vagal response. Administer analgesic prior to sheath removal. Maintain patent IV line. Instruct patient/family of activities that occur with sheath removal.

When sheaths are removed, pressure devices may be used to achieve hemostasis.

Increase fluid intake (usually 8 ounces per hour for several hours).

Monitor for signs and symptoms of retroperitoneal bleed.

Observe for complications:
- dissection
- acute occlusion
- MI
- cardiac tamponade
- hematoma
- hypotension
- dysrhythmias
- retroperitoneal bleeding

Interventional Cardiology Interdisciplinary Outcome Pathway (continued)

NUTRITION

Diagnosis/Stabilization Phase		Acute Management Phase		Recovery Phase	
Outcome	Interventions	Outcome	Interventions	Outcome	Interventions
Patient will be NPO after midnight the night before the procedure.	NPO after midnight. If procedure is scheduled for late afternoon, patient may have a light breakfast (usually liquids). Patient may take cardiac medications and others according to protocol with a small sip of water. Maintain at least two patent IV lines. If patient becomes dehydrated, IV fluids may be given.	Patient will remain NPO during the procedure. Patient will restart fluids after the procedure.	Patient will remain NPO during the procedure, however may take certain medications during the procedure with a small sip of water (i.e., platelet inhibitors, calcium channel blockers, aspirin). Patient may restart fluids immediately after the procedure. Progress DAT and monitor response. Increase fluid intake for first week after procedure. Advance to heart healthy diet (low fat, low cholesterol, low sodium if indicated) as tolerated. Monitor response to diet.	Patient will be adequately nourished as evidenced by: • stable weight • weight not >10% below or >20% above IBW • albumin >3.5 g/dL • total protein 6–8 g/dL • cholesterol <200 mg/dL	Continue monitoring response to diet. Continue increased fluid intake for at least a week after the procedure. Teach patient/family about heart healthy diet: • total fat <30% of daily intake • total saturated fat <10% of daily intake • total cholesterol intake <300 mg/day • caloric reduction if indicated • sodium reduction if indicated

MOBILITY

Diagnosis/Stabilization Phase		Acute Management Phase		Recovery Phase	
Outcome	Interventions	Outcome	Interventions	Outcome	Interventions
Patient will maintain mobility as before procedure.	Patient may be ambulatory prior to procedure if not contraindicated. Assess ambulation, mobility, and muscle strength prior to procedure. Instruct patient on need for bed rest for several hours after the procedure due to placement of femoral sheaths and pressure bandage.	Patient will lie still during the procedure. Patient will achieve optimal mobility after the procedure.	Instruct patient to lie as still as possible during the procedure due to placement of the femoral sheaths and intracoronary catheters. Place arms in comfortable position for patient without obstructing view of camera. Administer analgesics as necessary for comfort for back pain during the procedure. Administer sedatives as necessary to ensure compliance with instructions during the procedure.	Patient will achieve optimal mobility.	Continue to monitor response to activity. Continue to teach patient/family about any limitations at home after discharge: • no lifting over 10 pounds for at least 1 week • stairs may be taken slowly • notify physician should chest discomfort occur, or seek entry into the medical system • if bleeding occurs, apply pressure and call physician, or seek entry into the medical system

Refer to outpatient cardiac rehabilitation program.

After the procedure:
- patient will remain on bed rest for several hours (according to hospital protocol)
- patient must keep involved extremity (usually a leg) still while femoral sheaths are in place. Sheaths are usually removed 4–6h after the last dose of heparin or ACT <150.
- patient must keep involved extremity still with pressure bandage in place
- HOB may be elevated 30 degrees approximately 3 h after the procedure. Follow hospital protocol.
- patient will remain on bed rest after femoral sheath removal for several hours (according to hospital protocol but usually 4–6h).

After bed rest is completed, progress activity as tolerated. Dangle at bedside. Ambulate with assistance the first time up. Patient may have bathroom privileges.

Monitor response to increased activity. Decrease if adverse events occur (i.e., tachycardia, chest discomfort, bleeding, dyspnea, ectopy).

Provide physical assistance as necessary.

Begin teaching patient/family about exercise program after discharge.

OXYGENATION/VENTILATION

Diagnosis/Stabilization Phase		Acute Management Phase		Recovery Phase	
Outcome	Interventions	Outcome	Interventions	Outcome	Interventions
Patient will have adequate gas exchange as evidenced by: • SaO_2 >90% • $SpO_2,2$ >92% • ABGs WNL	Conduct respiratory assessment prior to cardiac intervention. Note any adventitious breath sounds and notify physician. Apply supplemental oxygen as needed.	Patient will have adequate gas exchange.	Monitor and treat oxygenation/ventilation status per ABGs and pulse oximetry. Utilize pulse oximetry during the entire procedure and afterward as indicated.	Patient will have adequate gas exchange.	Instruct patient/family to report any dyspnea that may occur after discharge.

Interventional Cardiology Interdisciplinary Outcome Pathway (continued)

OXYGENATION/VENTILATION (continued)

Diagnosis/Stabilization Phase		Acute Management Phase		Recovery Phase	
Outcome	Interventions	Outcome	Interventions	Outcome	Interventions
• respiratory rate, depth, and rhythm WNL • CXR WNL	Monitor pulse oximetry. Instruct patient he or she may be asked to cough or take a deep breath and hold during the procedure.		Apply supplemental oxygen during the procedure. Assess need for supplemental oxygen after the procedure and continue if necessary to keep SpO$_2$ >92%. While patient is on bed rest, encourage coughing and deep breathing at least q2h. Elevate HOB approximately 30 degrees 3h after procedure if tolerated.		

COMFORT

Diagnosis/Stabilization Phase		Acute Management Phase		Recovery Phase	
Outcome	Interventions	Outcome	Interventions	Outcome	Interventions
Patient will be as comfortable and pain free as possible as evidenced by: • no objective indicators of discomfort • no complaints of discomfort	Anticipate need for analgesics and provide as needed. Use visual analogue tool or pain scale. Should patient complain of chest discomfort prior to procedure, obtain 12 lead EKG immediately and notify physician. Encourage patient to report any discomfort before and during the procedure. Instruct patient some chest discomfort may occur during the cardiac procedure (i.e., when balloon is inflated, when atherectomy device is activated). Assure him or her this is normal but to report any discomfort. Analgesics will be available to help control the discomfort.	Patient will be as relaxed and comfortable as possible during the procedure. Patient will be as relaxed and comfortable as possible immediately after the procedure.	Administer conscious sedation according to hospital protocol before the procedure. Be prepared to administer analgesics and sedatives as necessary during the procedure. Assess patient's response to cardiac intervention and treat accordingly (i.e., treat life-threatening dysrhythmias, chest discomfort). Assist patient with relaxation techniques (deep breathing, pursed-lip breathing, imagery). After procedure, continue to monitor for any chest discomfort. Should chest discomfort occur:	Patient will be as relaxed and comfortable as possible.	Progress analgesics as needed and assess response. Teach patient/family about analgesic administration after discharge and how to monitor for adverse events. Continue alternative methods to promote relaxation. Teach patient/family about stress management. Teach patient/family what measures to take should chest discomfort recur.

Administer conscious sedation. Instruct patient that numbing of entry site will burn for approximately 30 seconds. Inform him or her to notify physician if any further discomfort at groin site.

- obtain 12 lead EKG immediately
- apply supplemental oxygen
- administer sublingual nitroglycerin as ordered
- notify physician
- provide reassurance

After procedure, monitor cardiac rate and rhythm. Note any rate or rhythm changes in addition to ST segment elevation. Should ST segment elevation occur, obtain 12 lead EKG immediately. Monitor at least two leads if at all possible. Monitor leads that reflect area of the heart involved: RCA, II, III, aVF; LAD, $V_1–V_4$; LCx, I, aVL, V_5, V_6. Utilize continuous ST segment monitoring equipment if available.

Encourage patient to report any discomfort (back, entry site) and treat accordingly. Monitor response to analgesics. Administer analgesics before uncomfortable procedures such as sheath removal.

SKIN INTEGRITY

Diagnosis/Stabilization Phase		Acute Management Phase		Recovery Phase	
Outcome	Interventions	Outcome	Interventions	Outcome	Interventions
Patient will have intact skin without abrasions or pressure ulcers.	Assess all bony prominences prior to procedure and apply protective mechanism if needed.	Patient will have intact skin without abrasions, pressure ulcers, wound infection, or hematoma.	Assess all bony prominences at least q4h and treat if needed. Place mattress overlay on bed. Assess entry site according to hospital protocol (usually every 15 minutes for 1 hour, every 30 minutes for 2 hours, and every hour for 4 hours). Observe for signs of infection and bleeding. If noted, take appropriate measures.	Patient will have intact skin without abrasions, pressure ulcers, wound infection, or hematoma.	Assess entry site for signs and symptoms of infection, bleeding, and hematoma. Teach patient/family care of incision after discharge.

Interventional Cardiology Interdisciplinary Outcome Pathway (continued)

PROTECTION/SAFETY

Diagnosis/Stabilization Phase		Acute Management Phase		Recovery Phase	
Outcome	Interventions	Outcome	Interventions	Outcome	Interventions
Patient will be protected from possible harm.	Keep side rails of stretcher up at all times. Provide conscious sedation and monitor response. Provide sedatives/antianxiety agents as needed and monitor response. Instruct patient to lie as still as possible during the procedure.	Patient will be protected from possible harm.	Monitor continuously while in cardiac cath lab. Remind patient to remain as still as possible during the procedure. Provide conscious sedation and monitor response. Provide sedatives/antianxiety agents as needed and monitor response. Instruct patient to lie quietly several hours after the procedure keeping the involved extremity as still as possible. A loose restraint may be needed on the involved extremity. Provide support with ambulation at least the first time up after the procedure.	Patient will be protected from possible harm.	Provide support with ambulation. Teach patient/family about physical limitations after discharge such as no lifting over 10 pounds for 1 week and to take stairs slowly. If patient is on anticoagulants or platelet-inhibiting agents, instruct on safety measures to prevent bleeding and actions to take should bleeding occur. If patient is on ticlopidine, instruct him or her to have WBC checked at 2 and 4 weeks.

PSYCHOSOCIAL/SELF-DETERMINATION

Diagnosis/Stabilization Phase		Acute Management Phase		Recovery Phase	
Outcome	Interventions	Outcome	Interventions	Outcome	Interventions
Patient will maintain psychophysiologic stability. Patient will demonstrate a decrease in anxiety as evidenced by: • VS WNL • subjective report of anxiety	Assess physiologic effect of critical care and cardiac cath lab environment on patient (hemodynamic parameters, psychological status, signs of increased sympathetic activity). Provide sedatives as ordered and monitor response. Provide conscious sedation as indicated and monitor response.	Patient will maintain psychophysiologic stability. Patient will demonstrate a decrease in anxiety.	Continue conscious sedation as indicated and monitor response. Administer sedatives as indicated and monitor response. Continue to instruct patient on activities to expect during and after the cardiac intervention. After the cardiac procedure, provide adequate rest periods. Continue to assess coping ability to patient/family and take measures as indicated.	Patient will maintain psychophysiologic stability. Patient will demonstrate a decrease in anxiety. Patient will verbalize understanding of need for risk factor modification.	Provide adequate periods of rest. Continue to assess coping ability of patient and family. Provide information on stress management and coping mechanisms for use after discharge. Refer to appropriate outside agencies as needed (i.e., home health, cardiac rehabilitation). Involve patient/family in decisions concerning care.

Use calm, caring, competent, and reassuring approach with patient and family.

Allow family to visit prior to cardiac intervention.

Determine emotional impact and coping ability of patient and take appropriate measures to meet needs.

Instruct patient on what to expect during and after the cardiac intervention.

Allow family to see patient as soon as possible after the procedure.

Discuss results of procedure with patient and family.

Allow flexible visitation after the procedure to meet the needs of the patient and family.

Involve patient/family in health care decisions.

Provide instruction on pertinent risk factor modification.

Remind patient of a 20–50% restenosis rate with these procedures and that risk modification is critical to recovery.

Minimally Invasive Cardiac Surgery Interdisciplinary Outcome Pathway

COORDINATION OF CARE

Diagnosis/Stabilization Phase		Acute Management Phase		Recovery Phase	
Outcome	Interventions	Outcome	Interventions	Outcome	Interventions
Plan for surgical intervention will be presented to patient and family. All appropriate team members and disciplines will be involved in the plan of care.	Develop plan of care with patient/family, primary physician, cardiologist, cardiac surgeon, RN, advanced practice nurse, and other appropriate disciplines.	Plan of care will be changed appropriately according to input from all team members.	Patient's status and progress will be continuously assessed. Changes in care made after input from appropriate team members. Assess patient's discharge/home needs. Initiate plans for discharge: teach family/patient home care, expectations, and home health if needed. Assess social support systems.	Patient will have a basic understanding of surgery and how to provide self-care. Patient will understand how to maintain optimal health at home.	Give postdischarge care guidelines to patient. Provide phone numbers of resources to call if questions after discharge. Arrange postop visit with surgeon.

DIAGNOSTICS

Diagnosis/Stabilization Phase		Acute Management Phase		Recovery Phase	
Outcome	Interventions	Outcome	Interventions	Outcome	Interventions
Patient will understand any tests or procedures that must be completed (VS, I & O, hemodynamic monitoring, chest tubes, lab work, coughing and deep breathing).	Explain all tests and procedures to patient/family. Be sensitive to individualized needs of patient/family for information. Establish effective communication technique with intubated patient.	Patient will understand any tests or procedures that must be completed (VS, removal of indwelling lines and chest tubes, removal of pacing wires, use of antithrombotic hose, increased ambulation, echocardiogram).	Continue as in Diagnosis/Stabilization Phase. Explain procedures and tests needed to assess recovery. Be prepared to repeat information frequently.	Patient will understand meaning of diagnostic tests in relation to continued health (lab tests, results of surgery, need for follow-up).	Review with patient the results of the surgery and pertinent lab values. Discuss any abnormal findings and appropriate measures patient can take to help return to normal (i.e., hypercholesterolemia). Provide guidelines concerning: • when to call physician • care of incision • diet • medications • activity • follow-up visits • smoking cessation • risk factor modification Inform patient that nurses may call periodically to check on his or her condition.

FLUID BALANCE

Diagnosis/Stabilization Phase		Acute Management Phase		Recovery Phase	
Outcome	Interventions	Outcome	Interventions	Outcome	Interventions
Patient will achieve optimal hemodynamic stability as evidenced by: • MAP > 70 mmHg • hemodynamic parameters WNL • UO > 0.5 mL/kg/hr • return to normothermic state • free of dysrhythmias	Monitor and treat cardiac and hemodynamic parameters: • HR, rhythm, and EKG changes • MAP • PA pressures • CO/CI • SVR/PVR • evidence of tissue perfusion • LOC Rewarm slowly to 38°C. Rewarming methods include head covering, radiant lights, thermal rewarming units, and warm blankets. Use epicardial pacing as needed. Monitor electrolytes, BUN, creatinine, glucose, and hematology values and treat appropriately. Assess chest tube drainage levels every 15 minutes. Watch for equalization of filling pressures, hypotension, and pulsus paradoxus. Monitor for complications: hypotension, bleeding, tamponade, dysrhythmias, MI. Treat atrial and/or ventricular dysrhythmias according to hospital protocol (i.e., calcium antagonist drip, antidysrhythmic medication). Institute an atrial fibrillation protocol.	Patient will achieve optimal fluid balance and hemodynamic function.	Assess patient daily: • weight • I & O • physical exam to determine need for diuresis Assist with indwelling line and chest tube removal. Monitor patient after chest tube, hemodynamic pressure monitoring lines, pacemaker wires, and urinary catheter are removed. Monitor blood chemistries. Assist patient in early mobilization. Involve patient/family in care, especially mobilization. Start teaching patient/family about surgical procedure, expected patient progress, and teaching for discharge. Continue to monitor for potential complications as listed earlier.	Patient will maintain optimal fluid balance and hemodynamic function.	Continue cardiac teaching with patient and family. Instruct patient/family on: • proper use of medications • monitoring of pulse • anticoagulant use • weight monitoring • weight management Provide information to patient/family.

Minimally Invasive Cardiac Surgery Interdisciplinary Outcome Pathway (continued)

NUTRITION

Diagnosis/Stabilization Phase		Acute Management Phase		Recovery Phase	
Outcome	Interventions	Outcome	Interventions	Outcome	Interventions
Patient will be adequately nourished as evidenced by: • stable weight • weight not >10% below or >20% above IBW • albumin >3.5 g/dL • total protein 6–8 g/dL • total lymphocyte count 1,000–3,000 • cholesterol <200 mg/dL	Keep patient NPO until extubation. Begin sips of clear liquids after extubation. Monitor for full airway clearance after swallowing liquids initially. Begin alternative nutritional therapy when patient has prolonged intubation (>24h). Assess patient's nutritional status by physical exam and patient's history. Assess protein, albumin, cholesterol, triglycerides, and lymphocyte counts. Administer all medications affecting GI/nutritional status appropriately (i.e., H$_2$ blockers, antiemetics).	Patient will be adequately nourished. Patient will maintain an appropriate intake of calories at this level of recovery.	Assess patient's ability to eat and process food. Adjust DAT. Monitor bowel sounds and function q4h and PRN. Administer laxatives as needed. Continue progressive early mobilization and ambulation: dangle, OOB for meals, ambulate 200 feet in hall TID to QID. Weigh daily. Involve dietitian for: • unanticipated weight loss • albumin <3.0 • eating less than half of food on tray • counseling on heart healthy diet	Patient will be adequately nourished. Patient will have a good understanding of appropriate diet for his or her needs.	Teach patient and family about diet appropriate to patient's needs incorporating activity/exercise: • total fat intake <30% per day • total saturated fat intake <10% per day • total cholesterol intake <300 mg/day • weight reduction if needed • foods affecting anticoagulation • diabetes diet if indicated Teach patient about dietary supplements (i.e., antioxidants, oat bran, fiber, vitamins and minerals).

MOBILITY

Diagnosis/Stabilization Phase		Acute Management Phase		Recovery Phase	
Outcome	Interventions	Outcome	Interventions	Outcome	Interventions
Patient will maintain normal ROM. Patient will experience minimal decline of muscle strength.	Turn and position q2h once hemodynamically stable. OOB to chair once awake and extubated or hemodynamically stable. Passive/active-assist ROM exercises while still on bed rest.	Patient will achieve optimal balance, mobility, and strength. Patient will experience reduced musculoskeletal discomfort.	Ambulate (on water seal if chest tube still in) in room night of surgery if extubated or the next morning. Progressive ambulation QID. Start with 50 feet and progress as tolerated. OOB for meals. Shower after chest tube out for 24h and pacemaker wires removed. Active-assist ROM exercises.	Patient will achieve optimal balance, mobility, and strength. Patient will experience reduced musculoskeletal discomfort.	Provide home exercise program with progressive ambulation, full ROM exercises, and progressive strengthening exercises. Teach this to patient/family. Assess for understanding. Assist patient in referral to outpatient cardiac rehabilitation program if feasible.

OXYGENATION/VENTILATION

Diagnosis/Stabilization Phase		Acute Management Phase		Recovery Phase	
Outcome	Interventions	Outcome	Interventions	Outcome	Interventions
Patient will maintain adequate respiratory status as evidenced by: • SaO₂ >90% • SpO₂ >92% • ABGs WNL • clear breath sounds • respiratory rate, depth, and rhythm WNL	Monitor ABGs, hemodynamic status, ET tube placement, breath sounds, O₂ saturations, tissue oxygenation, Hgb, and Hct. Treat when appropriate. Check CXR upon arrival to recovery and as needed. Monitor CXR for need for diuresis, atelectasis, and pneumothorax. Begin ventilator weaning when appropriate. Adjust as necessary, then extubate when appropriate. Use supplemental oxygen after extubation and monitor with pulse oximetry. Continue to monitor all respiratory and cardiovascular parameters for adequate oxygenation and ventilation. Use IS with patient and instruct on its proper use. Have patient give a return demonstration. Dangle, then up in chair as soon as patient is hemodynamically stable. Monitor patient's response to increased activity and decrease if adverse events occur (tachycardia, dyspnea, hypo/hypertension, ectopy, syncope). Monitor HR, SpO₂, and discomfort with activity. Initiate inpatient cardiac rehabilitation program. Begin teaching patient/family about home activity and restrictions and expected progression with exercise.	Patient will achieve optimal respiratory status.	Monitor oxygenation/ventilation by physical exam, CXR, and SpO₂. Wean from nasal oxygen when hemodynamically stable, no serious dysrhythmia present, Hgb >8.0 g and SpO₂ >90%. Continue use of IS, cough and deep breathing, and aggressive mobilization. Provide chest splint pillow. Instruct patient and family on its use. Have patient give return demonstration. Maintain adequate pain control with analgesics and NSAIDs. Monitor chest tube output. Report increase/decrease in levels. Discontinue as soon as possible. Watch for air leaks or resolution of air leak and report to physician. Initiate discussion of smoking cessation if appropriate.	Patient will maintain optimal respiratory status.	Continue to reinforce use of IS. Have patient give return demonstration. Assess patient for clear breath sounds before discharge. Continue discussion of smoking cessation if appropriate. Refer to support groups as needed.

Minimally Invasive Cardiac Surgery Interdisciplinary Outcome Pathway (continued)

COMFORT

Diagnosis/Stabilization Phase		Acute Management Phase		Recovery Phase	
Outcome	Interventions	Outcome	Interventions	Outcome	Interventions
Patient will be as comfortable and pain free as possible as evidenced by: • no objective indicators of discomfort • no complaints of discomfort • normal VS	Assess response to analgesics and effect on ability to wean from ventilator. Anticipate need for analgesics and administer as appropriate. Assess response. Use a pain scale or visual analogue tool. Establish effective communication technique with intubated patient with which he or she can communicate need for analgesia.	Patient will be as relaxed and comfortable as possible.	Anticipate need for analgesics and assess response. Progress to oral analgesics. Teach patient proper use of PCA pump, if used. Provide analgesics before removal of chest tubes. Provide uninterrupted periods of rest. Assist patient with relaxation exercises. Have patient give return demonstration. Use touch therapy, humor, imagery, and music therapy to potentiate effects of analgesics.	Patient will be as relaxed and comfortable as possible.	Continue alternative methods to promote relaxation. Have patient/family demonstrate these techniques. Monitor response to analgesics. Teach patient/family about analgesic administration at home and potential adverse effects. Reinforce need for uninterrupted periods of rest.

SKIN INTEGRITY

Diagnosis/Stabilization Phase		Acute Management Phase		Recovery Phase	
Outcome	Interventions	Outcome	Interventions	Outcome	Interventions
Patient will have intact skin without abrasions or pressure ulcers. Patient will return to normothermic state.	Examine for pressure points and interruption of skin integrity from positioning in surgery. Treat as needed. Turn and position q2h when hemodynamically stable. Assess drainage on dressings. Change or reinforce as needed using appropriate type of tape for patient's skin type. Incision is approximately 6 cm long. Consider elderly, patients on corticosteroid therapy, and those with poor nutritional status to be at high risk for developing	Patient will have no abrasions, pressure ulcers, or wound infection. Patient will have healing wounds.	Change surgical dressings after first 24h. Remove dressings entirely after 48h unless patient has excessive drainage. Use bacteriostatic soap for bathing. Shower once pacemaker wires removed. Assess all incision lines at least q8h for drainage, erythema, and integrity. Use antithrombotic hose on patients who have leg incisions. Encourage patient to elevate legs when in sitting position.	Patient will have no wound infection. Patient will have healing wounds.	Assess all wounds before discharge for progress in healing. Remove all sutures according to protocol. Reinforce suture lines with steri-strips as needed. Reinforce wound assessment and care with patient and family (signs and symptoms of infection, proper hygiene). Assess understanding. Provide numbers to call if drainage, pain at wound edges, or new redness develops.

Diagnosis/Stabilization Phase — Interventions	Acute Management Phase — Interventions	Recovery Phase — Interventions
pressure ulcers. Use preventive pressure reducing devices for high-risk patients. Treat pressure ulcers according to hospital protocol. Assess incision for drainage, erythema, and induration. Use sterile technique when changing bandages.	Teach patient/family wound care for discharge.	Arrange home health care as needed for assessment, dressing changes, and home antibiotic therapy. Antithrombotic hose may be worn up to 2 weeks if saphenous vein harvesting is done.

PROTECTION/SAFETY

Diagnosis/Stabilization Phase		Acute Management Phase		Recovery Phase	
Outcome	Interventions	Outcome	Interventions	Outcome	Interventions
Patient will be protected from possible harm.	Soft wrist restraints to be used until patient extubated. Assess areas near wrist for skin integrity and alteration to circulation q1h. Explain need for restraints to family and patient when awake. Remove restraints once patient is extubated and able to follow directions appropriately. Follow hospital protocol for restraint use. Use pharmacologic agents as needed as anesthesia wears off to control anxiety, delirium, and hallucination. Isolate pacing wires.	Patient will be protected from possible harm.	Assist patient with getting OOB and ambulation until he or she can achieve safely by self. Instruct family on proper support for patient. Provide assistance with showering (i.e., sturdy shower seat use). Monitor for changes in patients after receiving analgesics. Reduce dose if patient too sedated. Isolate pacing wires until removed.	Patient will be protected from possible harm.	Instruct patient and family on home activity, limitations, and expectations: • bathing • housework • driving • returning to work • social activities Provide support with ambulation and climbing stairs. Review signs and symptoms of infection and when to call the physician.

PSYCHOSOCIAL/SELF-DETERMINATION

Diagnosis/Stabilization Phase		Acute Management Phase		Recovery Phase	
Outcome	Interventions	Outcome	Interventions	Outcome	Interventions
Patient will achieve baseline psychophysiologic status. Patient will demonstrate a decrease in anxiety as evidenced by:	Reduce sensory overload when able. Provide uninterrupted rest periods. Provide sedatives as indicated and monitor response.	Patient will achieve baseline psychophysiologic stability. Patient will demonstrate a decrease in anxiety.	Reduce sensory overload. Address alarms on equipment as soon as possible. Monitor timing of various team member visits. Some visits may have to be postponed to allow adequate rest periods.	Patient will achieve baseline psychophysiologic status. Patient will be introduced to other coping skills for anxiety.	Facilitate referral to outpatient cardiac rehabilitation program. Provide verbal and written information for home care. Provide phone numbers for questions after discharge.

Minimally Invasive Cardiac Surgery Interdisciplinary Outcome Pathway *(continued)*

PSYCHOSOCIAL/SELF-DETERMINATION (continued)

Diagnosis/Stabilization Phase		Acute Management Phase		Recovery Phase	
Outcome	Interventions	Outcome	Interventions	Outcome	Interventions
• VS WNL • subjective report of decreased anxiety	Develop effective interventions for communication with intubated patient such as writing tablet, board, or letter board. Reduce anxiety by offering reassurance about condition, using easy to understand terminology, and answering questions. Allow flexible visitation to meet patient/family needs.		Assess coping abilities of patient and family. Provide assistance when needed for discharge plans: • home health care • education concerning surgery and recovery Explain current patient progress with patient and family and expectations for discharge. Continue to include family in all aspects of care.		Continue to assess coping ability of patient and family. Provide information on coping mechanisms. Address concerns patient may have about impact on daily life: ADLs, recreation, sexual functioning, return to work, and driving.

Myocardial Infarction Interdisciplinary Outcome Pathway

COORDINATION OF CARE

Diagnosis/Stabilization Phase		Acute Management Phase		Recovery Phase	
Outcome	Interventions	Outcome	Interventions	Outcome	Interventions
All appropriate team member and disciplines will be involved in the plan of care.	Develop the plan of care with the patient, family, primary physician(s), cardiologist, RN, advanced practice nurse, social services, chaplain, and other specialists as needed.	All appropriate team members and disciplines will be involved.	Update the plan of care with patient, family, other team members, PT, dietitian, discharge planner, interventional cardiologist, cardiovascular surgeon, and cardiac rehabilitation. Initiate planning for anticipated discharge and call home health as indicated. Begin teaching patient/family about care at home.	Patient will understand how to maintain optimal health at home.	Continue cardiac rehabilitation and plan for outpatient cardiac rehabilitation if possible. If not, plan an in-home exercise program. Provide guidelines concerning care at home and any necessary follow-up. Provide patient/family with phone number of resources available to answer questions.

DIAGNOSTICS

Diagnosis/Stabilization Phase		Acute Management Phase		Recovery Phase	
Outcome	Interventions	Outcome	Interventions	Outcome	Interventions
Patient will understand any tests or procedures that must be completed (VS, I & O, hemodynamic monitoring, cardiac monitor, CXR, supplemental oxygen, IV lines, pulse oximetry, lab work, emergency cardiac catheterization, and EKGs).	Explain all procedures and tests to patient/family. Be sensitive to individualized needs of patient/family for information.	Patient will understand any tests or procedures that must be completed (cardiac enzymes, cardiac troponin, daily EKG, increase in activity, cardiac monitoring, pulse oximetry, supplemental oxygen, coagulation studies, cardiac catheterization). Patient will understand any further treatment plans (i.e., PTCA, atherectomy, stent, CABG).	Explain procedures and tests needed to assess recovery from acute MI. Anticipate need for further diagnostic tests such as cardiac catheterization and any interventions that may result. Provide information on patient's role concerning diagnostic procedures, such as keeping leg straight and increased fluid intake after cardiac catheterization. Be sensitive to individualized needs of patient/family for information. Provide information about further treatment (i.e., PTCA, atherectomy, stent, CABG).	Patient will understand meaning of diagnostic tests in relation to continued health (lab tests, EKGs, echocardiogram).	Review with patient before discharge results of EKGs and lab tests. Discuss any abnormal values and appropriate measures patient can take at home to help return to normal (i.e., low cholesterol diet for hypercholesterolemia). Anticipate need for any further diagnostic tests such as stress testing or cardiac catheterization and any possible interventions that may result. Explain need to recognize symptoms of further myocardial ischemia in a timely manner and how to respond. Cardiac teaching with patient/family:

Myocardial Infarction Interdisciplinary Outcome Pathway (continued)

DIAGNOSTICS (continued)

Diagnosis/Stabilization Phase		Acute Management Phase		Recovery Phase	
Outcome	Interventions	Outcome	Interventions	Outcome	Interventions
					• risk factor modification • signs and symptoms of MI • signs and symptoms of angina • measures to take should discomfort occur • diet • activity • medications • cardiac rehabilitation • signs and symptoms of CHF • follow-up visits

FLUID BALANCE

Diagnosis/Stabilization Phase		Acute Management Phase		Recovery Phase	
Outcome	Interventions	Outcome	Interventions	Outcome	Interventions
Patient will achieve optimal hemodynamic status as evidenced by: • MAP >70 mmHg • hemodynamic parameters WNL • UO >0.5 mL/kg/hr • free of cardiac dysrhythmias Patient will maintain a normal cardiac output and SvO_2.	Monitor and treat cardiac parameters: • dysrhythmias • SvO_2 • BP • I & O • PA pressures • SV/SI • left and right ventricular stroke work index • LOC • CO/CI • evidence of tissue perfusion Anticipate need for pacing and/or pharmacologic interventions for dysrhythmias. Monitor lab values (electrolytes, Mg^{++}, PT, PTT, ACT if available, cardiac isoenzymes, cardiac troponin).	Patient will maintain optimal hemodynamic status. Patient will maintain normal cardiac output and SvO_2.	Continue to monitor and treat cardiac parameters. Monitor and treat dysrhythmias. Monitor lab values: PT, PTT, ACT if available, cardiac isoenzymes, electrolytes, Mg^{++}, cardiac troponin. Monitor EKG for evolutionary changes consistent with MI. Continue to assess for complications associated with acute MI. Assess response to any vasopressors, anticoagulants, or antiplatelet agents given. Begin patient/family teaching on cardiac system, current cardiac problems, current treatment, and expected clinical course. Monitor EKG for signs of myocardial ischemia.	Patient will maintain optimal hemodynamic status.	Continue as in Acute Management Phase. Teach patient/family signs of fluid overload (edema, SOB, sudden weight gain, rapid HR). Continue cardiac teaching. Assess for understanding and reinforce as needed.

Monitor for signs of fluid overload or deficit.

Anticipate need for vasopressor agents and assess response.

Observe for signs of bleeding while patient is receiving thrombolytic and anticoagulation therapy and treat accordingly. Keep antidotes for anticoagulants on unit.

Monitor for signs of reperfusion if thrombolytic agents are administered:
- reperfusion dysrhythmias
- ST segment return to baseline
- early rise and peak in CK
- relief of pain

Monitor for signs of complications that can occur following an acute MI: CHF, cardiogenic shock, ventricular septal defect, mitral regurgitation, papillary muscle dysfunction/rupture, cardiac tamponade, and dysrhythmias.

Assess heart sounds q4h and as needed. Assess breath sounds q4h and as needed.

Be prepared to initiate counterpulsation if indicated.

Be prepared to administer antiplatelet agents and observe response.

NUTRITION

Diagnosis/Stabilization Phase		Acute Management Phase		Recovery Phase	
Outcome	Interventions	Outcome	Interventions	Outcome	Interventions
Patient will be adequately nourished as evidenced by: • stable weight • weight not > 10% below or > 20% above IBW	Light diet as tolerated first 24h. Monitor response to diet. Monitor protein and albumin values. Determine lipid profile.	Patient will be adequately nourished.	Advance to heart healthy diet as tolerated (low fat, low cholesterol; low sodium if indicated) and monitor response. Weigh daily. Consult dietitian as needed for diet counseling.	Patient will be adequately nourished.	Teach patient/family about heart healthy diet: • total fat < 30% of daily intake • total saturated fat < 10% of daily intake • total daily cholesterol intake < 300 mg

Myocardial Infarction Interdisciplinary Outcome Pathway (continued)

NUTRITION (continued)

Diagnosis/Stabilization Phase		Acute Management Phase		Recovery Phase	
Outcome	Interventions	Outcome	Interventions	Outcome	Interventions
• albumin > 3.5 g/dL • total protein 6–8 g/dL • total lymphocyte count 1,000–3,000 • cholesterol < 200 mg/dL					• caloric reduction if indicated • sodium restriction if indicated Teach patient/family about any dietary supplements (i.e., antioxidants, oat bran, fiber, vitamins and minerals).

MOBILITY

Diagnosis/Stabilization Phase		Acute Management Phase		Recovery Phase	
Outcome	Interventions	Outcome	Interventions	Outcome	Interventions
Patient will rest to decrease myocardial workload and oxygen demand.	Bed rest with bedside commode privileges first 6h. Teach patient physiologic basis for rest. Assist with activities to meet basic needs. Plan adequate rest periods.	Patient will achieve optimal mobility.	Progress exercise as tolerated: dangle, OOB for meals, up in chair TID to QID while in critical care environment. Monitor response to increased activity. Decrease activity if adverse events occur (tachycardia, dyspnea, ectopy, syncope, hypotension, chest discomfort). Allow patient to begin light ADLs: partial bathing and brushing teeth. Initiate Phase I Cardiac Rehabilitation. Teach patient gradual exercise principles. Plan adequate rest periods.	Patient will achieve optimal mobility.	Continue to progress exercise as tolerated and monitor response. Walk at least 200 to 300 feet TID to QID. Walk up and down one flight of stairs prior to discharge. Teach patient/family about home exercise program.

OXYGENATION/VENTILATION

Diagnosis/Stabilization Phase		Acute Management Phase		Recovery Phase	
Outcome	Interventions	Outcome	Interventions	Outcome	Interventions
Patient will have adequate gas exchange as evidenced by: • $SaO_2 > 90\%$ • $SpO_2 > 92\%$ • ABGs WNL • clear breath sounds • respiratory rate, depth, and rhythm WNL • CXR WNL Patient will have increased myocardial oxygen supply with a decrease in myocardial oxygen demand.	Apply supplemental oxygen for at least the first 24h. Monitor SpO_2 with pulse oximetry. Assess respiratory functioning, including lung sounds, respiratory rate and depth, and CXR. Encourage coughing and deep breathing while on bed rest. Assess evidence of tissue perfusion. Monitor lab values: Hgb, ABGs.	Patient will have adequate gas exchange.	Assess respiratory functioning and intervene as indicated. Assess need for continued supplemental oxygen with use of pulse oximetry. Observe for complications of MI that may impair oxygenation/ventilation: CHF, mitral regurgitation, pulmonary embolus, cardiac tamponade, cardiogenic shock. Initiate discussion of smoking cessation if applicable.	Patient will have adequate gas exchange.	Continue as in Acute Management Phase. Teach patient/family to report dyspnea to physician. Continue discussion of smoking cessation if applicable. Refer to appropriate support group.

COMFORT

Diagnosis/Stabilization Phase		Acute Management Phase		Recovery Phase	
Outcome	Interventions	Outcome	Interventions	Outcome	Interventions
Patient will be as comfortable and pain free as possible as evidenced by: • no objective indicators of discomfort • no complaints of discomfort	Assess quantity and quality of discomfort. Administer narcotics (IV morphine is drug of choice) and monitor response. Avoid IM injections. Initiate nitroglycerin drip and monitor response. Titrate according to hemodynamic parameters and report of pain. Provide a quiet environment to potentiate analgesia. Provide supplemental oxygen. Provide reassurance in a calm, caring, competent manner.	Patient will be relaxed and pain free.	Continue as in Diagnosis/Stabilization Phase. Observe for complications of MI that may cause discomfort: pericarditis, pulmonary embolus, angina, extension of MI. Provide uninterrupted periods of rest. Teach patient/family use of other methods to promote relaxation: imagery, deep breathing, music therapy, humor therapy, and touch therapy.	Patient will be relaxed and pain free.	Continue alternative methods to promote relaxation as listed earlier. Teach patient/family alternative methods to promote relaxation at home. Have patient/family give return demonstration. Discuss techniques for stress management. Teach patient/family what to do at home if chest discomfort recurs and the importance of taking timely action.

Myocardial Infarction Interdisciplinary Outcome Pathway (continued)

COMFORT (continued)

Diagnosis/Stabilization Phase		Acute Management Phase		Recovery Phase	
Outcome	Interventions	Outcome	Interventions	Outcome	Interventions
	Teach patient importance of reporting chest discomfort and how to quantify. Use a pain analogue scale. Administer sedatives as needed. Allow flexible visitation to meet the needs of patient and family.				

SKIN INTEGRITY

Diagnosis/Stabilization Phase		Acute Management Phase		Recovery Phase	
Outcome	Interventions	Outcome	Interventions	Outcome	Interventions
Patient will have intact skin without abrasions.	Assess all bony prominences at least q4h if needed according to hospital protocol. Assess skin integrity surrounding all invasive sites.	Patient will have intact skin without abrasions.	Continue as in Diagnosis/Stabilization Phase.	Patient will have intact skin without abrasions.	Teach patient/family proper skin care at home after discharge.

PROTECTION/SAFETY

Diagnosis/Stabilization Phase		Acute Management Phase		Recovery Phase	
Outcome	Interventions	Outcome	Interventions	Outcome	Interventions
Patient will be protected from possible harm.	Assess need for wrist restraints if patient is intubated, has a decreased LOC, is restless or agitated, is unable to follow commands, has counterpulsation device in place, or is on a ventricular assist system. Explain need for restraints to patient/family. If restrained, assess response to restraints and check q1–2h for skin	Patient will be protected from possible harm.	Provide support when dangling or getting OOB, and monitor response.	Patient will be protected from possible harm.	Provide support with ambulation and climbing stairs. Teach patient/family about any physical limitations in activity after discharge.

integrity and impairment to circulation. Follow hospital protocol for use of restraints. Provide sedatives as needed.

PSYCHOSOCIAL/SELF-DETERMINATION

Diagnosis/Stabilization Phase		Acute Management Phase		Recovery Phase	
Outcome	Interventions	Outcome	Interventions	Outcome	Interventions
Patient will achieve psychophysiologic stability. Patient will demonstrate a decrease in anxiety as evidenced by: • VS WNL • LOC WNL • subjective report of decreased anxiety • objective report of decreased anxiety Patient will begin acceptance process for MI.	Assess physiologic effects of critical care environment on patient (hemodynamic variables, psychological status, signs of increased sympathetic response). Take measures to reduce sensory overload. Provide uninterrupted periods of rest. Use calm, caring, competent, and reassuring approach with patient and family. Allow flexible visitation to meet the needs of the patient and family. Determine coping ability of patient/family and take appropriate measures to meet their needs (i.e., explain condition, equipment, and medications; provide frequent condition reports; use easy to understand terminology; repeat information as needed; answer all questions).	Patient will achieve psychophysiologic stability. Patient will demonstrate a decrease in anxiety. Patient will continue acceptance of MI.	Continue as in Diagnosis/Stabilization Phase. Teach other methods to promote relaxation. Continue to assess coping ability of patient/family and take measures as indicated (family conferences, support services, verbalization of concerns/fears).	Patient will achieve psychophysiologic stability. Patient will demonstrate a decrease in anxiety. Patient will continue acceptance of MI and implications.	Provide instruction on coping mechanisms. Continue cardiac teaching. Assess understanding. Reinforce as needed. Communicate teaching goals to cardiac rehabilitation. Refer to outside services or agencies as appropriate (chaplain, social services, home health, cardiac rehabilitation). Address concerns patient may have about impact on daily life: ADLs, recreation, sexual functioning, return to work, and driving.

Peripheral Vascular Disease
Interdisciplinary Outcome Pathway

COORDINATION OF CARE

	Diagnosis/Stabilization Phase		Acute Management Phase		Recovery Phase
Outcome	**Interventions**	**Outcome**	**Interventions**	**Outcome**	**Interventions**
All appropriate team members and disciplines will be involved in the plan of care.	Develop the plan of care with the patient/family, primary physician(s), family practitioner, vascular surgeon, RN, advanced practice nurse, and other specialists as needed. Obtain cardiac consult if possible before any surgical intervention.	All appropriate team members and disciplines will be involved in the plan of care.	Initiate planning for anticipated discharge and call home health as indicated. Involve other disciplines as needed: chaplain, social worker, RCP, vascular rehabilitation staff, dietitian. Begin teaching patient/family about care at home. Initiate vascular rehabilitation program if available. Obtain pulmonary consult if patient has history of smoking.	Patient will understand how to maintain optimal health at home.	Provide guidelines concerning care at home and any follow-up visits. • diet • medications • smoking cessation • medical management • care of incision(s) if surgical management • exercise program Provide patient/family with phone numbers of resources available to answer questions.

DIAGNOSTICS

	Diagnosis/Stabilization Phase		Acute Management Phase		Recovery Phase
Outcome	**Interventions**	**Outcome**	**Interventions**	**Outcome**	**Interventions**
Patient will understand any tests or procedures that need to be completed (VS, I & O, hemodynamic monitoring, angiography, CO, CXR, echocardiogram, Doppler studies, lab work, ultrasound, EKG, plethysmography, CT scan, MRI, and any surgical procedures including angioplasty and stent placement).	Explain all interventions and tests to patient/family. Be sensitive to individualized needs of patient/family for information. Establish effective communication techniques with intubated patient.	Patient will understand any tests or procedures that need to be completed (removal of indwelling lines and ET tube, lab work, angiography, CXR, coughing and deep breathing, ROM, increase in activity, pulse oximetry).	Explain procedures and tests needed to assess recovery. Be sensitive to individualized needs of patient/family for information. Anticipate need for further diagnostic tests and any interventions that may result.	Patient will understand meaning of diagnostic tests in relation to continued health (lab tests, increase in activity, coughing and deep breathing, vascular rehabilitation program).	Review with patient before discharge the results of lab tests, Doppler studies, angiography, angioplasty, stent placement, and surgery. Discuss any abnormal findings and appropriate measures patient can take to help return to normal or to improve. Provide patient with guidelines concerning follow-up care. Provide instructions on care at home: • when to call doctor • care of healing wounds or incisions • activity limitations

- diet
- medications
- smoking cessation
- follow-up visits

FLUID BALANCE

Diagnosis/Stabilization Phase		Acute Management Phase		Recovery Phase	
Outcome	Interventions	Outcome	Interventions	Outcome	Interventions
Patient will achieve optimal hemodynamic status as evidenced by: • MAP > 70 mmHg • hemodynamic parameters WNL • UO > 0.5 mL/kg/hr • absence of dysrhythmias • adequate LOC • clear lung sounds • absence of JVD • good peripheral pulses • normal skin turgor	Monitor and treat cardiac parameters: • dysrhythmias • BP • PAP • PCWP • CO/CI • stroke volume/stroke index • SVR/PVR • SvO$_2$ • LOC • evidence of tissue perfusion • EKG Monitor lab values: electrolytes, Mg^{++}, Hgb, Hct, PT, PTT, ACT, platelets, CK, CK-MB, cardiac troponin, creatinine. Assess for fluid overload or deficit and treat accordingly. Anticipate need for vasopressor agents and assess response. Titrate accordingly. Assess neurologic status q1h and PRN, particularly if carotid vessels are involved. Prepare for surgery with peripheral vascular emergencies (i.e., arterial thrombus occlusion). Monitor for complications that can occur with peripheral vascular disease (PVD): thrombus formation, embolus formation, infection. Check all peripheral pulses, skin temperature, and color q1h and PRN.	Patient will maintain optimal hemodynamic status.	Continue as in Diagnosis/Stabilization Phase except decrease assessments to q2–4h and PRN. Check cardiac parameters q2–4h and PRN. Weigh daily. Continue to assess for complications. Monitor for signs and symptoms of fluid overload or deficit.	Patient will maintain optimal hemodynamic status.	Continue assessments as in Acute Management Phase except decrease to q4–8h and PRN. Begin teaching patient/family signs and symptoms of inadequate tissue perfusion and when to seek medical attention: tingling, numbness, discoloration, wounds that will not heal, discomfort with activity, claudication. Teach patient/family signs and symptoms of fluid overload or deficit and measures to take should they occur.

Peripheral Vascular Disease Interdisciplinary Outcome Pathway (continued)

FLUID BALANCE (continued)

Diagnosis/Stabilization Phase		Acute Management Phase		Recovery Phase	
Outcome	Interventions	Outcome	Interventions	Outcome	Interventions
	Assess capillary refill q1h and PRN. If postop: • keep systolic BP 100–120 mmHg • check peripheral pulses, skin temperature, color, and capillary refill q1h and PRN • monitor for complications of surgery (hypotension, hypertension, thrombus formation, hemorrhage) • cardiac monitoring • monitor renal status closely • keep patient well hydrated both before and after surgery • maintain NG tube if used and assess drainage Monitor anticoagulation if used. Monitor PT, PTT, and/or ACT as indicated. Monitor for bleeding complications. Fibrinolytic agents may be used for acute occlusions. Monitor for reperfusion and complications of fibrinolytic therapy (intracranial hemorrhage, hematoma, distal embolus, retroperitoneal hemorrhage, and allergic reaction).				

NUTRITION

Diagnosis/Stabilization Phase		Acute Management Phase		Recovery Phase	
Outcome	Interventions	Outcome	Interventions	Outcome	Interventions
Patient will be adequately nourished as evidenced by: • stable weight	Assess bowel sounds, abdominal distension, abdominal pain and tenderness q4h and PRN. Initiate heart healthy diet and monitor response.	Patient will be adequately nourished.	Assess bowel sounds, abdominal distension, abdominal pain and tenderness q4h and PRN. If on clear liquids, advance DAT and monitor response.	Patient will be adequately nourished.	Teach patient/family about heart healthy diet: • total fat <30% of daily intake

- weight not >10% below or >20% above IBW
- albumin >3.5 g/dL
- total protein 6–8 g/dL
- cholesterol <200 mg/dL

If patient has had surgery, initiate clear liquids and monitor response.
Assess nutritional status.
If patient is intubated >24h, initiate alternative methods of nutrition.

Monitor protein and albumin lab values.
Assess patient risk of hypercholesterolemia and hyperlipidemia and begin assessment of patient's diet.
Involve dietitian as needed:
- if eating less than half of food on tray
- for albumin <3.0
- for instruction on heart healthy diet
- for unanticipated weight loss

- total saturated fat <10% of daily intake
- total daily cholesterol intake <300 mg
- calorie restriction if indicated
- sodium restriction if indicated

MOBILITY

Diagnosis/Stabilization Phase		Acute Management Phase		Recovery Phase	
Outcome	Interventions	Outcome	Interventions	Outcome	Interventions
Patient will achieve optimal mobility.	Turn at least q2h if hemodynamically stable and monitor response. If intubated >24h, institute ROM exercises and consult PT if necessary. Begin passive/active-assist ROM exercises. Monitor for complaints of discomfort in lower extremities with activity, and decrease activity if claudication occurs. Monitor peripheral pulses with activity. Involve PT, particularly in setting of amputation or prolonged intubation (>24h). PT to assess ambulation mobility; muscle flexibility, strength, and tone. OT to assess functional abilities. PT/OT to help determine and direct activity goals.	Patient will achieve optimal mobility.	Progress exercise as tolerated: dangle, OOB TID to QID, and walking 50–100 feet several times a day. Monitor response to increased activity and decrease if adverse events occur (tachycardia, dyspnea, syncope, hypo/hypertension, dysrhythmias, decreased peripheral pulses, severe discomfort in lower extremities). Provide physical assistance or assistive devices as necessary. Initiate vascular rehabilitation program. Take measures to prevent embolus formation such as ROM, antithrombotic hose, and antiplatelet agents. Assess for claudication with increased activity. Assess peripheral nerve damage that will appear as loss of motor and/or sensory function. Assess skin for temperature, color, and cyanosis.	Patient will achieve optimal mobility.	Continue to progress exercise as tolerated and monitor response. Continue physical therapy in home if needed. Walk at least 200–300 feet TID to QID. Assess ability to negotiate stairs if part of home environment. Decrease activity if tachycardia, discomfort, hypo/hypertension, or dyspnea occurs. Teach patient/family about signs of decreased circulation to lower extremities and actions to take (nonhealing wounds, mottling, discoloration, numbness, tingling, claudication). Refer to outpatient vascular rehabilitation or physical therapy program.

Peripheral Vascular Disease Interdisciplinary Outcome Pathway (*continued*)

OXYGENATION/VENTILATION

Diagnosis/Stabilization Phase		Acute Management Phase		Recovery Phase	
Outcome	Interventions	Outcome	Interventions	Outcome	Interventions
Patient will have adequate gas exchange as evidenced by: • SaO$_2$ >90% • SpO$_2$ >92% • ABGs WNL • clear breath sounds • respiratory rate, depth, and rhythm WNL • CXR WNL • absence of dyspnea, cyanosis, and secretions • Hbg and Hct WNL	Monitor SvO$_2$ with pulse oximetry and apply supplemental oxygen as needed. Continue to monitor pulse oximetry. Keep SpO$_2$ >92%. If vascular surgery is done, patient may be on a mechanical ventilator. If so, monitor ventilator settings before, during, and after weaning. Monitor for patient response to weaning: • wean FIO$_2$ to keep SpO$_2$ >92% • monitor effects of anesthesia and wean ventilator accordingly Assess respiratory functioning, including lung sounds, respiratory muscle strength, respiratory rate and depth, coughing ability, and CXR. Assess evidence of tissue perfusion. Monitor lab values: Hgb, Hct, ABGs. If history of smoking, obtain pulmonary consult.	Patient will have adequate gas exchange.	Monitor and treat oxygenation/ventilation disturbances. Wean oxygen therapy as tolerated. Monitor with pulse oximetry. Keep SpO$_2$ >92%. Observe effects of increased activity on respiratory status (dyspnea, adventitious breath sounds). Observe for complications of PVD that may impair oxygenation/ventilation: pulmonary embolus, atelectasis, pneumonia. If applicable, begin discussion on smoking cessation.	Patient will have adequate gas exchange.	Continue as in Acute Management Phase. Continue discussion on smoking cessation. Refer to smoking cessation groups, American Lung Association, American Cancer Society, and other support groups. Teach patient appropriate use of nicotine control pharmaceutical agents.

COMFORT

Diagnosis/Stabilization Phase		Acute Management Phase		Recovery Phase	
Outcome	Interventions	Outcome	Interventions	Outcome	Interventions
Patient will be as comfortable and pain free as possible as evidenced by:	Assess quantity and quality of pain using pain scale. Remember the concept of "phantom pain" in setting of amputation.	Patient will be as relaxed and pain free as possible.	Continue as in Diagnosis/Stabilization Phase. Provide uninterrupted periods of rest.	Patient will be as relaxed and pain free as possible.	Progress analgesics to oral medications as needed. Assess response. Use sedatives as indicated and assess response.

Outcome	Interventions	Outcome	Interventions	Outcome	Interventions
• no objective indicators of discomfort • no complaints of discomfort Patient will be aware of subtle signs of discomfort due to peripheral neuropathy.	Administer narcotics and monitor response. Anticipate need for analgesics and provide as needed. If patient is intubated, establish effective communication technique with which patient can communicate discomfort and need for analgesics. Provide a quiet environment to potentiate analgesia. Provide reassurance in a calm, caring, and competent manner. Assess other symptoms of discomfort: paresthesia, numbness, tingling. Assess for claudication at rest and with activity. Assess for acute pain that may be associated with acute thrombosis. In same cases, this may appear as only mild claudication.	Patient will be aware of subtle signs of discomfort.	Teach patient relaxation exercises. Have patient give return demonstration. Use touch therapy, humor, music therapy, and imagery to promote relaxation. Involve family in techniques. Use sedatives as indicated. Observe for complications of PVD that may cause discomfort: pulmonary embolus, acute arterial occlusion, ulcers, emboli, MI, infection, angina.	Patient will be aware of subtle signs of discomfort.	Continue alternative methods to promote relaxation. Teach patient/family alternative methods to promote relaxation to use at home. Teach self-medication for after discharge. Continue to teach patient/family about potential signs of discomfort with PVD: paresthesia, numbness, tingling, acute pain, mild discomfort, mottling, cyanosis, and hair loss.

SKIN INTEGRITY

Diagnosis/Stabilization Phase		Acute Management Phase		Recovery Phase	
Outcome	Interventions	Outcome	Interventions	Outcome	Interventions
Patient will have intact skin without abrasions or pressure ulcers. Patient will have healing wounds/incisions.	Check temperature q4h and PRN. Begin passive/active-assist ROM exercises. Assess all bony prominences at least q4h and treat if needed. Treat any wounds according to orders or hospital protocol. Monitor response to therapy. Monitor for signs and symptoms of infection q4h and PRN (incision, wounds, respiratory, renal). Use preventive pressure-reducing devices if patient is at high risk for developing or already has pressure ulcers.	Patient will have intact skin without abrasions or pressure ulcers. Patient will have healing wounds/incisions.	Continue as in Diagnosis/Stabilization Phase. If surgery is done, keep surgical site covered for 24h. Then open the area to air unless actively draining. Assess incision sites for signs and symptoms of infection q4h and PRN. Cleanse incisions daily proximally to distally with sterile soap and water. Assess skin adjacent to surgical wounds for tape burns, allergic reactions. Continue preventive pressure-reducing devices if used.	Patient will have intact skin without abrasions or pressure ulcers. Patient will have healing wounds/incisions.	Assess all bony prominences at least q4h and treat if needed. Assess and cleanse wounds and/or incisions as described earlier. Teach patient/family importance of assessing all areas of skin for lesions every day, particularly feet and lower extremities. Teach patient/family proper skin care for at home: • foot care • care of incisions/wounds • appropriately fitting shoes and garments

Peripheral Vascular Disease Interdisciplinary Outcome Pathway (continued)

SKIN INTEGRITY (continued)

Diagnosis/Stabilization Phase		Acute Management Phase		Recovery Phase	
Outcome	Interventions	Outcome	Interventions	Outcome	Interventions
	Treat pressure ulcers according to hospital protocol. Assess skin for ulcers, gangrene, paleness, mottled appearance, turgor, and trophic changes.				• diet • avoidance of tight and restricting garments Provide information concerning wound infection as needed.

PROTECTION/SAFETY

Diagnosis/Stabilization Phase		Acute Management Phase		Recovery Phase	
Outcome	Interventions	Outcome	Interventions	Outcome	Interventions
Patient will be protected from possible harm.	Assess need for wrist restraints if patient is intubated, has a decreased LOC, and is agitated or restless. Explain need for restraints to patient/family. Assess response to restraints, if used; check q1–2h for skin integrity and impairment to circulation. Remove restraints as soon as patient is able to follow instructions. Follow hospital protocol for use of restraints. Provide sedatives as needed.	Patient will be protected from possible harm.	If wrist restraints still needed, check q1–2h for skin integrity and impairment to circulation. Provide support when dangling, getting OOB, and ambulating. Monitor response. Use gait belt as indicated for ambulation. In case of amputation, ask PT to start instructions with crutches, wheelchairs, and so on. Consider OT for teaching correct movement and appropriate functional skills to prevent joint stress, strain, or injury.	Patient will be protected from possible harm.	Teach patient/family about any physical limitations in activity after discharge. Continue with PT/OT as outpatient if needed. Refer to vascular rehabilitation program if feasible.

PSYCHOSOCIAL/SELF-DETERMINATION

Diagnosis/Stabilization Phase		Acute Management Phase		Recovery Phase	
Outcome	Interventions	Outcome	Interventions	Outcome	Interventions
Patient will achieve psychophysiologic stability. Patient will demonstrate a decrease in anxiety as evidenced by: • VS WNL • subjective reports of decreased anxiety • objective signs of decreased anxiety Patient will begin acceptance process of PVD.	Assess physiologic effects of critical care environment on patient (hemodynamic variables, psychological status, signs of increased sympathetic response). Provide sedatives as needed. Take measures to reduce sensory overload. If patient is intubated, develop effective interventions to communicate with patient. Use calm, caring, competent, and reassuring approach with patient and family. Arrange for flexible visitation to meet needs of patient/family. Determine coping ability of patient and family and take appropriate measures to meet those needs (i.e., explain condition, explain equipment, provide frequent condition reports, use easy to understand terminology, repeat information as needed, allow family to visit, answer all questions). Begin teaching patient/family about PVD. Allow patient/family to verbalize their fears and concerns.	Patient will achieve psychophysiologic stability. Patient will demonstrate a decrease in anxiety. Patient will continue acceptance process of PVD.	Continue as in Diagnosis/Stabilization Phase. Provide adequate rest periods. Continue to include family in all aspects of care. Continue to assess coping ability of patient/family and take appropriate measures. Maintain quiet environment. Continue to teach patient/family about self-care with PVD. Continue to encourage patient/family to discuss their feelings about PVD.	Patient will achieve psychophysiologic stability. Patient will demonstrate a decrease in anxiety. Patient will continue acceptance process of PVD.	Provide instruction on coping mechanisms to use after discharge. Refer to outside services or agencies as appropriate (chaplain, social services, home health care, vascular rehabilitation program). Address concerns patient may have about impact on daily life: ADLs, recreation, sexual functioning, return to work, and driving.

Thrombolytic Therapy Interdisciplinary Outcome Pathway

COORDINATION OF CARE

Diagnosis/Stabilization Phase		Acute Management Phase		Recovery Phase	
Outcome	Interventions	Outcome	Interventions	Outcome	Interventions
All emergency team members and disciplines will be involved in the plan of care.	Develop plan of care with patient/family, primary physician, cardiologist, RN, advanced practice nurse, RCP, chaplain, and social services.	All appropriate team members will be involved in the plan of care.	Revise and update plan of care with patient/family, other team members, dietitian, discharge planner, and cardiac rehabilitation. Initiate planning for anticipated discharge.	Patient/family will understand how to maintain optimal health at home.	Provide guidelines concerning follow-up care to patient and family (i.e., bleeding precautions, medication). Provide patient/family with phone numbers of resources available to answer questions.

DIAGNOSTICS

Diagnosis/Stabilization Phase		Acute Management Phase		Recovery Phase	
Outcome	Interventions	Outcome	Interventions	Outcome	Interventions
Patient will understand all tests and procedures that are needed (laboratory tests, frequent VS taken by automatic BP cuff, cardiac monitor, intravenous lines, oxygen per nasal cannula, pulse oximeter, and counter pulsation if indicated).	Explain all procedures and tests to patient/family. If thrombolytic therapy is contraindicated, begin standard medical treatment for AMI or consider mechanical reperfusion. Determine whether patient is candidate for thrombolytic therapy: • identify acute myocardial infarction (AMI), from STAT 12 lead EKG • at least 1 mm of ST segment elevation in 2 contiguous limb leads • at least 2 mm ST segment elevation in 2 contiguous precordial leads • new onset bundle branch block • less than 12h since onset of symptoms	Patient will understand need for thrombolytic therapy and the MI process and have questions answered.	Explain procedures and tests needed to give thrombolytic therapy. Explain the acute MI process. Be available to answer questions of patient/family. Administer thrombolytic therapy as ordered. Observe closely for bleeding Observe closely for signs of reperfusion: • relief of chest pain • ST segment returns to baseline • reperfusion dysrhythmias	Patient will understand the expectations of thrombolytic therapy and the MI process and have questions answered. Patient will follow healthy heart diet, exercise, and stop smoking. Patient will know the signs and symptoms of recurrent MI, what treatment steps to take (nitroglycerin for chest pain, emergency care if pain unrelieved with sublingual nitroglycerin × 3).	Give patient literature on MI process and thrombolytic therapy. Provide patient/family teaching of home care, when to call the physician, when to return to the ER, signs and symptoms of MI, angina, CHF, risk factor modification, increasing activities, importance of medication regimen, and type of thrombolytic agent used.

Patient will understand need for follow-up therapy and doctor's office visits to maintain optimal health.

Patient will know which thrombolytic agent he or she received.

No absolute contraindications:

- active internal bleeding
- altered level of consciousness
- recent head trauma
- known previous hemorrhagic cerebral vascular accident (CVA)
- intracranial or intraspinal surgery within 2 months
- trauma or surgery within 2 weeks
- blood pressure greater than 200/120 mmHg
- known bleeding disorder
- pregnancy
- suspected aortic dissection
- previous allergy to thrombolytic agent
- known spinal cord or cerebral arteriovenous malformation or tumor
- diabetic hemorrhagic retinopathy or other ophthalmic conditions

Evaluate relative contraindications and weigh risk/benefit ratio:

- active ulcer disease
- major trauma or surgery greater than 2 weeks, less than 2 months
- history of recent ischemic or embolic cerebrovascular accident
- current use of oral anticoagulants
- history of chronic severe hypertension (diastolic greater than 100 mmHg), with or without drug therapy

Be aware of using words that patient/family may not understand.

Be sensitive to patient/family's individualized needs for information.

Thrombolytic Therapy Interdisciplinary Outcome Pathway (continued)

DIAGNOSTICS (continued)

Diagnosis/Stabilization Phase		Acute Management Phase		Recovery Phase	
Outcome	Interventions	Outcome	Interventions	Outcome	Interventions
	Explain inclusion criteria for thrombolytics. ER physician should explain all risks from thrombolytic therapy (nosebleeds, venipuncture bleeds, gastrointestinal bleeds, and cerebral bleeds).				

FLUID BALANCE

Diagnosis/Stabilization Phase		Acute Management Phase		Recovery Phase	
Outcome	Interventions	Outcome	Interventions	Outcome	Interventions
Patient will achieve optimal hemodynamic status as evidenced by: • MAP greater than 70 mmHg • hemodynamic parameters WNL • free of life-threatening dysrhythmias • normal cardiac output/CI • urine output >0.5 mL/kg/hr • return of ST segments to baseline • clear lung sounds	Monitor and treat cardiac parameters: • dysrhythmias • BP • PA pressures, CVP, PCWP • CO/CI • SVR/PVR • SV/SI • I & O • left and right ventricular stroke work index • evidence of tissue perfusion Establish two twincath 18/20 intravenous lines. Anticipate need for pacing, defibrillation, and/or pharmacologic interventions as needed for dysrhythmias. Monitor laboratory values: cardiac enzymes, PT, PTT, Mg^{++}, electrolytes, cardiac troponin. Monitor and treat to maintain HR and reduce oxygen demand (metoprolol 3–5 mg dose administered every 2 minutes).	Patient will maintain normal cardiac output. Patient will maintain optimal hemodynamic status.	Administer thrombolytic agent according to hospital protocol or physician orders. Administer aspirin (to reduce platelet aggregation). Administer nitroglycerin drip to decrease preload. Administer heparin according to weight-based dosing. Monitor EKG and ST segment trends (graphs). Continue to monitor and treat cardiac parameters. Monitor and treat dysrhythmias. Monitor lab values and treat any electrolyte abnormalities. Continue to assess for complications associated with AMI. Begin patient/family teaching on cardiac system, current cardiac problems, treatments, and expected clinical course. Do not administer IM injection. Perform neurologic checks q2–4h. Follow Glascow Coma Scale.	Patient will maintain optimal hemodynamic status.	Continue to monitor and treat cardiac parameters and dysrhythmias. Monitor lab values. Monitor EKG for evolutionary changes consistent with MI. Assess for complications. Teach patient/family signs of fluid overload (SOB, sudden weight gain, rapid heartbeat). Continue cardiac teaching and assess for understanding. Reinforce as needed. Teach patient and family how to maintain optimal fluid balance at home (decrease salt intake, weigh weekly, drink 8 glasses of water per day).

Anticipate need for vasopressor agents and assess response.
Observe for signs of bleeding while patient is receiving thrombolytics and treat accordingly.
Keep antidotes for anticoagulants on unit.
Monitor for signs of complications that can occur following an acute MI:
- CHF
- cardiogenic shock
- dysrhythmias
- cardiac tamponade
- mitral regurgitation
- papillary muscle dysfunction/rupture
  - coronary atherosclerosis and arterial dissection
Keep lidocaine and atropine at bedside.

Observe for signs and symptoms of increased intracranial bleeding including change in mental status, decreased LOC, pupil changes, headache, or weakness in arms or legs.

NUTRITION

Diagnosis/Stabilization Phase		Acute Management Phase		Recovery Phase	
Outcome	Interventions	Outcome	Interventions	Outcome	Interventions
Patient will be adequately nourished as evidenced by: • stable weight not >10% below or >20% above IBW • albumin 3.5–4.5 g/dL • total protein 6–8 g/dL • total lymphocyte count 1,000–3,000	NPO the first 6h; advance as condition dictates and assess response. Clear liquids to full liquids first 24h; monitor response and change as needed.	Patient will be adequately nourished.	Advance to heart healthy diet as tolerated (low fat, low cholesterol, low sodium) and monitor for response. Weigh daily. Consult dietitian to help determine and direct nutritional support.	Patient will be adequately nourished.	Teach patient/family about heart healthy diet: • total fat <30% of daily intake • total saturated fat <10% of daily intake • total daily cholesterol intake <300 mg • caloric reduction as indicated • sodium restriction as indicated Teach patient about dietary supplements (i.e., anitoxidants, oat bran, fiber, vitamins and minerals).

Thrombolytic Therapy Interdisciplinary Outcome Pathway (continued)

MOBILITY

Diagnosis/Stabilization Phase		Acute Management Phase		Recovery Phase	
Outcome	Interventions	Outcome	Interventions	Outcome	Interventions
Patient will achieve optimal mobility.	Complete bed rest first 6h following thrombolytic therapy. Bed rest with bedside commode privileges first 24h. Teach patient physiologic basis for rest.	Patient will achieve optimal mobility.	Progress exercise as tolerated: • dangle • OOB for meals • up in chair TID and QID while in CCU environment Assess response to increased activity. Decrease activity as needed if adverse events occur (tachycardia, dyspnea, ectopy, syncope, hypotension, chest discomfort). Encourage patient to begin light activities (brushing teeth and partial bathing). Teach patient gradual exercise principles. Initiate Phase I Cardiac Rehabilitation. Consult PT/OT as needed to help determine and direct activity goals.	Patient will achieve optimal mobility.	Continue to progress exercises as tolerated and monitor response. Walk at least 200–300 feet TID to QID. Walk up and down one flight of stairs. Teach patient/family about home exercise program. Refer to outpatient cardiac rehabilitation program if feasible.

OXYGENATION/VENTILATION

Diagnosis/Stabilization Phase		Acute Management Phase		Recovery Phase	
Outcome	Interventions	Outcome	Interventions	Outcome	Interventions
Patient will have adequate gas exchange as evidenced by: • SaO_2 > 90% • SpO_2 > 92% • ABGs WNL • clear breath sounds • respiratory rate, depth, and rhythm WNL • CXR normal	Apply supplemental oxygen for at least 24h. Monitor SpO_2. Assess respiratory functioning including lung sounds, respiratory rate and depth, and CXR. Consult RCP as needed. Encourage coughing and deep breathing while on bed rest. Assess evidence of tissue perfusion: • LOC • UO > 0.5 mL/kg/hr	Patient will have adequate gas exchange.	Assess respiratory functioning and intervene as indicated. Involve RCP as needed. Assess need for continued supplemental oxygen with use of pulse oximetry. Observe for complications of MI that may impair oxygenation/ventilation: • CHF • pulmonary embolus • mitral regurgitation	Patient will maintain adequate gas exchange.	Continue to assess oxygenation and respiratory functions while increasing activity. Intervene as indicated. Assess need for oxygen therapy at home. Teach patient/family about oxygen demand and how to maintain normal oxygenation at home (if increased SOB, call physician).

- cardiac tamponade
- cardiogenic shock

- normal liver enzymes
- peripheral pulses

Monitor lab values: ABGs, Hgb, PT, PTT, ACT.

COMFORT

Diagnosis/Stabilization Phase		Acute Management Phase		Recovery Phase	
Outcome	Interventions	Outcome	Interventions	Outcome	Interventions
Patient will be as comfortable as possible as evidenced by: • no objective indicators of discomfort • no complaints of discomfort • return of ST segment to baseline	Assess quantity and quality of pain. Administer narcotics (morphine drug of choice) and monitor response and respirations. Administer nitroglycerin drip; monitor response. Titrate according to hemodynamic parameters and report of pain (scale 1–10). Monitor BP closely. Provide a quiet environment. Provide reassurance in a calm, caring, competent manner. Teach the importance of reporting chest pain. Administer sedatives as needed.	Patient will be as pain free and relaxed as possible.	Continue as in Diagnosis/Stabilization Phase. Administer medication to alleviate pain. Advance to oral medications as tolerated and monitor response. Observe for complications of MI that may cause discomfort (chest pain, SOB, increased anxiousness). Instruct patient on relaxation techniques. Have patient give return demonstration. Obtain 12 lead EKG with complaints of chest pain. Teach patient/family alternative methods to promote relaxation at home (imagery, deep breathing, music).	Patient will be as relaxed as possible.	Teach patient/family what to do at home if chest discomfort recurs (sublingual nitroglycerin × 3, cessation of exertional activity). Continue alternative methods to promote relaxation.

SKIN INTEGRITY

Diagnosis/Stabilization Phase		Acute Management Phase		Recovery Phase	
Outcome	Interventions	Outcome	Interventions	Outcome	Interventions
Patient will have intact skin and maintain hemostasis.	Assess skin integrity surrounding all invasive sites. Assess all bony prominences at least q4h and treat if needed according to hospital protocol. Assess all venipunctures as sites of potential bleeding due to anticoagulants.	Patient will have intact skin.	Continue as in Diagnosis/Stabilization Phase. Assess gingiva for any evidence of bleeding (frequent assessment of the mouth and gums will minimize potential complications from blood loss, allow for early intervention should bleeding occur, and help to differentiate bleeding from GI tract).	Patient will have intact skin.	Teach patient/family proper skin care at home and actions to take should bleeding occur.

Thrombolytic Therapy Interdisciplinary Outcome Pathway (continued)

SKIN INTEGRITY (continued)

Diagnosis/Stabilization Phase		Acute Management Phase		Recovery Phase	
Outcome	Interventions	Outcome	Interventions	Outcome	Interventions
	If bleeding occurs from venipuncture, direct manual pressure should be applied for 15–30 minutes, or until hemostasis has been achieved. If hematoma does develop, the area should be marked, dated, and timed for future assessment of any increase in size. Apply pressure dressing to all venipunctures to maintain hemostasis. Assess for evidence of superficial wounds or abrasions. Attempt to establish all peripheral IV lines (at least two) prior to initiation of thrombolytic therapy. Avoid all IM injections during and following thrombolytic therapy. Avoid all noncompressible assess sites (subclavian vein, internal jugular vein). If central venous access becomes necessary, utilize femoral or brachial vein approach.		Use an electric razor during the first 24h following the thrombolytic therapy. Inform the patient not to brush too vigorously during the first 24h. Place a sign at the bedside stating "Bleeding Precautions" to alert to potential danger of bleeding.		

PROTECTION/SAFETY

Diagnosis/Stabilization Phase		Acute Management Phase		Recovery Phase	
Outcome	Interventions	Outcome	Interventions	Outcome	Interventions
Patient will be protected from possible harm.	Assess need for wrist restraints if patient is intubated, has a decreased LOC, is restless or agitated, is unable to follow commands, or has counterpulsation device	Patient will be protected from possible harm.	Continue as in Diagnosis/Stabilization Phase. Provide physical support when dangling or getting OOB, and monitor response.	Patient will be protected from possible harm.	Provide physical support with ambulation and climbing stairs. Teach patient/family about any physical limitations in activity after discharge.

PSYCHOSOCIAL/SELF-DETERMINATION

Diagnosis/Stabilization Phase		Acute Management Phase		Recovery Phase	
Outcome	Interventions	Outcome	Interventions	Outcome	Interventions
Patient will achieve psychophysiologic stability. Patient will demonstrate a decrease in anxiety as evidenced by: • vital signs WNL • subjective report of decreased anxiety • objective report of decreased anxiety Patient will begin acceptance process for MI.	Assess physiologic effects of emergency care environment on patient (hemodynamic variables, psychological status, signs of increased sympathetic response). Take measures to reduce sensory overload. Use calm, caring, competent, and reassuring approach with patient/family. Determine coping ability of patient/family and take appropriate measures to meet their needs. Explain all procedures, equipment, condition in words that are easy to understand, and be available to answer all questions as they arise. Provide sedatives as needed. Monitor RR. in place. Explain need for restraints to patient/family. If restrained, assess response to restraints and check according to hospital protocol for skin integrity and impairment to circulation. Provide sedatives as needed. Post sign stating "Thrombolytic Therapy Given." Avoid unnecessary venipuncture. Do not give any IM injections. For laboratory work, use placement of saline lock for samples.	Patient will begin to accept diagnosis of MI. Patient will achieve psychophysiologic stability. Patient will demonstrate objective and subjective decrease in anxiety.	As in Diagnosis/Stabilization Phase, assess for possible depression due to diagnosis of MI. Allow family to visit in small numbers and for short periods of time. Be as flexible as possible. Initiate cardiac teaching. Assess understanding by listening to patient verbalize about condition. Continue to assess coping ability of patient/family and take measures as indicated (family conferences, support services, verbalization of concerns/fears).	Patient will achieve psychophysiologic stability. Patient will demonstrate a decrease in anxiety. Patient will continue acceptance of MI and implications.	Provide instructions on coping mechanisms. Refer to outside services or agencies as appropriate (chaplain, social services, home health, cardiac rehabilitation). Address concerns patient may have about impact of MI on daily life: recreation, return to work, ADLs, sexual functioning.

Valve Replacement
Interdisciplinary Outcome Pathway

COORDINATION OF CARE

Diagnosis/Stabilization Phase		Acute Management Phase		Recovery Phase	
Outcome	Interventions	Outcome	Interventions	Outcome	Interventions
All appropriate team members and disciplines will be involved in the plan of care.	Develop plan of care with patient/family, primary physician(s), cardiovascular surgeon, cardiologist, pulmonologist, hematologist, anesthesiologist, RN, advanced practice nurse, perfusionist, and RCP.	All appropriate team members and disciplines will be involved in the plan of care.	Update the plan of care with patient/family, other team members, PT, cardiac rehabilitation staff, discharge planner, dietitian, social services, and chaplain. Assess social support systems at home. Initiate planning for anticipated discharge and call home health as indicated. Begin teaching patient/family about care at home. Assess ability to manage at home versus extended care.	Patient will understand how to maintain optimal health at home.	Provide guidelines concerning care at home: • follow-up visits • diet • activity limitations • medications • care of incision Arrange first postop visit for patient prior to discharge. Assist with travel arrangements if necessary. Provide patient/family with phone number of resources available to answer questions. Arrange home health care if needed. Refer to outpatient cardiac rehabilitation program.

DIAGNOSTICS

Diagnosis/Stabilization Phase		Acute Management Phase		Recovery Phase	
Outcome	Interventions	Outcome	Interventions	Outcome	Interventions
Patient will understand any tests or procedures that must be completed (VS, I & O, CO, hemodynamic monitoring, CXR, lab work, hyper/hypothermia unit, chest tubes, invasive devices, EKG).	Explain all procedures and tests to patient/family. Be sensitive to individualized needs of patient/family for information. Establish effective communication technique with intubated patient.	Patient will understand any tests or procedures that must be completed (removal of indwelling lines and chest tubes, lab work, CXR, IS, coughing and deep breathing).	Explain procedures and tests needed to assess recovery. Be sensitive to individualized needs of patient/family for information. Be prepared to repeat information frequently.	Patient will understand meaning of diagnostic tests in relation to continued health (lab tests, increase in activity, coughing and deep breathing, IS).	Review with patient before discharge the results of lab tests, CXR, and surgery. Discuss any abnormal values and appropriate measures patient can take to help return to normal (i.e., hypercholesterolemia). Provide patient with guidelines concerning follow-up care. Provide instruction on care at home: • when to call physician

- care of incision
- activity limitations
- medications
- diet
- cardiac rehabilitation
- late complications (pericarditis, infection, CHF)
- antibiotic prophylaxis
- anticoagulation

FLUID BALANCE

Diagnosis/Stabilization Phase		Acute Management Phase		Recovery Phase	
Outcome	Interventions	Outcome	Interventions	Outcome	Interventions
Patient will achieve optimal hemodynamic status as evidenced by: • MAP >70 mmHg • hemodynamic parameters WNL • UO >0.5 mL/kg/hr • return to normothermic state • free from abnormal EKG changes • free of dysrhythmias Patient will remain free from bleeding.	Monitor and treat cardiac parameters as needed: • HR • BP • PA pressures • PCWP • CO/CI • SV/SI • SVR/PVR • ST segment • I & O • LOC • peripheral pulses • evidence of tissue perfusion • dysrhythmias Rewarm slowly and monitor temperature and signs of shivering. Methods of rewarming include head covering, radiant light, warmed circulating air blanket, warmed convective air blanket, and/or vasodilators. Monitor IABP and VAD if used. Observe for complications associated with these devices: infection, thrombus, distal embolus, pulmonary embolus, CVA, bleeding, vascular. Anticipate need for epicardial pacing and/or pharmacologic agents.	Patient will maintain optimal hemodynamic status. Patient will remain free from dysrhythmias.	Monitor and treat cardiac parameters. Assist with chest tube and indwelling line removal and monitor patient afterward. In some facilities, nurses may remove chest tubes and indwelling lines. Follow hospital protocol. Monitor for potential complications of valve replacement surgery: CVA, tamponade, bleeding, embolic events, hypotension. Monitor and treat potentially life-threatening dysrhythmias: supraventricular tachycardia, ventricular tachycardia, ventricular fibrillation, and bradycardia. Consider need for dysrhythmia prophylaxis. Be prepared to institute temporary cardiac pacing either transvenous or transcutaneous. Begin patient/family teaching on cardiovascular system, current treatment, and expected clinical course. Monitor lab values: Hgb, Hct, BUN, creatinine, platelets, PT, PTT.	Patient will maintain optimal hemodynamic state.	Continue to monitor and treat cardiac parameters as needed. Continue cardiac teaching. Assess for understanding and reinforce as needed. Assist with pacing wire removal and monitor patient after pacing wires removed. Teach patient about long-term anticoagulation (at least 6 weeks for porcine or bovine valves; lifelong for mechanical valves).

Valve Replacement Interdisciplinary Outcome Pathway (continued)

FLUID BALANCE (continued)

Diagnosis/Stabilization Phase		Acute Management Phase		Recovery Phase	
Outcome	Interventions	Outcome	Interventions	Outcome	Interventions
	Assess patient for signs and symptoms of CHF: JVD, peripheral edema, S3, S4, rales, tachycardia. Notify physician. Monitor for cardiac tamponade: decreased CO, decreased CVP, pulsus paradoxus, widened cardiac silhouette, distant heart sounds. Notify physician. Monitor lab values: K^+, Mg^{++}, Hgb, Hct, PT, PTT, ACT, platelets, CK, CK-MB, cardiac troponin, glucose, BUN, creatinine. Assess for sudden increase/decrease in chest tube drainage, equalization of filling pressures, widening mediastinum, decrease in BP, and pulsus paradoxus. Notify physician.		Monitor weight, I & O, and signs of peripheral edema. Assess need for diuretics and/or potassium repletion.		

NUTRITION

Diagnosis/Stabilization Phase		Acute Management Phase		Recovery Phase	
Outcome	Interventions	Outcome	Interventions	Outcome	Interventions
Patient will be adequately nourished as evidenced by: • stable weight • weight not >10% below or >20% above IBW • albumin >3.5 g/dL	Keep patient NPO until extubation. If extubation is delayed >24h, assess need for alternative nutritional therapy. Monitor response to clear liquids. Remove NG tube (if utilized) once extubated. Monitor protein and albumin lab values.	Patient will be adequately nourished. Patient will remain free from nausea. Patient will demonstrate return of appetite.	Advance to heart healthy diet (low fat, low cholesterol) as tolerated. Monitor response to diet. Weigh daily. Assess bowel sounds q4h and PRN. Administer laxatives/stool softeners as needed.	Patient will be adequately nourished.	Teach patient/family about heart healthy diet: • total fat <30% of daily intake • total saturated fat <10% of daily intake • total daily cholesterol intake <300 mg • calorie restriction if indicated

- total protein 6–8 g/dL
- prealbumin 15 g/dL
- total lymphocyte count 1,000–3,000
- cholesterol <200 mg/dL

Administer antiemetics, H$_2$ blockers, and/or antacids as needed.

Involve dietitian for:
- unanticipated weight loss
- albumin <3.0
- eating less than half of food on tray
- diet counseling for heart healthy diet

- sodium restriction

Continue laxatives/stool softeners if needed.

MOBILITY

Diagnosis/Stabilization Phase		Acute Management Phase		Recovery Phase	
Outcome	Interventions	Outcome	Interventions	Outcome	Interventions
Patient will maintain normal ROM and muscle strength.	Bed rest until extubation unless extubation delayed >24h. If extubation is delayed, start passive/active-assist ROM and consult PT. Begin passive/active-assist ROM exercises. Dangle after extubation.	Patient will achieve optimal mobility.	PT to assess ambulation mobility, muscle strength, flexibility, and tone. OT to assess functional ability. PT/OT to help determine and direct activity goals. Progress exercise as tolerated: dangle, bathroom privileges, OOB for meals, and walking 50 feet. Monitor response to increased activity. Decrease if adverse events occur (tachycardia, chest discomfort, dyspnea, ectopy, bleeding). Provide physical assistance or assistive devices as necessary. Begin patient/family teaching on principles of a gradual exercise program. Initiate inpatient cardiac rehabilitation.	Patient will achieve optimal mobility.	Walk at least 200–300 feet TID to QID. Walk up and down one flight of stairs, particularly if stairs at home. Teach patient/family about home exercise program. Refer to outpatient cardiac rehabilitation program.

Valve Replacement Interdisciplinary Outcome Pathway (continued)

OXYGENATION/VENTILATION

Diagnosis/Stabilization Phase		Acute Management Phase		Recovery Phase	
Outcome	Interventions	Outcome	Interventions	Outcome	Interventions
Patient will have adequate gas exchange as evidenced by: • SaO_2 >90% • SpO_2 >92% • ABGs WNL • clear breath sounds • respiratory rate, depth, and rhythm WNL • CXR WNL	Monitor ventilator settings and determine wakefulness and readiness to wean. Determine if patient meets early extubation criteria. Monitor hemodynamic variables before, during, and after weaning. Wean ventilator and monitor response: • wean FIO_2 to keep SpO_2 >92% • monitor effects of anesthesia and wean accordingly • after extubation, apply supplemental oxygen Assess respiratory functioning, including lung sounds, respiratory muscle strength, respiratory rate and depth, coughing ability, and CXR. Monitor pulse oximetry. Use supplemental oxygen to keep SpO_2 >92%. Teach patient how to use IS (with inspiratory hold) when extubated.	Patient will have adequate gas exchange.	Monitor and treat oxygenation/ventilation status per ABGs, SpO_2, chest assessment, and CXR. Monitor closely for hypoxemia or dyspnea related to atelectasis and/or pleural effusion. Evaluate need for thoracentesis. Assess chest tubes for drainage/presence of air leaks. Support patient with oxygen therapy as indicated. Reinforce use of IS. Have patient give return demonstration. Monitor for complications that may impair oxygenation/ventilation: pneumonia, atelectasis, pulmonary embolus, CHF. Provide chest splint pillow and instruct on proper use. Have patient give return demonstration.	Patient will have adequate gas exchange.	Reinforce use of IS and chest splint pillow at home. Have patient give return demonstration. Teach patient/family signs and symptoms of respiratory infection and when to call the physician.

COMFORT

Diagnosis/Stabilization Phase		Acute Management Phase		Recovery Phase	
Outcome	Interventions	Outcome	Interventions	Outcome	Interventions
Patient will be as comfortable and pain free as possible as evidenced by: • no objective indicators of discomfort	Anticipate need for analgesia and provide as needed. Use a pain scale or visual analogue tool. Assess response to all analgesics and effects on ability to wean from ventilator when indicated. Use newer NSAIDs with fewer sedative effects.	Patient will be as relaxed and comfortable as possible.	Anticipate need for analgesics and provide as needed. Assess response. Teach patient proper use of PCA pump, if used. Provide chest splint pillow and instruct on proper use. Have patient give return demonstration.	Patient will be as relaxed and comfortable as possible.	Progress analgesics to oral medications as needed and monitor response. Teach patient/family regarding analgesic administration and potential side effects for post-discharge.

Outcome (continued)	Diagnosis/Stabilization Phase Interventions	Acute Management Phase Interventions	Recovery Phase Interventions
• no complaints of discomfort • normal VS	Establish effective communication technique with intubated patients with which he or she can communicate discomfort and need for analgesics.	Provide uninterrupted periods of rest. Assist patient with relaxation techniques. Use touch therapy, humor, music therapy, and imagery to promote relaxation. Provide analgesics as needed before chest tube removal, ambulation, and any other procedures.	Continue alternative methods to promote relaxation. Teach patient/family alternative methods to promote relaxation at home. Have patient/family give return demonstration. Provide uninterrupted periods of rest.

SKIN INTEGRITY

Diagnosis/Stabilization Phase		Acute Management Phase		Recovery Phase	
Outcome	Interventions	Outcome	Interventions	Outcome	Interventions
Patient will have intact skin without abrasions or pressure ulcers. Patient will have healing wounds/incisions. Patient will return to normothermic state.	Rewarm slowly; monitor temperature and signs of shivering. Methods of rewarming include warmed air or water blankets, radiant lighting, head covering. In some institutions, the degree of hypothermia is decreasing. Adapt rewarming techniques to need of patient. Assess all bony prominences at least q4h and treat if needed. Maintain integrity of all dressings. Consider mattress overlay.	Patient will have intact skin without abrasions, pressure ulcers, or wound infections. Patient will have healing wounds/incisions.	Assess all bony prominences at least q4h and treat if needed. Use preventive pressure-reducing devices if patient is at high risk for developing pressure ulcers. Assess sternotomy incision for drainage, erythema, and induration. Use sterile technique when changing bandages. Teach patient/family proper skin care at home (care of incision, signs and symptoms of infection).	Patient will have intact skin without abrasions, pressure ulcers, or wound infections. Patient will have healing wounds/incisions.	Assess all wounds/incisions for signs and symptoms of infection. Culture if necessary. Reinforce importance of proper hygiene and wound care at home. Continue patient/family teaching on skin care at home. Assess understanding and reinforce as needed.

PROTECTION/SAFETY

Diagnosis/Stabilization Phase		Acute Management Phase		Recovery Phase	
Outcome	Interventions	Outcome	Interventions	Outcome	Interventions
Patient will be protected from possible harm.	Assess need for wrist restraints while patient is intubated, has a decreased LOC, or is agitated and restless. Explain need for restraints to patient/family. Assess response to restraints and check q1–2h for skin integrity and impairment to circulation.	Patient will be protected from possible harm.	Provide physical assistance when dangling or getting OOB; monitor response. Isolate pacing wires. Begin teaching patient/family about anticoagulation and safety measures.	Patient will be protected from possible harm.	Provide support with ambulation and climbing stairs. Teach patient/family: • physical limitations such as no lifting/pulling objects over 10–15 pounds for 2–3 months

Valve Replacement Interdisciplinary Outcome Pathway (continued)

PROTECTION/SAFETY (continued)

Diagnosis/Stabilization Phase		Acute Management Phase		Recovery Phase	
Outcome	Interventions	Outcome	Interventions	Outcome	Interventions
	Remove restraints as soon as patient is awake from anesthesia and able to follow instructions. Follow hospital protocol for use of restraints. Provide sedatives as needed. Isolate pacing wires.				• no driving until approved by surgeon • prophylactic antibiotic therapy for any surgical or dental procedure • signs and symptoms of infection; infection can occur up to 21 days postop • when to call the physician • anticoagulation (at least 6 weeks with porcine or bovine valve; lifelong with mechanical valves) Isolate pacing wires until removed.

PSYCHOSOCIAL/SELF-DETERMINATION

Diagnosis/Stabilization Phase		Acute Management Phase		Recovery Phase	
Outcome	Interventions	Outcome	Interventions	Outcome	Interventions
Patient will achieve psychophysiologic stability. Patient will demonstrate a decrease in anxiety as evidenced by: • VS WNL • LOC WNL • subjective reports	Assess physiologic effects of critical care and/or open heart recovery environment on patient (hemodynamic variables, psychological status, signs of increased sympathetic response). Provide sedatives as indicated. Take measures to reduce sensory overload. Develop effective interventions to communicate with intubated patient. Use calm, caring, competent, and reassuring approach with patient and family. Allow flexible visitation to meet patient and family needs.	Patient will achieve psychophysiologic stability. Patient will demonstrate a decrease in anxiety. Patient will begin acceptance of lifelong medical condition.	Take measures to decrease sensory overload. Provide adequate rest periods. Provide sedatives as needed. Continue to include family in aspects of care. Continue to assess coping ability of patient/family and take measures as indicated. Involve patient/family in health care decisions.	Patient will achieve psychophysiologic stability. Patient will demonstrate a decrease in anxiety. Patient will continue acceptance of lifelong medical condition.	Provide adequate rest periods. Continue to assess coping ability of patient and family. Provide information on coping mechanisms for use after discharge. Refer to outside services or agencies as appropriate (chaplain, social services, support group, home health). Include patient/family in decisions concerning care. Encourage patient/family to verbalize feelings about condition. Some patients have difficulty adjusting to the fact that they may hear their mechanical

Determine emotional impact and coping ability of patient and take appropriate measures to meet needs (provide frequent condition reports, repeat information, use easy to understand terminology, answer questions, allow to verbalize feelings).

Conduct a family needs assessment and employ measures to meet identified concerns.

valve "clicking." Provide support as needed. Refer to an open heart support group. If feasible, have a person with a mechanical valve visit the patient before surgery.

Address concerns patient may have about impact on daily life: ADLs, recreation, sexual functioning, return to work, and driving.

Vascular Emergencies
Interdisciplinary Outcome Pathway

COORDINATION OF CARE

Diagnosis/Stabilization Phase		Acute Management Phase		Recovery Phase	
Outcome	Interventions	Outcome	Interventions	Outcome	Interventions
All appropriate team members and disciplines will be involved in the plan of care.	Develop the plan of care with the patient/family, primary physician, vascular surgeon, cardiologist, RN, advanced practice nurse, perfusionist (if used), RCP, and other specialists as needed.	All appropriate team members and disciplines will be involved in the plan of care.	Initiate planning for anticipated discharge to home, SNF, or rehabilitation facility. Call home health if necessary. Begin teaching patient/family about care at home. Consult other disciplines (i.e., chaplain, social services) as needed. Initiate vascular rehabilitation program if available.	Patient will understand how to maintain optimal health at home, SNF, or rehabilitation facility.	Provide guidelines concerning care: • dietary restrictions • activity limitations • medications • follow-up visits • signs and symptoms of infection • when to call physician Provide patient/family with phone number of resources available to answer questions.

DIAGNOSTICS

Diagnosis/Stabilization Phase		Acute Management Phase		Recovery Phase	
Outcome	Interventions	Outcome	Interventions	Outcome	Interventions
Patient will understand any tests or procedures that need to be completed (VS, I & O, hemodynamic monitoring, angiography, echocardiography, Doppler studies, lab work, ultrasounds, CT scan, x-rays, MRI, EKG, transesophageal echocardiography).	Explain all tests and procedures to patient/family. Be sensitive to individualized needs of patient/family for information. Establish effective communication technique with intubated patient.	Patient will understand any tests or procedures that need to be completed (removal of indwelling lines and chest tubes, lab work, x-rays, IS).	Explain tests and procedures needed to assess and aid recovery. Be sensitive to individualized needs of patient/family for information. Anticipate need for further diagnostic tests such as ultrasound, angiography, or transesophageal echocardiography, and any intervention that may result.	Patient will understand meaning of diagnostic tests in relation to continued health (lab tests, increase in activity, IS).	Review with patient before discharge the results of all tests. Discuss any abnormal values and measures to help return to normal (i.e., hypercholesterolemia). Provide instructions on care after discharge: • when to call physician • care of incision(s) • activity limitations • risk factor modification (smoking, hypertension, diabetes, obesity, hypercholesterolemia) • vascular rehabilitation program Discuss medications with patient: name, dosage, how to take, potential side effects. Stress compliance with medical regimen.

FLUID BALANCE

Diagnosis/Stabilization Phase		Acute Management Phase		Recovery Phase	
Outcome	Interventions	Outcome	Interventions	Outcome	Interventions
Patient will achieve optimal hemodynamic status as evidenced by: • MAP > 70 mmHg • hemodynamic parameters WNL • UO > 0.5 mL/kg/hr • absence of dysrhythmias • adequate LOC • clear lung sounds • absence of JVD • normal CO	Monitor and treat hemodynamic parameters: • dysrhythmias • BP • PA pressures • PCWP • CO/CI • SVR/PVR • I & O • LOC Monitor lab values: electrolytes, Mg^{++}, Hgb, Hct, PT, PTT, ACT, platelets, CK, CK-MB, cardiac troponin. Assess for fluid overload or deficit and treat accordingly. Assess neurologic status q1h and PRN. If used, assess intracranial pressure q1h and PRN. Observe for signs of bleeding and administer blood products as needed. Assess response. Also monitor for signs of internal bleeding. Insert urinary catheter and monitor renal function. Monitor for evidence of tissue perfusion q1h. Check for: • pain • pulselessness • paresthesia • pallor • temperature Assess capillary refill time in seconds q1h. If appropriate, monitor heparin drip. Monitor clotting time with PTT and/or ACT. Administer fibrinolytic therapy as ordered and observe response. Assess response to vasopressor therapy and titrate as needed.	Patient will maintain optimal hemodynamic status.	Assess neurologic status q2–4h and PRN. If used, assess intracranial pressure q2–4h and PRN. Continue to assess for complications associated with vascular emergencies. Monitor and treat cardiac parameters. Monitor lab values. Weigh daily.	Patient will maintain optimal hemodynamic status.	Assess neurologic status q4–8h and PRN. Continue to monitor and treat hemodynamic parameters. Begin teaching patient/family signs and symptoms of inadequate tissue perfusion and when to seek medical attention (pain, numbness, discoloration, cool to touch, cyanosis).

Vascular Emergencies Interdisciplinary Outcome Pathway (continued)

FLUID BALANCE (continued)

Diagnosis/Stabilization Phase		Acute Management Phase		Recovery Phase	
Outcome	Interventions	Outcome	Interventions	Outcome	Interventions
	Monitor for signs of complications that can occur with vascular emergencies: • hypovolemic shock • aneurysm dissection • aortic dissection • embolism • thrombus formation • CVA • GI complications • cerebral hemorrhage • acute renal failure • colon ischemia • spinal cord ischemia • MI • infection • hypertension • aortic regurgitation • mesenteric infarction • compartment syndrome • heparin-induced thrombocytopenia • dysrhythmias • ileus • ARDS Assess heart and bowel sounds q4h and PRN.				

NUTRITION

Diagnosis/Stabilization Phase		Acute Management Phase		Recovery Phase	
Outcome	Interventions	Outcome	Interventions	Outcome	Interventions
Patient will be adequately nourished as evidenced by: • stable weight • weight not >10% below or 20% above IBW	NPO until extubation, if applicable. If extubation delayed >24h, initiate alternative nutritional therapy. Initiate clear liquids and monitor response.	Patient will be adequately nourished.	Assess bowel sounds, abdominal distension, abdominal pain and tenderness q4h and PRN. Continue alternative nutritional therapy as needed. Advance to DAT and monitor response.	Patient will be adequately nourished.	Teach patient/family about heart healthy diet: • total fat <30% of daily intake • total saturated fat <10% of daily intake

- albumin >3.5 g/dL
- total protein 6–8 g/dL
- total lymphocyte count 1,000–3,000
- cholesterol <200 mg/dL

Assess bowel sounds, abdominal distension, abdominal pain and tenderness q4h and PRN.
Monitor UO q1h with urinary catheter.
Monitor NG tube and record drainage.

Involve dietitian if:
- albumin <3.0
- unanticipated weight loss
- eating less than half of food on tray
- diet counseling needed for heart healthy diet

Monitor protein and albumin levels.
Assess patient for hypercholesterolemia and hyperlipidemia and begin assessment of patient's usual diet.
Remove urinary catheter as soon as possible.
Maintain NG tube to low intermittent suction until bowel sounds are present.

- total daily cholesterol intake <300 mg
- caloric restriction if needed
- sodium restriction if needed

Teach patient about dietary supplements (i.e., anitoxidants, oat bran, fiber, vitamins and minerals).

MOBILITY

Diagnosis/Stabilization Phase		Acute Management Phase		Recovery Phase	
Outcome	Interventions	Outcome	Interventions	Outcome	Interventions
Patient will achieve optimal mobility.	Turn at least q2h if hemodynamically stable and monitor response. If not stable, consider other methods to assist with mobility (i.e., lateral rotational therapy, air mattress). Begin passive/active-assist ROM exercises.	Patient will achieve optimal mobility.	PT to assess ambulation mobility, muscle strength, flexibility, and tone. OT to assess functional ability. PT/OT to help determine and direct activity goals. Progress exercise as tolerated: dangle, OOB TID to QID, and walking 50 feet. Monitor response to increased activity and decrease if adverse events occur (tachycardia, dysrhythmias, syncope, hypotension, hypertension, dyspnea, dizziness, and bleeding). Provide physical assistance or assistive devices as necessary.	Patient will achieve optimal mobility.	Continue to progress exercise as tolerated and monitor response. Walk at least 200–300 feet TID to QID. Assess ability to negotiate stairs if part of home environment. Decrease activity if adverse events occur. Refer to outpatient vascular rehabilitation program if feasible. If discharged to inpatient rehabilitation program or SNF, send copy of activity guidelines with patient.

Vascular Emergencies Interdisciplinary Outcome Pathway (continued)

OXYGENATION/VENTILATION

Diagnosis/Stabilization Phase		Acute Management Phase		Recovery Phase	
Outcome	Interventions	Outcome	Interventions	Outcome	Interventions
Patient will have adequate gas exchange as evidenced by: • SaO_2 >90% • SpO_2 >92% • ABGs WNL • clear breath sounds • respiratory rate, depth, and rhythm WNL • CXR WNL • absence of dyspnea, cyanosis, and secretions • Hgb and Hct WNL	Monitor ventilator settings and hemodynamic variables before, during, and after weaning. Wean ventilator and monitor patient response: • wean FIO_2 to keep SpO_2 >92% • monitor effects of anesthesia and wean ventilator accordingly • extubate as soon as possible Assess respiratory functioning, including lung sounds, respiratory muscle strength, respiratory rate and depth, coughing ability, and CXR. If not intubated, apply supplemental oxygen. Monitor with pulse oximetry to keep SpO_2 >92%. Assess evidence of tissue perfusion q1h (pain, pulselessness, paresthesia, pallor, temperature).	Patient will have adequate gas exchange.	Monitor and treat oxygenation/ventilation disturbances. Wean oxygen therapy and/or mechanical ventilation as tolerated. Apply supplemental oxygen to keep SpO_2 >92%. Monitor with pulse oximetry. Use chest splint pillow or abdominal splint pillow with coughing and deep breathing. Have the patient give a return demonstration. Teach patient use of IS. Have patient give return demonstration. Observe effect of increased activity on respiratory status. Observe for complications of vascular emergencies that may impair oxygenation/ventilation: aortic dissection, thrombus formation, tamponade, shock, embolism. If applicable, begin discussion on smoking cessation.	Patient will have adequate gas exchange.	Continue to monitor for oxygenation/ventilation disturbances. Obtain CXR before discharge. Reinforce instruction to patient/family on IS and use of chest/abdominal pillow at home. Continue discussion on smoking cessation. Refer to Smokers Anonymous or other available support groups.

COMFORT

Diagnosis/Stabilization Phase		Acute Management Phase		Recovery Phase	
Outcome	Interventions	Outcome	Interventions	Outcome	Interventions
Patient will be as comfortable and pain free as possible as evidenced by:	Assess quantity and quality of pain using a pain scale or visual analogue scale. Anticipate need for analgesia and provide as needed.	Patient will be as relaxed and pain free as possible.	Continue as in Diagnosis/Stabilization Phase. Provide chest or abdominal pillow, if indicated, and instruct patient on proper use during	Patient will be as relaxed and pain free as possible.	Progress analgesics to oral medications as needed and assess response. Use sedatives as indicated and assess response.

- no objective indicators of discomfort
- no complaints of discomfort

Administer narcotics (usually morphine) and monitor response.

If patient is intubated, establish effective communication technique with which patient can communicate discomfort and need for analgesics.

Provide a quiet environment to potentiate analgesia.

Provide reassurance in a calm, caring, and competent manner.

coughing and deep breathing. Have patient give a return demonstration.

Provide uninterrupted periods of rest.

Teach patient relaxation exercises.

Use touch therapy, humor, music therapy, and imagery to promote relaxation. Involve family in strategies.

Provide analgesics as needed before uncomfortable or painful procedures (i.e., removal of chest tubes).

Use sedatives as indicated.

Observe for complications of vascular emergencies that may cause discomfort: graft thrombosis, thromboembolism, MI, compartment syndrome.

Continue alternative methods to promote relaxation.

Teach patient/family alternative methods to promote relaxation at home.

SKIN INTEGRITY

Diagnosis/Stabilization Phase		Acute Management Phase		Recovery Phase	
Outcome	Interventions	Outcome	Interventions	Outcome	Interventions
Patient will have intact skin without abrasions or pressure ulcers. Patient will be afebrile and without objective signs of infection. Patient will have healing wounds.	Preop shower/scrub with antibacterial agent. Temperature q4h and more frequently if elevated. Begin passive/active-assist ROM exercises. Assess all bony prominences at least q4h and treat if indicated. Use preventive pressure-reducing devices if patient is at high risk for developing pressure ulcers. Treat pressure ulcers according to hospital protocol.	Patient will have intact skin without abrasions or pressure ulcers. Patient will be afebrile and without objective signs of infection. Patient will have healing wounds.	Temperature q4h unless elevated, then more frequently as needed. Keep surgical site covered for 24h; then open to air unless actively draining. Assess incision sites for signs and symptoms of infection q4h and PRN. Wash incision sites proximally to distally with sterile soap and water. Continue to assess all bony prominences at least q4h and treat if indicated. Assess skin adjacent to surgical wounds for symptoms of tape burns, allergies.	Patient will have intact skin without abrasions or pressure ulcers. Patient will be afebrile and without objective signs of infection. Patient will have healing wounds.	Assess all bony prominences at least q4h and treat if needed. Assess and cleanse incisions as described earlier. Teach patient/family proper skin care at home: • foot care • care of incision • appropriately fitting shoes and garments • diet • avoidance of tape and restricting garments Provide information concerning wound infection as needed and when to call the physician.

Vascular Emergencies Interdisciplinary Outcome Pathway *(continued)*

SKIN INTEGRITY (continued)

Diagnosis/Stabilization Phase		Acute Management Phase		Recovery Phase	
Outcome	Interventions	Outcome	Interventions	Outcome	Interventions
			Take measures to protect any ischemic limb: • do not elevate the involved limb • bed cradle • lamb's wool • eggcrate mattress • no application of heat or cold		

PROTECTION/SAFETY

Diagnosis/Stabilization Phase		Acute Management Phase		Recovery Phase	
Outcome	Interventions	Outcome	Interventions	Outcome	Interventions
Patient will be protected from possible harm.	Assess need for wrist restraints if patient is intubated, has a decreased LOC, or is agitated and restless. Explain need for restraints to patient/family. Check q1–2h for skin integrity and impairment to circulation. Follow hospital protocol for use of restraints. Remove as soon as patient is able to follow instructions. Provide sedatives as needed.	Patient will be protected from possible harm.	If need still exists for restraints, check q1–2h for skin integrity and impairment to circulation. Provide support when dangling, getting OOB, and ambulating. Monitor response. Consider OT to teach correct movement and appropriate functional skills to prevent joint stress, strain, or injury. Use gait belt as indicated for ambulation.	Patient will be protected from possible harm.	Teach patient/family about any physical limitations in activity after discharge.

PSYCHOSOCIAL/SELF-DETERMINATION

Diagnosis/Stabilization Phase		Acute Management Phase		Recovery Phase	
Outcome	Interventions	Outcome	Interventions	Outcome	Interventions
Patient will achieve psychophysiologic stability. Patient will demonstrate a decrease in anxiety as evidenced by: • VS WNL • subjective report of decreased anxiety • objective signs of decreased anxiety	Assess physiologic effects of critical care environment on patient (hemodynamic variables, psychological status, signs of increased sympathetic response). Provide sedatives as indicated. Take measures to reduce sensory overload. Develop effective communication technique with intubated patient. Use calm, caring, and competent approach when providing care. Assess patient/family's ability to cope and provide appropriate measures (i.e., explain condition and equipment, provide frequent condition reports, use easy to understand terminology, repeat information as needed, flexible visitation, answer all questions). Pay particular attention to the patient who reports a feeling of impending doom.	Patient will achieve psychophysiologic stability. Patient will demonstrate a decrease in anxiety.	Continue as in Diagnosis/Stabilization Phase. Provide adequate rest periods. Continue to include family in all aspects of care. Continue to assess coping ability of patient/family and take measures as indicated. Maintain quiet environment. Start teaching risk factor modification. Discuss how surgery may impact patient's quality of life.	Patient will achieve psychophysiologic stability. Patient will demonstrate a decrease in anxiety.	Provide instruction on coping mechanisms after discharge. Refer to outside services or agencies as appropriate (chaplain, social services, home health). Continue teaching risk factor modification. Address concerns patient may have about impact on daily life: ADLs, recreation, sexual functioning, return to work, and driving.

CHAPTER 2

Pulmonary Pathways

Acute Respiratory Failure Interdisciplinary Outcome Pathway

COORDINATION OF CARE

Diagnosis/Stabilization Phase		Acute Management Phase		Recovery Phase	
Outcome	Interventions	Outcome	Interventions	Outcome	Interventions
All appropriate team members and disciplines will be involved in the plan of care.	Develop the plan of care with patient, family, primary physician, pulmonologist, intensivist, RN, advanced practice nurse, RCP, PT, OT, dietitian, and social services.	All appropriate team members and disciplines will be involved in the plan of care.	Update the plan of care with other team members, pulmonary care practitioners, and discharge planners. Begin home care teaching with patient and family. Consult pulmonary rehabilitation if indicated.	Patient will understand how to maintain optimal health at home.	Teach patient/family about need for follow-up health care visits. Coordinate home care with continuing care agency. Involve home care company for home equipment if needed. Provide guidelines concerning continuing care to patient/family. Provide patient/family with phone numbers of resources available to answer questions.

DIAGNOSTICS

Diagnosis/Stabilization Phase		Acute Management Phase		Recovery Phase	
Outcome	Interventions	Outcome	Interventions	Outcome	Interventions
Patient will understand tests and procedures that must be completed (VS, I & O, hemodynamic monitoring, intubation, mechanical ventilation, suctioning, lab work, EKG).	Explain all procedures and tests to patient/family. Be sensitive to patient and family's individualized needs for information. Establish effective communication technique with intubated patient.	Patient will understand tests and procedures that are needed (removal of ET tube, lab work, CXR, O_2 therapy, ABGs).	Explain procedures and tests needed to assess respiratory ability such as respiratory mechanics and PFTs.	Patient will understand tests and procedures that are needed (lab work, CXR, ABGs).	Review with patient/family before discharge results of tests and how the patient's baseline values compare to normal (ABGs, PFTs). Make sure patient has a copy of test results, which may be significant to continuing health care. Provide patient with guidelines concerning follow-up care.

FLUID BALANCE

Diagnosis/Stabilization Phase		Acute Management Phase		Recovery Phase	
Outcome	Interventions	Outcome	Interventions	Outcome	Interventions
Patient will achieve optimal hemodynamic status as evidenced by: • MAP > 70 mmHg • normal hemodynamic parameters • free from dysrhythmias • optimal hydration	Monitor and treat hemodynamic parameters: • BP • CO/CI • SV/SI • SVR/PVR • PA pressures • PCWP • CVP • SvO$_2$ • O$_2$ delivery • O$_2$ consumption Monitor lab values: electrolytes, ABGs, CBC. Monitor and treat dysrhythmias. Assess weight changes from daily weights. Determine hydration needs based on hemodynamics, I & O, viscosity of pulmonary secretions, VS, SaO$_2$, CXR, and electrolytes.	Patient will maintain optimal hemodynamic status.	Continue as in Diagnosis/Stabilization Phase. Maintain optimal hydration based on continued assessment.	Patient will maintain optimal hemodynamic status.	Teach patient/family: • patient's optimal fluid balance and how to maintain it • signs and symptoms of fluid overload and dehydration • importance of daily weights • importance of reporting any changes to physician • home medications

NUTRITION

Diagnosis/Stabilization Phase		Acute Management Phase		Recovery Phase	
Outcome	Interventions	Outcome	Interventions	Outcome	Interventions
Patient will be adequately nourished as evidenced by: • stable body weight not >10% below or >20% above IBW • albumin >3.5 g/dL • total protein 6–8 g/dL • total lymphocyte count 1,000–3,000	Assess nutritional status. Consult dietitian to determine and direct nutritional support. Monitor albumin, prealbumin, total protein, cholesterol, triglycerides, and lymphocyte count. If extubation delayed > 24h, initiate enteral nutrition.	Patient will be adequately nourished. Patient will be free of bowel and elimination problems.	Dietary consult if: • eating less than half of food on tray • albumin <3.0 • unanticipated weight loss Determine patient's resting energy expenditure. Estimate caloric need and type of intake required. Consider calorie count to ascertain if patient is meeting nutritional need. Monitor response to diet. Avoid high carbohydrate load in patients who retain CO$_2$.	Patient will be adequately nourished.	Assess effectiveness of patient/family teaching that began in Acute Management Phase. Reinforce information as needed. Consider dietitian follow-up after discharge.

Acute Respiratory Failure Interdisciplinary Outcome Pathway (continued)

NUTRITION (continued)

Diagnosis/Stabilization Phase		Acute Management Phase		Recovery Phase	
Outcome	Interventions	Outcome	Interventions	Outcome	Interventions
			Treat diarrhea, constipation, or ileus if needed. Teach patient/family about: • food pyramid and suggested servings per day • daily caloric requirements • safe weight-reducing or weight-gaining techniques if needed		

MOBILITY

Diagnosis/Stabilization Phase		Acute Management Phase		Recovery Phase	
Outcome	Interventions	Outcome	Interventions	Outcome	Interventions
Patient will achieve optimal mobility.	Consult PT to assess mobility, ambulation, flexibility, strength, and muscle tone. Consult OT to assess functional ability. Begin passive/active-assist ROM exercises.	Patient will achieve optimal mobility.	Assess physical limitations of mobility. Continue PT and/or OT for specific mobility limitations. Develop progressive activity program. Monitor response to activity and decrease if tachycardia, dyspnea, ectopy, syncope, or hypotension occurs. Provide physical support as necessary. Space activities to allow adequate rest periods. Consider assistive devices as needed.	Patient will achieve optimal mobility.	Continue PT/OT in home if needed. Assist patient in developing realistic goals for home exercise program. Determine a gradual increasing program of aerobic activity such as walking, swimming, water aerobics, treadmill, or exercise bicycle. Refer to outpatient pulmonary rehabilitation program if indicated. Have patient demonstrate proper use of assistive devices.

OXYGENATION/VENTILATION

Diagnosis/Stabilization Phase		Acute Management Phase		Recovery Phase	
Outcome	Interventions	Outcome	Interventions	Outcome	Interventions
Patient will have a patent airway and optimal ventilation as evidenced by: • normal CXR • respiratory rate, depth, and rhythm WNL • clear breath sounds bilaterally • SaO$_2$ > 90% • SpO$_2$ > 92% • ABGs, VS, mental status, and PFTs WNL for the patient • demonstrated ability to cough and clear secretions Patient will exhibit optimal gas exchange and tissue perfusion as evidenced by: • ABGs, VS, and mental status WNL for patient • normal Hgb • normal intrapulmonary shunting • UO > 0.5 mL/kg/hr • normal liver enzymes	Monitor breath sounds, respiratory pattern, SpO$_2$ q1h and PRN. Be prepared for intubation and mechanical ventilation. Involve RCP. Monitor quantity, color, and consistency of secretions. Monitor for signs and symptoms of respiratory distress: • weak ineffective cough • SOB, dyspnea • use of accessory muscles • adventitious breath sounds • alterations in LOC • PCO$_2$ > 50 mmHg or above normal for patient • SaO$_2$ < 90% • SpO$_2$ < 92% Monitor patients at high risk of inadequate ventilation (postop, on narcotics or sedation, anxious or in pain, CNS or metabolic disorders). Assist with placement and maintenance of artificial airway if needed. Maintain adequate humidification. Assist with monitoring or adjusting of ventilator settings to obtain appropriate level of assistance and minute ventilation. Assist in correction of underlying disorder. Provide chest physiotherapy as needed. Administer bronchodilators as indicated. Monitor patient for signs and symptoms of altered gas exchange: • dyspnea • restlessness • confusion	Patient will have a patent airway and optimal ventilation. Patient will exhibit optimal gas exchange and normal tissue perfusion.	Continue as in Diagnosis/Stabilization Phase. As patient improves, change aminophylline to oral agent and monitor response. Assess readiness to wean. Continue to involve RCP. Measure respiratory mechanics: MV, NIF, respiratory rate, TV, VC. Assess hemodynamic stability and factors that increase metabolic demand (fever, increased WBCs, bacteremia, sepsis, systemic inflammatory syndrome, hypo/hyperthyroidism). Monitor electrolytes including calcium, magnesium, and phosphate. Assess for improvement in breath sounds, thin white secretions, and adequate cough reflexes. Monitor ventilatory status and hemodynamic variables prior to, during, and after weaning from mechanical ventilation. Assist with extubation. Teach patient effective cough techniques such as cascade coughing. Have patient give return demonstration. Wean oxygen therapy as gas exchange improves. Begin patient/family teaching on the pulmonary system, current pulmonary problems, current treatment, and expected clinical course. Begin discussion of smoking cessation if appropriate.	Patient will have optimal ventilation and gas exchange.	Teach patient about home medications and treatments. Include the proper way to use metered dose inhalers with and without a spacer device. Teach patient/family signs and symptoms of respiratory infection and when to report symptoms. Refer to outpatient pulmonary rehabilitation program if indicated. Remind patient/family that energy may be low and susceptibility to other respiratory infections may be high for 2–3 months. Continue discussion of smoking cessation if appropriate. Consider need for RCP follow-up after discharge.

Acute Respiratory Failure Interdisciplinary Outcome Pathway (continued)

OXYGENATION/VENTILATION (continued)

Diagnosis/Stabilization Phase		Acute Management Phase		Recovery Phase	
Outcome	Interventions	Outcome	Interventions	Outcome	Interventions
	• HA				
	• central cyanosis (not peripheral)				
	• PaO_2 <50 mmHg on room air				
	• PaO_2/PAO_2 ratio <0.60				
	• PCO_2 >50 mmHg				
	• SaO_2 <90%				
	• SpO_2 <92%				
	• use of accessory muscles				
	• dysrhythmias				
	• hypotension				
	Administer oxygen therapy as needed to maintain SpO_2 >92%.				
	Assess intrapulmonary shunting by one of the following:				
	• classic shunt equation				
	• PaO_2/PAO_2 ratio				
	• PaO_2/FIO_2 ratio				
	• a-A gradient				
	Improve V/Q mismatch and shunt by:				
	• determining optimal PEEP and monitoring response to PEEP				
	• suctioning as needed				
	• chest physiotherapy				
	Optimize oxygen delivery by monitoring and treating CO, BP, HR, SaO_2, SvO_2, Hgb, and PaO_2.				
	Assess for evidence of adequate tissue perfusion in all organ systems (normal BP, LOC, UO, liver enzymes).				
	Monitor and treat complications: hypoxemia, hypercapnia, acid-base disturbances, HA, restlessness, tachycardia, and hypertension.				

COMFORT

Diagnosis/Stabilization Phase		Acute Management Phase		Recovery Phase	
Outcome	Interventions	Outcome	Interventions	Outcome	Interventions
Patient will be as comfortable and pain free as possible as evidenced by: • no objective indicators of discomfort • no complaints of discomfort	Plan interventions to provide optimal rest periods. Assess quantity and quality of discomfort. Administer analgesics when indicated. Provide reassurance in a calm, caring, and competent manner. Keep lights dim and a quiet environment to minimize catecholamine response. Keep HOB elevated to enhance breathing comfort. If intubated, establish effective communication techniques. Observe for complications of acute respiratory failure that can cause discomfort: dyspnea, SOB, bronchospasm.	Patient will be as comfortable and pain free as possible.	Teach patient relaxation techniques. Have patient give return demonstration. Consult PT/OT as needed. Use complementary therapies such as guided imagery, music, humor, or touch therapy to enhance patient comfort. Involve family in strategies.	Patient will be as comfortable and pain free as possible.	Instruct patient/family on alternative methods to promote relaxation after discharge.

SKIN INTEGRITY

Diagnosis/Stabilization Phase		Acute Management Phase		Recovery Phase	
Outcome	Interventions	Outcome	Interventions	Outcome	Interventions
Patient will have intact skin without abrasions or pressure ulcers.	Assess all bony prominences q4h. Use preventive pressure-reducing devices when patient is at high risk for developing pressure ulcers. Treat pressure ulcers according to hospital protocol.	Patient will have intact skin without abrasions or pressure ulcers.	Continue as in Diagnosis/Stabilization Phase.	Patient will have intact skin without abrasions or pressure ulcers.	Instruct patient/family on proper skin care interventions to be continued at home.

Acute Respiratory Failure Interdisciplinary Outcome Pathway (continued)

PROTECTION/SAFETY

Diagnosis/Stabilization Phase		Acute Management Phase		Recovery Phase	
Outcome	Interventions	Outcome	Interventions	Outcome	Interventions
Patient will be protected from possible harm.	Assess need for wrist restraints if patient is intubated. Balance the need to protect patient from dislodgement of ET with additional fear and anxiety that might be caused by restraints. Use sedatives as indicated (preferably short acting and/or those that have the least effect on respiratory drive). Allow family to remain with patient if they have a calming influence and can promote rest and safety.	Patient will be protected from possible harm.	Give appropriate physical support as patient increases mobility to prevent falls or injury. Consider use of assistive devices as needed.	Patient will be protected from possible harm.	Review with patient/family any physical limitations in activity before discharge home. Consult PT and/or OT for home follow-up if limitations are present.

PSYCHOSOCIAL/SELF-DETERMINATION

Diagnosis/Stabilization Phase		Acute Management Phase		Recovery Phase	
Outcome	Interventions	Outcome	Interventions	Outcome	Interventions
Patient will achieve psychophysiologic stability. Patient will demonstrate a decreased level of anxiety as evidenced by: • VS WNL • mental status WNL • patient reports feeling less anxious	Assess physiologic effect of environment on patient. Assess patient for appropriate level of stress. Assess personal responses (affective, feelings) of patient regarding critical illness. Observe patient's patterns of thinking and communicating. Use calm, competent, reassuring approach to all interventions. Take measures to reduce sensory overload such as providing uninterrupted periods of rest. Allow flexible visitation to meet the psychosocial needs of patient and family.	Patient will achieve psychophysiologic stability. Patient will demonstrate a decreased level of anxiety.	Continue as in Diagnosis/Stabilization Phase. Provide adequate rest periods. Continue to assess coping ability of patient and family. Take appropriate measures to assist patient and family in developing appropriate coping mechanisms. Include patient/family in all health care decisions.	Patient will achieve psychophysiologic stability. Patient will demonstrate a decreased level of anxiety.	Continue as in Acute Management Phase. Provide information on appropriate coping mechanisms for use after discharge. Address concerns patient may have about impact on life: ADLs, return to work, sexual functioning, recreation.

Adult Respiratory Distress Syndrome Interdisciplinary Outcome Pathway

COORDINATION OF CARE

Diagnosis/Stabilization Phase		Acute Management Phase		Recovery Phase	
Outcome	Interventions	Outcome	Interventions	Outcome	Interventions
All appropriate team members and disciplines will be involved in the plan of care.	Develop the plan of care with the patient, family, primary physician, pulmonologist, intensivist, other specialists as needed, RN, advanced practice nurse, RCP, dietitian, and chaplain.	All appropriate team members and disciplines will be involved in the plan of care.	Update the plan of care with patient, family, OT, PT, social services, discharge planner, and home health agency. Initiate planning for anticipated discharge.	Patient/family will understand how to maintain optimal health at home.	Provide guidelines concerning follow-up care to patient and family. Provide patient/family with phone numbers of resources available to answer questions.

DIAGNOSTICS

Diagnosis/Stabilization Phase		Acute Management Phase		Recovery Phase	
Outcome	Interventions	Outcome	Interventions	Outcome	Interventions
Patient/family will understand any tests or procedures that must be completed (VS, I & O, hemodynamic monitoring, x-rays, lab work, ABGs, EKG, cardiac monitoring, mechanical ventilation, PEEP, pulse oximetry, investigational treatments for ARDS).	Explain all procedures and tests to patient/family. Be sensitive to individualized needs of patient/family for information.	Patient/family will understand any tests or procedures that must be completed.	Explain procedures and tests necessary to assess progress and recovery of ARDS to patient/family. Anticipate need for further procedures such as ECMO, IVOX, extracorporeal CO_2 removal.	Patient/family will understand meaning of diagnostic tests in relation to continued health.	Review with patient/family results of tests prior to discharge (such as ABGs, PFTs). Discuss any abnormal findings and appropriate measures patient/family can take to return to normal if possible. Provide patient/family with guidelines concerning follow-up and/or home care: • when to call physician • physical restrictions • skin care • medications

Adult Respiratory Distress Syndrome Interdisciplinary Outcome Pathway (*continued*)

FLUID BALANCE

Diagnosis/Stabilization Phase		Acute Management Phase		Recovery Phase	
Outcome	Interventions	Outcome	Interventions	Outcome	Interventions
Patient will achieve optimal hemody-namic status as evi-denced by: • MAP > 70 mmHg • normal hemody-namic parame-ters • free from dys-rhythmias • optimal hydra-tion • adequate perfu-sion to vital organs	Monitor and treat hemodynamic parameters: • BP • CO/CI • PA pressures • PCWP • CVP • SVR/PVR • SvO_2 Note especially increases in pul-monary vascular resistance, widening of the PA diastolic and PCWP gradient, and changes in SvO_2 (may be nor-mal to elevated in sepsis, low in oxygen transport distur-bances). Monitor lab values: electrolytes, ABGs, CBC with differential, platelets, factor VIII, antithrombin III, and DIC pro-file (PT, PTT, thrombin time, fibrinogen level, FDP). Monitor and treat dysrhythmias. Monitor and treat predisposing conditions commonly associ-ated with ARDS: • sepsis • systemic inflammatory response syndrome (SIRS) • shock • trauma • drug overdose • pneumonias • multiple blood transfusions • anemia • thrombocytopenia • DIC • embolism (fat, amniotic fluid, thrombotic, or air)	Patient will maintain optimal hemody-namic status.	Continue as in Diagnosis/Stabi-lization Phase. Monitor and treat hemodynamic parameters. Maintain optimal fluid therapy based on cardiopulmonary assessment and daily weight.	Patient will maintain optimal hemody-namic status.	Continue as in Diagnosis/Stabi-lization and Acute Manage-ment phases. Teach patient/family: • home medication regimen • signs and symptoms of fluid overload • what to report to physician

• hemorrhagic pancreatitis
• cardiopulmonary bypass
• burns
• smoke inhalation
• toxemia in pregnancy
• aspiration
• oxygen toxicity
• near drowning

Monitor and treat complications of ARDS such as right-sided heart failure occurring from excessive PA pressures.

Administer fluid therapy to maintain adequate cardiac performance (based on hemodynamics WNL and SvO_2 of 60–75). Other complications of ARDS include renal failure, fluid retention, gastrointestinal bleeding, ileus, liver failure, and neurologic/endocrine disorders.

Administer vasodilators and inotropic agents as indicated and monitor response.

Assess weight changes from baseline and weigh daily. Assess need for diuretics based on weight increases, CXR, or increased dependent crackles in lung sounds.

NUTRITION

Diagnosis/Stabilization Phase		Acute Management Phase		Recovery Phase	
Outcome	Interventions	Outcome	Interventions	Outcome	Interventions
Patient will be adequately nourished as evidenced by: • stable body weight not >10% below or >20% above IBW • albumin >3.5 g/dL	Assess nutritional status. Monitor albumin, prealbumin, total protein, and lymphocyte count. Consult dietitian to determine and direct nutritional support.	Patient will be adequately nourished.	Continue as in Diagnosis/Stabilization Phase. Estimate caloric need. Assess caloric count to determine if patient is meeting nutritional goals. Continue DAT and monitor response. Dietary needs will change as patient condition changes.	Patient will be adequately nourished.	Continue as in Diagnosis/Stabilization and Acute Management phases. Teach patient/family: • food pyramid and suggested servings per day • daily caloric intake needed • safe weight-reducing or weight-gaining techniques as indicated

Adult Respiratory Distress Syndrome Interdisciplinary Outcome Pathway *(continued)*

NUTRITION *(continued)*

Diagnosis/Stabilization Phase		Acute Management Phase		Recovery Phase	
Outcome	Interventions	Outcome	Interventions	Outcome	Interventions
• total protein 6–8 g • total lymphocyte count 1,000–3,000	Anticipate increased protein/calorie needs without excessive carbohydrates. In undernourished patients, pulmonary defense mechanisms become impaired, including an altered ventilatory response to hypoxemia. Initially NPO. Advance DAT and monitor response. Patient may receive enteral or parenteral nutrition. If extubation delayed > 24h, initiate alternate nutritional therapy. Maintain a positive protein balance.		Assess bowel sounds and tenderness q4h and PRN.		

MOBILITY

Diagnosis/Stabilization Phase		Acute Management Phase		Recovery Phase	
Outcome	Interventions	Outcome	Interventions	Outcome	Interventions
Patient will achieve optimal mobility.	Consult PT to assess degree of mobility, ambulation, flexibility, strength, and muscle tone. Consult OT to assess functional ability. Begin passive/active-assist ROM exercises. Bed rest if hemodynamically unstable.	Patient will achieve optimal mobility.	Continue as in Diagnosis/Stabilization Phase. Continue PT/OT for specific mobility or functional ability limitations. Monitor response to increased activity. Decrease activity if adverse events occur (tachycardia, discomfort, dyspnea, or hypo/hypertension). Provide physical support as necessary.	Patient will achieve optimal mobility.	Teach patient/family home exercise program. Have patient demonstrate proper use of assistive devices. Consider need for OT/PT follow-up after discharge.

OXYGENATION/VENTILATION

Diagnosis/Stabilization Phase		Acute Management Phase		Recovery Phase	
Outcome	Interventions	Outcome	Interventions	Outcome	Interventions
Patient will have adequate ventilation, gas exchange, and tissue perfusion as evidenced by: • ABGs, pulse oximetry, VS WNL for the patient • respiratory rate, depth, and rhythm WNL for the patient • normal intrapulmonary shunting • UO > 0.5 mL/kg/hr • normal liver enzymes • mental status normal • ability to cough and clear secretions	Constantly monitor respiratory rate, depth, pattern, pulse oximetry, ABGs, lung sounds, and CXR. Be prepared for intubation and mechanical ventilation. Involve RCP. Assist with monitoring and adjusting of ventilator settings to maintain appropriate level of assistance and minute ventilation. Monitor peak airway pressures and pulmonary compliance to assess patient's progress. Monitor patient for signs and symptoms of altered gas exchange: • dyspnea • increased work of breathing • restlessness • confusion • tachypnea • apprehension • headache • central cyanosis (not peripheral) • refractory hypoxemia (PaO_2 < 60 mmHg with an FIO_2 > 0.50) • PaO_2/PAO_2 ratio < 0.25 Qs/Qt > 20%	Patient will have adequate ventilation, gas exchange, and tissue perfusion.	Continue to monitor patient's response to mechanical ventilation. Assess readiness to wean: 1. Measure respiratory mechanics: • minute ventilation (VE) • NIF • respiratory rate • TV • VC 2. Assess hemodynamic stability and factors that increase metabolic demand: • fever • increased WBC count • bacteremia • sepsis or SIRS • thyroid dysfunction 3. Monitor electrolytes including Ca^{++}, Mg^{++}, and PO_4^{+++}. 4. Assess for improvement in breath sounds. Monitor ventilatory/oxygenation status and hemodynamic variables before, during, and after weaning patient from mechanical ventilation. Involve RCP as needed.	Patient will have adequate ventilation, gas exchange, and tissue perfusion.	Continue patient/family teaching. Assess understanding and reinforce as needed. Teach patient: • home medications • signs and symptoms of respiratory distress • when to contact physician • how to avoid respiratory infections • measures to assist with smoking cessation Refer to outpatient pulmonary rehabilitation program when indicated. Consider RCP follow-up after discharge.
	Space activities to allow adequate rest periods. Provide assistive devices as necessary. Allow patient to assist in ADLs as tolerated. Instruct on proper breathing technique with activity. Involve RCP as needed.				

Adult Respiratory Distress Syndrome Interdisciplinary Outcome Pathway (continued)

OXYGENATION/VENTILATION (continued)

Diagnosis/Stabilization Phase		Acute Management Phase		Recovery Phase	
Outcome	Interventions	Outcome	Interventions	Outcome	Interventions
	• PCO_2 > 50 mmHg • SaO_2 < 0.90 • use of accessory muscles • dysrhythmias • hypotension Assess intrapulmonary shunting by one of the following: • classical shunt equation • PaO_2/PAO_2 ratio (normal is > 0.60. Many times with ARDS, the a/A ratio is < 0.25.) • PaO_2/FIO_2 ratio Administer oxygen therapy as ordered when intrapulmonary shunt present. Utilize lowest FIO_2 to attain adequate arterial blood oxygen content level. Assist in determining optimal level of PEEP and monitor response (improve V/Q matching yet not compromise alveolar expansion and/or CO). Assess hemodynamic parameters with any change in PEEP therapy. Consider use of continuous lateral rotational therapy if severe intrapulmonary shunt present (Qs/Qt > 30% and/or PaO_2/PAO_2 ratio < 0.25). Optimize O_2 delivery by monitoring and treating CO, BP, HR, SaO_2, SvO_2, Hgb, PaO_2, DO_2, VO_2, and O_2 extraction ratio. Assess for adequate tissue perfusion in all organ systems (normal BP, LOC, UO, liver enzymes). Monitor and treat complications of ARDS that can affect oxygenation/ventilation: • bronchoconstriction • interstitial edema		Assist with extubating patient from mechanical ventilation. Wean O_2 therapy as gas exchange improves. Monitor with pulse oximetry. Provide supplemental oxygen to keep SpO_2 > 92%. Consider positioning of patient to enhance gas exchange (i.e., good lung dependent if unilateral lung disease or prone position if bilateral lung involvement). Begin teaching on the pulmonary system, current pulmonary problems, current treatment, and expected clinical course. Start discussion on smoking cessation if appropriate.		

- decreased pulmonary compliance
- atelectasis
- dysrhythmias
- pulmonary microemboli
- barotrauma (pneumomediastinum, pneumothorax, subcutaneous emphysema)
- decreased CO
- increased PVR
- oxygen toxicity
- pulmonary fibrosis

Monitor CXR closely (diffuse bilateral interstitial and alveolar infiltrates seen early and later fibrotic changes seen).

Administer medications as ordered: antibiotics, NSAIDs (inhibit thromboxane production), prostacyclins (PGE_1) (oppose thromboxane action).

Maintain adequate humidification.

COMFORT

Diagnosis/Stabilization Phase		Acute Management Phase		Recovery Phase	
Outcome	Interventions	Outcome	Interventions	Outcome	Interventions
Patient will be as relaxed and pain free as possible as evidenced by: • no objective indicators of discomfort • no complaints of discomfort	Plan interventions to provide optimal rest periods. Assess quantity and quality of discomfort. Use a pain scale. Provide reassurance in a calm, caring, and competent manner. Keep lights dim and maintain a quiet environment to minimize catecholamine responses. While patient is intubated, establish effective communication technique so patient can communicate. Observe for complications of ARDS that can cause discomfort: dyspnea, breathlessness, bronchospasm. Implement nursing measures to decrease pain, anxiety, and shivering related to fever.	Patient will be as comfortable as possible.	Teach patient relaxation techniques. Have patient give return demonstration. Consult OT/PT as necessary. Use complementary therapies such as guided imagery, music, humor, or touch therapy to enhance patient's comfort. Involve family in strategies. Consider use of assistive devices as appropriate.	Patient will be as comfortable as possible.	Patient will demonstrate relaxation techniques to use at home. Patient will demonstrate proper use of assistive devices if needed. Consider need for PT/OT follow-up after discharge.

Adult Respiratory Distress Syndrome Interdisciplinary Outcome Pathway (continued)

SKIN INTEGRITY

Diagnosis/Stabilization Phase		Acute Management Phase		Recovery Phase	
Outcome	Interventions	Outcome	Interventions	Outcome	Interventions
Patient will have intact skin without abrasions or pressure ulcers.	Assess all bony prominences q4h. Use preventive pressure-reducing devices when patient is at high risk for developing pressure ulcers (based on scoring tool such as Gosnell). Treat pressure ulcers according to hospital protocol.	Patient will have intact skin without abrasions or pressure ulcers.	Continue as in Diagnosis/Stabilization Phase.	Patient will have intact skin without abrasions or pressure ulcers.	Teach patient/family proper skin care after discharge.

PROTECTION/SAFETY

Diagnosis/Stabilization Phase		Acute Management Phase		Recovery Phase	
Outcome	Interventions	Outcome	Interventions	Outcome	Interventions
Patient will be protected from possible harm.	Assess need for assistance with activities. Provide physical support as needed. Assess need for restraints if patient is intubated, has a decreased LOC, or is agitated and restless. Explain need for restraints to patient/family. Assess response to restraints when used and check q1h for skin integrity and impairment to circulation. Follow hospital protocol for use of restraints. Provide sedatives as needed and monitor response, especially to respiratory system. Monitor pulmonary effects of PEEP and high FIO_2 closely to minimize further pulmonary insults.	Patient will be protected from possible harm.	If need still exists for restraints, check q1–2h for skin integrity and impairment to circulation. Provide physical support when activity increases. Monitor response to activity. Consider use of assistive devices as needed.	Patient will be protected from possible harm.	Review with patient and family any physical limitations in activity before discharge home. Consult PT or OT for home follow-up if limitations present.

Monitor peak airway pressures and make ventilatory adjustments to minimize risk of barotrauma.

Allow family to remain with patient if they have a calming influence and can promote rest and safety.

PSYCHOSOCIAL/SELF-DETERMINATION

Diagnosis/Stabilization Phase		Acute Management Phase		Recovery Phase	
Outcome	Interventions	Outcome	Interventions	Outcome	Interventions
Patient will achieve psychophysiologic stability. Patient will demonstrate a decrease in anxiety as evidenced by: • VS WNL for the patient • subjective report of decreased anxiety • objective report of decreased anxiety	Assess physiologic effects of critical care environment on patient (i.e., hemodynamic variables, psychological status, signs of increased sympathetic response). Assess patient for appropriate level of stress. Assess personal responses (affective and/or feelings) of patient/family regarding critical illness. Take measures to reduce sensory overload. When patient is intubated, develop effective communication techniques. If unresponsive, use tactile and verbal stimuli. Use calm, caring, competent, and reassuring approach with patient/family. Allow flexible visitation to meet the needs of patient and family. Administer anxiolytics if indicated and monitor response. Involve patient/family care partner in health care decisions. Determine coping ability of patient/family and take measures to help patient cope (allow verbalization of concerns and fears, provide frequent explanations, hold family conferences, consult support services, etc.).	Patient will achieve psychophysiologic stability. Patient will demonstrate a decrease in anxiety.	Continue as in Diagnosis/Stabilization Phase. Instruct patient/family on alternative methods to promote relaxation: guided imagery, massage, humor, and deep breathing. Have patient/family give return demonstration of these techniques.	Patient will achieve psychophysiologic stability. Patient will demonstrate a decrease in anxiety.	Continue as in Diagnosis/Stabilization Phase. Continue to encourage alternative methods to promote relaxation. Address concerns patient may have about effect of ARDS on life: ADLs, return to work, sexual functioning, recreation.

Asthma
Interdisciplinary Outcome Pathway

COORDINATION OF CARE

Diagnosis/Stabilization Phase		Acute Management Phase		Recovery Phase	
Outcome	Interventions	Outcome	Interventions	Outcome	Interventions
All appropriate team members and disciplines will be involved in the plan of care.	Develop the plan of care with the patient/family, primary physician, pulmonologist, intensivist, RN, advanced practice nurse, and RCP.	All appropriate team members and disciplines will be involved in the plan of care.	Update the plan of care with other team members and discharge planners (i.e., RCP, OT, dietitian, social services). Consult asthma/allergy specialist if indicated. Encourage patient to become an active participant in plan of care. Begin home care teaching with patient and family. Consult pulmonary rehabilitation if indicated.	Patient will understand how to maintain optimal health at home.	Teach patient/family about need for follow-up health care visits. Involve home care company for home equipment if needed. Provide guidelines concerning continued care to patient/family. Provide patient/family with phone number of resources available to answer questions. Refer to outpatient pulmonary rehabilitation program if indicated. Refer to asthma support group if available. Emphasize to the patient/family that they play a very significant role in the day-to-day management of asthma. The patient must become an active partner with the health care providers in an effort to control his or her asthma. Teach patient self-care measures for asthma: • avoidance of triggers • monitoring of peak flow • proper use of medications • proper use of inhalers with and without spacer device • pursed-lip breathing • recognition of signs of impending attack • relaxation techniques • importance of follow-up visits • exercise program

- seek early treatment for colds, sinus infections, and coughs (especially nocturnal)
- dietary restrictions, if any
- actions to take for acute episodes

DIAGNOSTICS

Diagnosis/Stabilization Phase		Acute Management Phase		Recovery Phase	
Outcome	Interventions	Outcome	Interventions	Outcome	Interventions
Patient will understand tests and procedures that are needed (CXR, monitoring, SpO_2, sputum culture, lab work, peak flow).	Explain all procedures and tests to patient. Be sensitive to patient and family's individualized needs for information.	Patient will understand tests and procedures that are needed (PFTs, x-rays, nasal stain, lab work).	Explain procedures and tests needed to assess respiratory ability such as respiratory mechanics, peak flow, and PFTs. Explain tests needed to assess for triggers of asthma: respiratory infection, sinusitis, nasal polyps, gastroesophageal reflux.	Patient will understand tests and procedures that are needed to continue care (bronchial provocation, x-rays, allergy testing).	Review with patient/family before discharge the results of all tests and how the patient's baseline values compare to normal. Make sure patient has a copy of tests that may be significant to continuing care. Explain any tests the patient may have as an outpatient such as allergy testing, bronchial provocation, exercise stress test. Teach patient how to monitor peak flow at home. Patient should also know his or her normal values and actions to take when peak flow decreases. Give the patient written guidelines to follow based on peak flow: • green zone: peak flow 80–100% of predicted and/or personal best. Continue baseline medications. • yellow zone: peak flow 50–80% of predicted and/or personal best. Increase bronchodilator inhaler(s) to 2 puffs q4h or as directed by physician.

Asthma Interdisciplinary Outcome Pathway (continued)

DIAGNOSTICS (continued)

Diagnosis/Stabilization Phase		Acute Management Phase		Recovery Phase	
Outcome	Interventions	Outcome	Interventions	Outcome	Interventions
					• red zone: peak flow <50% of predicted and/or personal best. Take 2 puffs of bronchodilator inhaler(s) and repeat in 20 minutes. Repeat peak flow. If still less than 50% of predicted and/or personal best, contact physician or ER. Review with patient the need for environmental control and smoking cessation. Stress need for compliance with medical plan of treatment.

FLUID BALANCE

Diagnosis/Stabilization Phase		Acute Management Phase		Recovery Phase	
Outcome	Interventions	Outcome	Interventions	Outcome	Interventions
Patient will achieve optimal hemodynamic status as evidenced by: • MAP > 70 mmHg • normal hemodynamic parameters • free from dysrhythmias • optimal hydration • normal temperature	Monitor and treat hemodynamic parameters: • BP • HR • CO/CI • SV/SI • SVR/PVR • PA pressures • PCWP • CVP • SvO$_2$ • O$_2$ delivery and consumption Monitor lab values: electrolytes, CBC, ABGs, BUN, creatinine. Monitor and treat potentially life-threatening dysrhythmias.	Patient will maintain optimal hemodynamic status.	Continue as in Diagnosis/Stabilization Phase. Maintain optimal hydration based on continued assessment.	Patient will maintain optimal hemodynamic status.	Teach patient and family: • patient's optimal fluid balance and how to maintain • review signs and symptoms of fluid overload and dehydration and actions to take • importance of daily weights • importance of reporting any changes to physician • home medications • increased fluid intake to keep secretions thin if no contraindications

NUTRITION

	Diagnosis/Stabilization Phase		Acute Management Phase		Recovery Phase
Outcome	**Interventions**	**Outcome**	**Interventions**	**Outcome**	**Interventions**
Patient will be adequately nourished as evidenced by: • stable weight • weight not >10% below IBW or >20% above IBW • albumin >3.5 g/dL • total protein 6–8 g/dL • prealbumin at least 15 • total lymphocyte count 1,000–3,000	Assess nutritional status. Keep patient NPO until extubated. If extubation is delayed >24h, initiate alternate nutritional therapy. When patient is able, start clear liquids and monitor response. Monitor albumin, prealbumin, total protein, cholesterol, triglycerides, and lymphocyte count. Assess weight changes from daily weights. Determine hydration needs based on hemodynamics, I & O, viscosity of pulmonary secretions, breath sounds, VS, SaO$_2$, CXR, and electrolytes. Increase fluid intake to maintain thin pulmonary secretions if no contraindications. Assess temperature q4h and PRN.	Patient will be adequately nourished. Patient will be free of bowel and elimination problems.	Advance DAT and monitor response. Consult dietitian as needed to determine and direct nutritional support. Continue alternate nutritional therapy as indicated. Determine patient's resting energy expenditure. Estimate caloric need and type of intake required. Monitor response to diet. Avoid high carbohydrate diet if patient is retaining CO$_2$. Teach patient/family about: • food pyramid and suggested servings per day • daily caloric requirement • weight-reducing or weight-gaining techniques if needed • foods to avoid if they trigger an asthma episode	Patient will be adequately nourished.	Assess effectiveness of patient/family concerning diet. Reinforce information as needed. Teach patient to avoid foods that may trigger an exacerbation of asthma once identified (i.e., nuts, MSG, food dyes). Suggest allergy testing if appropriate. Teach patient about dietary supplements (i.e., antioxidants, vitamins and minerals). Teach patient to avoid dairy products if increased sputum production.

Asthma Interdisciplinary Outcome Pathway (continued)

MOBILITY

Diagnosis/Stabilization Phase		Acute Management Phase		Recovery Phase	
Outcome	Interventions	Outcome	Interventions	Outcome	Interventions
Patient will achieve optimal mobility. Patient will maintain ROM and muscle strength.	Assess ambulation, mobility, muscle flexibility, strength, and tone. Promote rest during acute episode.	Patient will achieve optimal mobility.	Assess physical limitations of mobility. Consult PT/OT for specific mobility or functional ability limitations. Develop progressive activity program. Monitor response to activity and decrease if tachycardia, dyspnea, bronchospasm, ectopy, syncope, wheezing, or hypotension occurs. Exercise with pulse oximetry. If SpO_2 <90%, apply supplemental oxygen. Allow uninterrupted periods of rest between activities.	Patient will achieve optimal mobility.	Assist patient in developing realistic goals for home exercise program. Determine a gradually increasing program of aerobic activity such as walking, swimming, water aerobics, treadmill, or bicycle. Continue to monitor with pulse oximetry and use supplemental oxygen as needed to keep SpO_2 >90%. Refer to outpatient pulmonary rehabilitation program if indicated. Determine if asthma is exercise induced. If so, develop treatment program with medications to prevent bronchospasm with activity. Teach patient to monitor effects of activity with peak flow.

OXYGENATION/VENTILATION

Diagnosis/Stabilization Phase		Acute Management Phase		Recovery Phase	
Outcome	Interventions	Outcome	Interventions	Outcome	Interventions
Patient will have a patent airway and optimal ventilation as evidenced by: • normal CXR • respiratory rate, depth, and rhythm WNL • clear breath sounds bilaterally • SaO_2 >90% • SpO_2 >92%	Continuously assess quality of breath sounds, respiratory pattern, and SpO_2. Involve RCP. Be prepared for intubation and mechanical ventilation. Remember, new techniques for mechanical ventilation may be used with the asthmatic patient, such as permissive hypercapnia. Remember, a quiet chest could indicate decreased air movement, not improvement.	Patient will have a patent airway and optimal ventilation. Patient will exhibit optimal gas exchange and normal tissue perfusion.	Continue as in Diagnosis/Stabilization Phase. As patient improves, change medications to oral form and monitor response. Assess readiness to wean. Monitor ventilatory status and hemodynamic variables prior to, during, and after weaning from mechanical ventilation. Assist with extubation. Continue to involve RCP.	Patient will have optimal ventilation and gas exchange.	Teach patient/family: • home medications and treatment (NSAIDs, corticosteroids, beta agonists) • proper use of inhalers, with and without a spacer device • possible asthma triggers and how to avoid • signs and symptoms of infection • when to report symptoms to physician • precipitating factors

- ABGS, VS, mental status, and PFTs normal for patient
- Demonstrates ability to cough and clear secretions

Patient will exhibit optimal gas exchange and tissue perfusion as evidenced by:

- ABGs, VS, and mental status WNL for patient
- normal Hgb
- normal intrapulmonary shunting
- UO >0.5 mL/kg/hr

Monitor quantity, color, and consistency of secretions.

Monitor for signs and symptoms of respiratory distress/status asthmaticus:

- weak ineffective cough
- dyspnea
- use of accessory muscles
- adventitious breath sounds
- alteration in LOC
- PCO_2 >50 mmHg or greater than normal for patient
- SaO_2 <90% or SpO_2 <92%
- respiratory rate >30 breaths per minute
- pulsus paradoxus >18 mmHg
- paresthesia
- fatigue
- prolonged forced exhalation
- inspiratory inward movement of intercostal muscles
- paradoxical movement of abdominal muscle with exhalation

Elevate HOB.

Rule out other potential causes of wheezing: mechanical obstruction of airway, laryngeal spasm, emphysema, chronic bronchitis, pulmonary embolus, cough secondary to medications such as beta-blockers and ACE inhibitors.

Assist with placement and maintenance of artificial airway if needed.

Maintain adequate humidification.

Assist with monitoring and adjustment of ventilator settings to obtain optimal oxygenation and ventilation.

Administer medications (bronchodilators, corticosteroids, continuous beta agonist therapy) as indicated.

Monitor patient for signs and symptoms of altered gas exchange:

- dyspnea
- restlessness

Measure respiratory mechanics: minute ventilation, negative inspiratory pressure, respiratory rate, tidal volume, and vital capacity.

Assess hemodynamic stability.

Instruct in pursed-lip breathing technique. Have patient give return demonstration.

Monitor electrolytes (including Ca^{++}, Mg^{++}, and PO_4^{+++}).

Assess for improvement in breath sounds, thin white secretions, and adequate cough reflexes.

Teach patient effective cough techniques (i.e., huff cough, cascade technique).

Begin teaching patient/family about the pulmonary system, asthma, current treatment, and expected clinical course.

Begin discussion about smoking cessation, if appropriate.

Refer to outpatient pulmonary rehabilitation program.

Have patient demonstrate pursed-lip breathing.

Refer to asthma support group.

Determine if patient is at risk for future episodes of status asthmaticus (several hospitalizations for status asthmaticus, chronic steroid use, history of noncompliance with medical regimen, excessive sick days from work or school).

Continue discussion on smoking cessation. Refer to support groups as needed. Advise patient about various methods of smoking cessation.

Asthma Interdisciplinary Outcome Pathway (continued)

OXYGENATION/VENTILATION (continued)

Diagnosis/Stabilization Phase		Acute Management Phase		Recovery Phase	
Outcome	Interventions	Outcome	Interventions	Outcome	Interventions
	• confusion				
	• HA				
	• central cyanosis				
	• PaO_2 < 50 mmHg on room air				
	• PaO_2/PAO_2 ratio < 0.6				
	• PCO_2 > 50 mmHg				
	• SaO_2 < 90%				
	• SpO_2 < 92%				
	• use of accessory muscles				
	• dizziness				
	• hypotension				
	Administer supplemental oxygen to keep SpO_2 > 92%. Monitor with pulse oximetry.				
	Assess intrapulmonary shunting by one of the following:				
	• classic shunt equation				
	• PaO_2/PAO_2 ratio				
	• PaO_2/FIO_2 ratio				
	Improve ventilation/perfusion mismatch and shunt by:				
	• determining optimal PEEP and monitoring response				
	• suctioning as needed				
	• chest physiotherapy				
	• monitoring shunt parameters				
	Optimize oxygen delivery by monitoring and treating CO, HR, respiratory rate, SaO_2, SpO_2, Hgb, and PaO_2.				
	Assess for evidence of adequate tissue perfusion in all organ systems (normal blood pressure, LOC, UO, liver enzymes).				
	Monitor and treat complications:				
	• hypoxemia				
	• hypercapnia				

- acid-base imbalances
- HA
- restlessness
- tachycardia
- hypertension
- pneumonia
- hypotension
- pneumothorax
- atelectasis
- dyspnea
- CHF

Monitor for signs and symptoms of further deterioration:

- increased dyspnea (may need to use a dyspnea scale similar to a pain scale)
- increased sleep disturbances
- chest tightness
- change in wheezing pattern
- decreased peak flow
- increased cough, especially nocturnal

COMFORT

Diagnosis/Stabilization Phase		Acute Management Phase		Recovery Phase	
Outcome	Interventions	Outcome	Interventions	Outcome	Interventions
Patient will be as comfortable as possible as evidenced by: • no objective indicators of discomfort • no subjective complaints of discomfort	Plan interventions to promote optimal rest periods. Administer analgesics when indicated. Provide reassurance in a calm, caring, and competent manner. Keep lights dim and maintain a quiet environment to minimize catecholamine response. Keep HOB elevated to enhance breathing comfort. If intubated, establish effective communication method. Observe for complications of status asthmaticus that can cause discomfort (pneumonia, pulmonary embolus, atelectasis, muscle strain).	Patient will be as comfortable as possible.	Continue as in Diagnosis/Stabilization Phase. Instruct patient on relaxation techniques. Have patient give return demonstration. Use complementary therapies such as guided imagery, music, humor, and touch therapy to enhance patient comfort.	Patient will be as comfortable as possible.	Have patient demonstrate relaxation techniques. Have patient demonstrate pursed-lip breathing.

Asthma Interdisciplinary Outcome Pathway (continued)

COMFORT (continued)

Diagnosis/Stabilization Phase		Acute Management Phase		Recovery Phase	
Outcome	Interventions	Outcome	Interventions	Outcome	Interventions
	Allow family to remain with patient when they are able to promote rest. Take a succinct history that patient can answer in monosyllables. Take a detailed history from the family/significant others. Conduct the physical examination quickly, paying particular attention to patient's report of the severity of the episode. Use sedatives/analgesics as ordered and assess effect on respiration.				

SKIN INTEGRITY

Diagnosis/Stabilization Phase		Acute Management Phase		Recovery Phase	
Outcome	Interventions	Outcome	Interventions	Outcome	Interventions
Patient will have intact skin without abrasions or pressure ulcers.	Assess all bony prominences q4h. Use preventive pressure-reducing devices when patient is at high risk for developing pressure ulcers. Treat pressure ulcers according to hospital protocol.	Patient will have intact skin without abrasions or pressure ulcers.	Continue as in Diagnosis/Stabilization Phase.	Patient will have intact skin without abrasions or pressure ulcers.	Instruct patient/family on proper skin care techniques to be used at home.

PROTECTION/SAFETY

Diagnosis/Stabilization Phase		Acute Management Phase		Recovery Phase	
Outcome	Interventions	Outcome	Interventions	Outcome	Interventions
Patient will be protected from possible harm.	Assess need for wrist restraints if patient is intubated, restless, or has altered LOC. Balance the need to protect the patient from dislodgement of ET tube with additional fear and anxiety that may be caused by restraints. Follow hospital protocol for use of restraints. Check skin integrity and circulation q1–2h. Remove restraints as soon as patient is able to follow instructions. Allow family to remain with patient if they have calming influence and can promote rest and safety. Use sedatives as indicated (preferably short acting and/or those that have the least effect on respiratory drive).	Patient will be protected from possible harm.	Give appropriate physical support as patient increases mobility to prevent falls and injuries. Continue to allow family to remain with patient.	Patient will be protected from possible harm.	Review with patient/family any physical limitations in activity before discharge. Consult PT or OT for home follow-up if limitations are present.

PSYCHOSOCIAL/SELF-DETERMINATION

Diagnosis/Stabilization Phase		Acute Management Phase		Recovery Phase	
Outcome	Interventions	Outcome	Interventions	Outcome	Interventions
Patient will achieve psychophysiologic stability. Patient will demonstrate a decreased level of anxiety as evidenced by: • VS WNL • mental status WNL • subjective report of decreased anxiety	Assess physiologic effect of environment on patient. Assess patient for appropriate level of stress. Assess personal response of patient regarding critical illness. Observe patient's patterns of thinking and communication. Use calm, competent, reassuring approach with all interventions.	Patient will achieve psychophysiologic stability. Patient will demonstrate a decreased level of anxiety. Patient will begin acceptance process of asthma.	Continue as in Diagnosis/Stabilization Phase. Include patient/family in all health care decisions. Encourage patient to become active participant in plan of care. Instruct patient/family on alternative methods to promote relaxation: guided imagery, massage, humor, deep breathing. Have patient/family give return demonstration.	Patient will achieve psychophysiologic stability. Patient will demonstrate a decreased level of anxiety. Patient will continue acceptance process of asthma.	Continue as in Diagnosis/Stabilization and Acute Management phases. Have patient/family give return demonstration of alternative methods to promote relaxation. Treat patient as an equal partner in the management of asthma. Discuss impact of asthma on quality of life, ADLs, return to work, sexual functioning, driving, and recreation.

Asthma Interdisciplinary Outcome Pathway *(continued)*

PSYCHOSOCIAL/SELF-DETERMINATION (continued)

Diagnosis/Stabilization Phase		Acute Management Phase		Recovery Phase	
Outcome	Interventions	Outcome	Interventions	Outcome	Interventions
	Take measures to reduce sensory overload such as providing uninterrupted periods of rest. Allow patient to verbalize concerns about asthma and acute episodes. Allow flexible visitation patterns to meet the psychosocial needs of patient and family.				

Chronic Obstructive Pulmonary Disease Interdisciplinary Outcome Pathway

COORDINATION OF CARE

Diagnosis/Stabilization Phase		Acute Management Phase		Recovery Phase	
Outcome	Interventions	Outcome	Interventions	Outcome	Interventions
All appropriate team members and disciplines will be involved in the plan of care.	Develop plan of care with patient, family, primary physician, pulmonologist, RN, advanced practice nurse, RCP, social services, chaplain, and outcome manager.	All appropriate team members and disciplines will be involved in the plan of care.	Update plan of care with patient, family, other staff members, PT, OT, recreational therapist, pulmonary rehabilitation staff (if available), dietitian, home health, medical equipment company (if home supplies necessary—e.g., home oxygen, nebulizer), and discharge planner. Assess social support systems. Initiate planning for anticipated discharge and arrange any equipment that may be needed at home. Assess ability to manage care at home. Begin teaching patient/family about COPD.	Patient will understand how to maintain optimal health at home.	Instruct patient/family about need for follow-up visits and/or pulmonary rehabilitation. Provide guidelines concerning care at home such as: • oxygen therapy • correct use of multidose inhalers and proper use of spacer, if used • medications (indication, dose, and potential side effects) • pursed-lip breathing and coordination with exercise for energy conservation • other breathing exercises (e.g., abdominal breathing) • cough techniques—cascade, huff (forced exhalation) • 6–8 glasses of water per day to keep secretions thin, white, watery (unless contraindicated due to other comorbidities, e.g., cardiovascular and/or renal disease) • energy conservation techniques to increase functioning and strengthening • postural drainage—if indicated • when to call physician—change in secretions, fever, increased shortness of breath Coordinate home care with continuing care agency.

Chronic Obstructive Pulmonary Disease Interdisciplinary Outcome Pathway (continued)

COORDINATION OF CARE (continued)

Diagnosis/Stabilization Phase		Acute Management Phase		Recovery Phase	
Outcome	Interventions	Outcome	Interventions	Outcome	Interventions
					Provide patient/family with phone number of resources available to answer questions and provide support. Refer to outpatient pulmonary rehabilitation program if indicated.

DIAGNOSTICS

Diagnosis/Stabilization Phase		Acute Management Phase		Recovery Phase	
Outcome	Interventions	Outcome	Interventions	Outcome	Interventions
Patient will understand any tests or procedures that must be completed (VS, I & O, CXR, hemodynamic monitoring, intubation, mechanical ventilation, suctioning, lab work, collection of sputum, blood, and/or urine culture, EKG, cardiac monitoring).	Explain all procedures and tests to patient and family. Be sensitive to individual needs of patient and family for information. Establish effective communication technique with patient while intubated.	Patient will understand any tests or procedures that must be completed (removal of ET, mechanical ventilation, removal of urinary catheter, lab work, CXR).	Explain procedures and tests needed to assess respiratory ability such as respiratory mechanics and PFTs.	Patient will understand any tests or procedures that must be completed (lab tests, CXR, follow-up PFTs, ABGs).	Review with patient/family prior to discharge the results of significant tests and how the patient's baseline values compare to normal (such as ABGs, SpO$_2$, PFTs). Make sure patient has a copy of tests that may be significant to continuing care. Provide patient with guidelines concerning follow-up care.

FLUID BALANCE

Diagnosis/Stabilization Phase		Acute Management Phase		Recovery Phase	
Outcome	Interventions	Outcome	Interventions	Outcome	Interventions
Patient will achieve optimal hemodynamic status as evidenced by:	Monitor and treat hemodynamic parameters: • BP • CO/CI	Patient will maintain optimal hemodynamic status.	Continue as in Diagnosis/Stabilization Phase. Monitor for complications that may occur such as paroxysmal	Patient will maintain optimal hemodynamic status.	Teach patient and family: • optimal fluid balance and how to maintain optimal balance

- signs/symptoms of fluid overload
- importance of daily weight
- importance of reporting changes in weight/fluid status to health care providers

- MAP >70 mmHg
- normal hemodynamic parameters
- free from dysrhythmias
- UO >0.5 mL/kg/hr

- SV/SI
- PA pressures
- PCWP
- CVP
- SvO_2
- O_2T/O_2 consumption
- I & O
- LOC
- evidence of tissue perfusion
- dysrhythmias

Weigh daily.
Determine hydration needs based on hemodynamics, I & O, viscosity of secretions, vital signs, CXR, breath sounds, SpO_2, and electrolytes.
Monitor lab values: SMA-7, ABGs, CBC.

atrial tachycardias, acute respiratory failure, pulmonary embolus, pneumonia or pneumothorax.
Maintain optimal hydration based on continued assessment.

NUTRITION

	Diagnosis/Stabilization Phase		Acute Management Phase		Recovery Phase	
	Outcome	Interventions	Outcome	Interventions	Outcome	Interventions
	Patient will be adequately nourished as evidenced by: • stable weight • weight not >10% below or >20% above IBW • albumin >3.5 g/dL • total protein 6–8 g/dL • prealbumin >15 g/dL • total lymphocyte count 1,000–3,000	Assess nutritional status. Monitor albumin, prealbumin, total protein, cholesterol, triglycerides, and lymphocytes.	Patient will be adequately nourished. Patient will be free of bowel and elimination problems.	Involve dietitian as needed: • if eating less than half of food on tray • for unanticipated weight loss • for albumin <3.0 • for instruction on general healthy nutrition and daily caloric requirements • safe weight-reducing and/or weight-gaining techniques if indicated Estimate patient's caloric need and type/amount of intake required. Monitor patient's response to diet. Avoid activity for a half hour to an hour before or after meals. Avoid high carbohydrate diet in patients who retain CO_2. Treat diarrhea, constipation, or ileus as indicated.	Patient will be adequately nourished and consuming at least three-quarters caloric need.	Assess effectiveness of patient/family teaching. Reinforce as needed. Teach patient/family about: • food pyramid • suggested servings per day • daily caloric requirements • weight-reducing or weight-gaining techniques if needed • dietary supplements (antioxidants, vitamins, minerals, and fiber)

Chronic Obstructive Pulmonary Disease Interdisciplinary Outcome Pathway(continued)

MOBILITY

Diagnosis/Stabilization Phase		Acute Management Phase		Recovery Phase	
Outcome	Interventions	Outcome	Interventions	Outcome	Interventions
Patient will achieve optimal mobility.	Consult PT to assess ambulation, mobility, muscle flexibility, strength, and tone. OT to assess functional ability for ADLs and IADLs. PT/OT to help determine and direct activity goals. Allow frequent rest periods between activities to help conserve energy. Begin passive/active-assist ROM exercises.	Patient will maintain optimal mobility.	Develop individualized progressive activity program and advance as tolerated. Use oxygen if necessary to enhance exercise capability. Avoid activity for a half hour to an hour before and after meals. Pulmonary rehabilitation consult if available and appropriate. Monitor response to increased activity. Decrease if adverse events occur (dyspnea, syncope, ectopy, tachycapnea, tachycardia, hypo/hypertension). Provide physical assistance and assistive devices as necessary. Teach energy conservation techniques to enhance increased functioning and strengthening.	Patient will maintain optimal mobility.	Continue PT/OT in home if indicated. Assist patient in developing realistic goals for home exercise plan. Refer to inpatient or outpatient pulmonary rehabilitation program if available.

OXYGENATION/VENTILATION

Diagnosis/Stabilization Phase		Acute Management Phase		Recovery Phase	
Outcome	Interventions	Outcome	Interventions	Outcome	Interventions
Patient will have a patent airway and optimal ventilation as evidenced by: • normal CXR • respiratory rate, depth, and rhythm WNL for patient • clear breath sounds bilaterally	Monitor breath sounds, respiratory pattern, SpO$_2$, and/or ABGs. Be prepared for intubation and mechanical ventilation. Monitor and adjust ventilator settings to obtain appropriate level of assistance and minute ventilation. Maintain adequate humidification. Monitor quantity, color, and consistency of secretions.	Patient will have a patent airway and optimal ventilation. Patient will exhibit optimal gas exchange and normal tissue perfusion.	Continue as in Diagnosis/Stabilization Phase. Assess for improvement in breath sounds, thin white secretions, and adequate cough reflexes. Assess readiness to wean from mechanical ventilation: • measure respiratory mechanics; minute ventilation, negative inspiratory force, RR, tidal volume, and vital capacity	Patient will have optimal ventilation and gas exchange.	Teach patient/family home medications, home treatments, correct use of multidose inhalers and spacers, oxygen therapy (if indicated), breathing exercises, relaxation exercises, energy conservation techniques (coordinating pursed-lip breathing with activity, eating small frequent meals), daily fluid intake requirements, and cough techniques.

- SaO_2 > 90%/ SpO_2 > 92%
- ABGs, vital signs, mental status, and pulmonary function tests WNL for patient
- demonstrated ability to cough and clear secretions

Patient will exhibit optimal gas exchange and tissue perfusion as evidenced by:
- ABGs, VS, and mental status WNL for the patient
- normal Hgb
- normal degree of intrapulmonary shunting or WNL for patient
- UO > 0.5 mL/kg/hr
- normal liver enzymes

Monitor for signs/symptoms of respiratory distress:
- weak ineffective cough
- dyspnea; SOB
- use of accessory muscles
- adventitious breath sounds
- alterations in level of consciousness
- PCO_2 > 50 mmHg or > normal limits for patient
- SaO_2 < 90% or SpO_2 < 92%

Administer bronchodilators, corticosteroids, and antibiotics as indicated.

Monitor patient for signs/symptoms of altered gas exchange:
- dyspnea
- restlessness
- confusion
- headache
- central cyanosis (not peripheral)
- PaO_2 < 50 mmHg on room air
- PaO_2/PAO_2 ratio < 60; PaO_2/FiO_2 < 300
- PCO_2 > 50 mmHg
- SaO_2 < 90% or SpO_2 < 92%
- use of accessory muscles
- dysrhythmias
- hypo/hypertension

Administer oxygen therapy as needed.

Optimize oxygen delivery by monitoring hemodynamic status, Hgb, ABGs, and minimizing oxygen expenditure.

Assess for evidence of adequate tissue perfusion in all organ systems (normal BP, LOC, UO, and liver enzymes).

Monitor and treat complications such as hypoxemia, hypercapnea, pneumonia, acid-base disturbances, headache, restlessness, tachycardia, and hypo/hypertension.

- assess hemodynamic stability and factors that increase metabolic demand (fever, increased WBCs, hypo/hyperthyroid)
- monitor electrolytes including calcium, magnesium, and phosphorous.

Monitor ventilatory and hemodynamic variables prior to, during, and after weaning from mechanical ventilation.

Assist with extubation.

Teach patient effective cough techniques such as cascade coughing, huff technique.

Change medications to oral route and monitor response.

Begin smoking cessation program if indicated. Determine motivation level of quitting (precontemplator, contemplator, or action) in order to provide appropriate support.

Wean oxygen therapy as gas exchange improves.

Begin teaching patient/family on pulmonary system, current condition and treatment, expected clinical course, and future health implications.

Begin to instruct on pursed-lip breathing technique. Have patient give return demonstration.

Teach patient/family signs and symptoms of respiratory infection and to report symptoms to health care provider.

Teach preventive strategies such as:
- avoidance of smoking areas, crowds in high flu seasons, and sudden change in climate
- obtaining adequate hydration
- importance of annual flu shot (influenza vaccine)
- obtaining a pneumonia shot (pneumococcal vaccine) every 5 years

Continue smoking cessation counseling if indicated.

Refer to pulmonary rehabilitation program if indicated.

Chronic Obstructive Pulmonary Disease Interdisciplinary Outcome Pathway (continued)

COMFORT

Diagnosis/Stabilization Phase		Acute Management Phase		Recovery Phase	
Outcome	Interventions	Outcome	Interventions	Outcome	Interventions
Patient will be comfortable and pain free as possible as evidenced by: • no objective indicators of discomfort • no complaints of discomfort	Plan interventions to provide optimal rest periods. Assess amount and degree of discomfort. Use visual analogue scale for objective assessment of pain. Administer analgesics/sedatives cautiously when indicated considering effect on respiratory system. Provide reassurance in a calm, caring, and competent manner. Keep HOB elevated to enhance breathing comfort. If intubated, establish effective communication methods. Observe for complications of COPD that can cause discomfort (dyspnea, SOB, bronchospasm, angina, or musculoskeletal discomfort).	Patient will be as comfortable as possible.	Continue as in Diagnosis/Stabilization Phase. Teach patient relaxation techniques. Use complementary therapies such as guided imagery, music, humor, or touch therapy to enhance patient's comfort. Involve family in strategies.	Patient will be as comfortable as possible.	Continue as in Acute Management Phase. Instruct patient/family on alternative methods to promote relaxation after discharge.

SKIN INTEGRITY

Diagnosis/Stabilization Phase		Acute Management Phase		Recovery Phase	
Outcome	Interventions	Outcome	Interventions	Outcome	Interventions
Patient will have intact skin without abrasions or pressure ulcers.	Assess all bony prominences q4h. Use preventative pressure-reducing devices when patients are at high risk for developing pressure ulcers. Treat pressure ulcers (if present) per hospital protocol.	Patient will have intact skin without abrasions or pressure ulcers.	Continue as in Diagnosis/Stabilization Phase.	Patient will have intact skin without abrasions or pressure ulcers.	Instruct patient/family on proper skin care post discharge.

PROTECTION/SAFETY

Diagnosis/Stabilization Phase		Acute Management Phase		Recovery Phase	
Outcome	Interventions	Outcome	Interventions	Outcome	Interventions
Patient will be protected from possible harm.	Assess need for wrist restraints if patient is intubated. Balance the need to protect patient from dislodgment of ET with additional fear and anxiety that might be caused by restraints. If indicated, assess response to restraints. Follow hospital protocol for use of restraints. Check skin integrity and potential for impairment to circulation q1–2h. Explain need for restraints to family. Use sedatives as indicated (preferably short acting and/or those that have the least effect on respiratory drive). Allow family to remain with patient if they have calming influence and can promote rest and safety.	Patient will be protected from possible harm.	Support patient as indicated as mobility increases to avoid falls or injuries. Continue to allow family to remain with patient.	Patient will be protected from possible harm.	Review with patient/family any physical limitations in activity prior to discharge. Consult PT and/or OT for home follow-up if indicated.

PSYCHOSOCIAL/SELF-DETERMINATION

Diagnosis/Stabilization Phase		Acute Management Phase		Recovery Phase	
Outcome	Interventions	Outcome	Interventions	Outcome	Interventions
Patient will achieve psychophysiologic stability. Patient will demonstrate a decrease in anxiety as evidenced by: • VS WNL • subjective report of decreased anxiety • objective signs of decreased anxiety	Assess physiologic effect of environment on patient/family. Assess patient for appropriate level of stress. Assess personal responses (affective, feelings) of patient regarding critical illness. Observe patient's patterns of thinking and communicating. Use calm, competent, reassuring approach to all interventions. Take measures to reduce sensory overload such as providing uninterrupted periods of rest.	Patient will achieve psychophysiologic stability. Patient will demonstrate a decrease in anxiety. Patient will continue acceptance process for chronic illness.	As in Diagnosis/Stabilization Phase. Provide adequate rest periods. Continue to include family in aspects of care and involve patient/family in health care decisions. Continue to assess coping ability of patient and family and take measures as indicated. Obtain psychological/psychiatric consult as needed.	Patient will achieve psychophysiologic stability. Patient will demonstrate a decrease in anxiety. Patient will continue acceptance process for chronic illness.	Continue to assess coping ability of patient and family. Provide information on coping mechanisms for use after discharge. Have patient/family give return demonstration of alternative method to promote relaxation. Refer to outside agencies (Better Breathers Club, American Lung Association) or services as appropriate.

Chronic Obstructive Pulmonary Disease Interdisciplinary Outcome Pathway*(continued)*

PSYCHOSOCIAL/SELF-DETERMINATION (continued)

Diagnosis/Stabilization Phase		Acute Management Phase		Recovery Phase	
Outcome	Interventions	Outcome	Interventions	Outcome	Interventions
Patient will begin/continue acceptance process for chronic illness.	Allow flexible visiting patterns to meet the psychosocial needs of patient and family. Provide psychological support for dealing with chronic illness. Include emphasis on dyspnea/inactivity cycle. Discuss with patient that panic during breathlessness often increases muscle tension and oxygen need, which may lead to more dyspnea.	Patient will achieve psychophysiologic stability. Patient will demonstrate a decrease in anxiety. Patient will continue acceptance process for chronic illness.	Encourage progressive increase toward IADLs to increase independence and self-esteem. Involve recreational therapists to help deal with quality of life issues.	Patient will achieve psychophysiologic stability. Patient will demonstrate a decrease in anxiety. Patient will continue acceptance process for chronic illness.	Include patient/family in decisions concerning care. Address concerns patient may have about impact on daily life.

Chronic Ventilator-Dependent Patients Interdisciplinary Outcome Pathway

COORDINATION OF CARE

Diagnosis/Stabilization Phase		Acute Management Phase		Recovery Phase	
Outcome	Interventions	Outcome	Interventions	Outcome	Interventions
All appropriate team members and disciplines will be involved in the plan of care.	Develop the plan of care with patient, family, primary physician, pulmonologist, thoracic surgeon (for tracheostomy), RN, advanced practice nurse, RCP, PT, OT, SP, recreational therapist, chaplain, and social services.	All appropriate team members and disciplines will be involved in the plan of care.	Update the plan of care with patient/family, other team members, dietitian, discharge planner, and home health agency. Initiate planning for anticipated discharge. Begin teaching patient/family about home care: • medications • ventilator care and maintenance • care of tracheostomy tube • diet • skin care	Patient/family will understand how to maintain optimal health at home.	Provide guidelines concerning home care for patient/family. Provide patient/family with phone numbers of resources available to answer questions.

DIAGNOSTICS

Diagnosis/Stabilization Phase		Acute Management Phase		Recovery Phase	
Outcome	Interventions	Outcome	Interventions	Outcome	Interventions
Patient/family will understand any tests or procedures that must be completed (VS, I & O, cardiac monitoring, x-rays, lab work, EKG, ABGs, SpO$_2$, IV lines, PFT, end tidal CO$_2$ levels, bronchoscopy, or swallowing studies).	Explain all tests and procedures to patient/family. Be sensitive to individual's needs for information.	Patient/family will understand any tests or procedures that must be completed.	Continue as in Diagnosis/Stabilization Phase.	Patient/family will understand meaning of diagnostic tests in relation to continued health.	Review with patient/family results of tests before discharge. Discuss abnormal findings and appropriate measures patient/family can take to return to prehospital condition if possible. Provide guidelines concerning follow-up care and care at home for patient/family.

Chronic Ventilator-Dependent Patients Interdisciplinary Outcome Pathway (*continued*)

FLUID BALANCE

Diagnosis/Stabilization Phase		Acute Management Phase		Recovery Phase	
Outcome	Interventions	Outcome	Interventions	Outcome	Interventions
Patient will achieve and maintain optimal hemodynamic status as evidenced by: • MAP > 70 mmHg • hemodynamic parameters WNL for the patient • UO >0.5 mL/kg/hr • free from dysrhythmias • VS WNL for the patient	Monitor and treat evidence of abnormal hemodynamic status such as tachycardia, hypertension, hypotension, increased respiratory distress, increased crackles or wheezes, murmurs, or presence of S3 and/or S4. Monitor lab values: electrolytes, ABGs, SpO₂, BUN, and CBC with differential. Monitor and treat dysrhythmias. Assess and monitor fluid balance. Assess weight changes from baseline and weigh daily. Determine hydration needs based on hemodynamics, I & O, cardiopulmonary assessment, viscosity of pulmonary secretions, VS, and electrolytes. Monitor and treat complications of chronic ventilator dependence such as cor pulmonale resulting in right-sided heart failure from prolonged hypoxemia, causing decreased left ventricular filling, CO, and BP; CHF or hyper/hypovolemia. Administer vasodilators and inotropic agents as indicated and monitor response.	Patient will maintain optimal hemodynamic status.	Continue as in Diagnosis/Stabilization Phase. Maintain optimal hydration based on cardiopulmonary assessment.	Patient will maintain optimal hemodynamic status.	Continue as in Acute Management Phase. Teach patient/family about the following: • patient's optimal fluid balance and how to maintain it. Review signs and symptoms of fluid overload and dehydration. Remind patient to weigh daily and report sudden changes to physician. • antidysrhythmic agents and/or other cardiac medications that will be taken at home

NUTRITION

Diagnosis/Stabilization Phase		Acute Management Phase		Recovery Phase	
Outcome	Interventions	Outcome	Interventions	Outcome	Interventions
Patient will be adequately nourished and/or regain nutritional balance as evidenced by: • stable weight • weight not >10% below or >20% above IBW • albumin >3.5 g/dL • prealbumin >15 g/dL • total protein 6–8 g/dL • total lymphocyte count 1,000–3,000 • positive nitrogen balance	Consult dietitian to help determine and direct nutritional support. Assess nutritional status. Monitor for albumin, prealbumin, total protein, nitrogen balance, PO_4^{+++}, Mg^{++}, Ca^{++}, and lymphocyte count. Assess skin turgor and inspect oral mucous membranes.	Patient will be adequately nourished. Patient will be free of bowel or elimination problems.	Assess caloric requirements via indirect calorimetry. In undernourished patients, response to hypoxemia/hypercapnia is impaired. Avoid high carbohydrate load that may result in increased CO_2 production. Initiate DAT and monitor response (enteral feedings, parenteral nutrition, oral foods as able). Consult SP when indicated for swallowing studies. If patient is eating, deflate cuff of tracheostomy tube to facilitate swallowing function when patient is off positive pressure ventilation. Consult OT when functional ability to feed self is impaired. OT to determine special equipment needs when eating such as built-up handles or lightweight utensils. Treat diarrhea, constipation, or ileus as indicated. Weigh every other day and report changes of ±3 pounds. Consider calorie count to determine if patient meeting caloric need.	Patient will be adequately nourished.	Teach patient/family about: • food pyramid and recommended daily allowances • daily calorie intake needed • safe weight-reducing or weight-gaining techniques as indicated • dietary supplements for cachectic patients

MOBILITY

Diagnosis/Stabilization Phase		Acute Management Phase		Recovery Phase	
Outcome	Interventions	Outcome	Interventions	Outcome	Interventions
Patient will achieve optimal mobility.	PT to assess ambulation, mobility, muscle flexibility, strength, and tone. Include assessment of respiratory muscle function. OT to assess functional abilities for ADLs. PT/OT to help determine and direct activity goals.	Patient will achieve optimal mobility.	Assess physical limitations of mobility. Nursing/PT to perform ROM at least BID.	Patient will maintain optimal mobility. Patient will develop home exercise plan.	Continue PT/OT in home if indicated. Assist patient in developing realistic goals for home exercise plan. Determine a gradually increasing program of aerobic activity such as walking.

Chronic Ventilator-Dependent Patients Interdisciplinary Outcome Pathway (continued)

MOBILITY (continued)

Diagnosis/Stabilization Phase		Acute Management Phase		Recovery Phase	
Outcome	Interventions	Outcome	Interventions	Outcome	Interventions
			Develop progressive activity program (sitting on side of bed, transferring from bed to chair, gradual increase in walking, and gradual increase in active ROM/stretching exercises). Monitor response to activity and decrease if adverse events occur (tachycardia, dyspnea, ectopy, syncope, or hypotension).		Refer to outpatient pulmonary rehabilitation program if indicated.

OXYGENATION/VENTILATION

Diagnosis/Stabilization Phase		Acute Management Phase		Recovery Phase	
Outcome	Interventions	Outcome	Interventions	Outcome	Interventions
Patient will have a patent airway and optimal ventilation as evidenced by: • respiratory rate, depth, and rhythm WNL for the patient • CXR WNL • clear airways • ABGs, VS, mental status, and PFTs WNL for the patient • demonstrated ability to cough and clear secretions • optimal oxygenation/ventilation on positive pressure ventilation	Monitor and treat abnormal breath sounds, respiratory pattern (rate, depth, rhythm, and WOB), and CXR. Monitor and treat signs/symptoms of respiratory distress: • weak ineffective cough • SOB, dyspnea • use of accessory muscles/respiratory alternans • presence of adventitious breath sounds • alterations in LOC • $PCO_2 > 50$ mmHg and/or above normal for patient Monitor quantity, color, and consistency of pulmonary secretions. Maintain artificial airway. Provide humidification. Monitor cuff inflation pressure every	Patient will have a patent airway, optimal ventilation, and gas exchange. Patient will have adequate tissue perfusion.	Continue as in Diagnosis/Stabilization Phase. Continue to monitor patient's response to mechanical ventilation. Assess readiness to wean per Burns weaning assessment program (Burns, 1994): **General Assessment** • free from factors that increase or decrease metabolic rate (seizures, temperature, sepsis, bacteremia, hypo/hyperthyroid) • Hct > 25% (or baseline) • electrolytes WNL including Ca^{++}, Mg^{++}, PO_4^{+++} • CXR improving **Respiratory Assessment** • eupneic respiratory rate and pattern	Patient will have adequate ventilation and gas exchange. Patient will have adequate tissue perfusion.	Continue as in Diagnosis/Stabilization Phase. Teach patient/family the following if partial or full mechanical ventilatory support will be used at home: • portable home ventilator care, function, and maintenance • how to troubleshoot three most common alarms: high pressure, low pressure, and low exhaled volume • how to perform clean tracheal suction technique • how to perform tracheostomy tube care • how to maintain minimal occlusive pressure in tracheostomy tube cuff • how to breathe with manual resuscitator bag

Patient will exhibit optimal gas exchange and tissue perfusion as evidenced by:
- ABGs, VS, and mental status WNL for the patient
- SaO_2 >90%
- SpO_2 >92%
- normal Hgb
- UO >0.5 mL/kg/hr

shift and monitor for complications of artificial airways such as tracheal stenosis, tracheomalacia, or granulomas causing obstructions.

Suction only as often as necessary. Beware of complications of suctioning such as hypoxemia, dysrhythmias, discomfort, vagal stimulation causing bradycardia, bronchospasm, and airway trauma. Avoid routine use of saline instillation when suctioning (associated with many adverse effects).

Assist with monitoring and adjusting of ventilator settings to maintain appropriate level of assistance and minute ventilation.

Administer chest physiotherapy q4h when indicated.

Administer bronchodilators as indicated.

Monitor and treat complications that can occur in chronic ventilator-dependent patients such as acute acid-base disturbances, HA, restlessness, hypertension, bronchopleural air leak, or patient/ventilator asynchrony.

Monitor and treat patient for signs and symptoms of altered gas exchange:
- dyspnea
- restlessness
- tachycardia
- tachypnea
- confusion
- HA
- central cyanosis (not peripheral)
- PaO_2 <50 mmHg on room air
- PaO_2/PAO_2 ratio <0.6
- SaO_2 <90%
- use of accessory muscles

- absence of adventitious breath sounds (assess for improvement in breath sounds)
- absence of neuromuscular disease/deformity
- absence of abdominal distension/obesity/ascites
- oral ET tube >7.5 cm or tracheal tube >7.0
- cough and swallowing reflexes adequate
- negative inspiratory pressure at least –20 mmHg
- positive expiratory pressure > + 30 mmHg
- spontaneous tidal volume >5 cc/kg
- vital capacity >10–15 mL/kg
- pH 7.30–7.45
- $PaCO_2$ approximately 40 mmHg (or baseline) with minute ventilation <10 L/minute
- PaO_2 >60 mmHg on FIO_2 <40%

Monitor ventilatory/oxygenation status and hemodynamic variables during the weaning process.

Use consistent, calm approach to weaning strategy. Provide psychological support and encouragement to allay fears, avoiding increased inspiratory WOB.

Wean FIO_2/PEEP as oxygenation improves.

Consider positioning patient to enhance gas exchange (i.e., good lung dependent if unilateral lung disease or prone position if bilateral lung involvement). Encourage patient to sit up to ease chest expansion.

- how to reinsert tracheostomy tube if it becomes displaced
- when to call physician
- how to use backup battery power in cases of power failure
- energy conservation techniques to enhance increased functioning and strengthening
- teach also to monitor energy level so as not to overdo and exhaust patient and/or caregivers

Organize weekly Interdisciplinary discharge rounds to coordinate patient's discharge. Determine which company will supply equipment, be responsible for follow-up care, and contact utility companies, fire department, and police department regarding use of home mechanical ventilator. Teach patient about home medications and signs and symptoms of respiratory distress.

Refer to outpatient pulmonary rehabilitation program when indicated.

Chronic Ventilator-Dependent Patients Interdisciplinary Outcome Pathway (continued)

OXYGENATION/VENTILATION (continued)

Diagnosis/Stabilization Phase		Acute Management Phase		Recovery Phase	
Outcome	Interventions	Outcome	Interventions	Outcome	Interventions
	• dysrhythmias • hypotension Change FIO$_2$ or PEEP as indicated and monitor response. Observe for potential complications such as barotrauma or decreased CO. Optimize O$_2$ delivery by monitoring and treating CO, BP, HR, SaO$_2$, Hgb, and PaO$_2$. Assess for evidence of adequate tissue perfusion in all organ systems (normal BP, LOC, UO, liver enzyme levels).		Begin patient/family teaching on pulmonary system, current pulmonary problems, current treatment, and expected clinical course.		

COMFORT

Diagnosis/Stabilization Phase		Acute Management Phase		Recovery Phase	
Outcome	Interventions	Outcome	Interventions	Outcome	Interventions
Patient will be as comfortable and pain free as possible as evidenced by: • no objective signs of discomfort • no complaints of discomfort	Plan interventions to provide optimal uninterrupted rest periods. Assess patient's perspective of adequacy of rest. Assess quantity and quality of discomfort or pain and treat as indicated. Use visual analogue scale or pain scale. Provide reassurance in a calm, caring, and competent manner. Keep lights dim and a quiet environment to minimize catecholamine responses. While patient is intubated, establish effective communication technique. Encourage patient	Patient will be as comfortable as possible.	Teach patient about relaxation techniques. Use complementary therapies such as guided imagery, music, humor, or touch therapy to enhance patient's comfort. Involve family in strategies. Use diversional therapies such as pet therapy, reading, and listening to book tapes, especially during weaning trials.	Patient will be as comfortable as possible.	Patient will demonstrate relaxation techniques to use at home.

to write message or use a magic slate, alphabet board, flash cards, or computer to express needs and feelings. Use a Passy-Muir speaking valve, talking tracheostomy tube, or cuffed fenestrated tracheostomy tube when patient is able. Value of voicing is very significant to recovery. Observe for complications of prolonged ventilator dependence that can cause discomfort: dyspnea, breathlessness, bronchospasm.

SKIN INTEGRITY

Diagnosis/Stabilization Phase		Acute Management Phase		Recovery Phase	
Outcome	Interventions	Outcome	Interventions	Outcome	Interventions
Patient will have intact skin without abrasions or pressure ulcers.	Assess all bony prominences q4h. Use preventive pressure-reducing devices when patient is at high risk for developing pressure ulcers. Treat pressure ulcers according to hospital protocol.	Patient will have intact skin without abrasions or pressure ulcers.	Continue as in Diagnosis/Stabilization Phase.	Patient will have intact skin without abrasions or pressure ulcers.	Teach patient/family interventions to be continued at home for proper skin care.

PROTECTION/SAFETY

Diagnosis/Stabilization Phase		Acute Management Phase		Recovery Phase	
Outcome	Interventions	Outcome	Interventions	Outcome	Interventions
Patient will be protected from possible harm.	Monitor cuff pressures to prevent trauma to airway and keep pressure lower than 25 cm H_2O. Monitor peak inspiratory pressures. If peak airway pressure is excessive, may need to adjust ventilator settings. Evaluate breath sounds, ABGs, and CXR. Make sure	Patient will be protected from possible harm.	Provide support when dangling, getting OOB, and with increasing activity and monitor response. OT consult for splinting, positioning of extremities, or teaching of correct movement and appropriate functional skills to prevent joint stress, strain, or injury.	Patient will be protected from possible harm.	Provide support as needed with ambulation. Teach patient/family about any physical limitations patient might have.

Chronic Ventilator-Dependent Patients Interdisciplinary Outcome Pathway (continued)

PROTECTION/SAFETY (continued)

Diagnosis/Stabilization Phase		Acute Management Phase		Recovery Phase	
Outcome	Interventions	Outcome	Interventions	Outcome	Interventions
	tracheostomy tube is held/tied securely to avoid trauma/inflammation at the stoma. Deflate cuff of tracheostomy tube if patient is to eat and is off positive pressure ventilation. Assess for adequate swallowing function. Have patient perform oral motor exercises if swallowing is impaired. Change tracheostomy tube every 4–6 weeks. Assess need for restraints while patient is intubated, has a decreased LOC, or is agitated and restless. Explain need for restraints to patient/family. Assess response to restraints and check q1–2h for skin integrity and impairment to circulation. Follow hospital protocol for use of restraints. Provide sedatives/anxiolytics as needed.				

PSYCHOSOCIAL/SELF-DETERMINATION

Diagnosis/Stabilization Phase		Acute Management Phase		Recovery Phase	
Outcome	Interventions	Outcome	Interventions	Outcome	Interventions
Patient will achieve psychophysiologic stability. Patient will demonstrate a decrease in anxiety as evidenced by: • vital signs WNL	Assess physiologic effects of critical care environment on patient (hemodynamic variables, psychological status, signs of increased sympathetic response). Use calm, caring, competent, and reassuring approach with	Patient will achieve psychophysiologic stability. Patient will be as relaxed as possible. Patient will continue acceptance process of long-term ventilator needs.	Continue as in Diagnosis/Stabilization Phase. OT to teach progressive increase in ADLs and IADLs to increase independence and enhance self-esteem.	Patient will achieve psychophysiologic stability. Patient will be as relaxed as possible. Patient will continue acceptance process of long-term ventilator needs.	Provide instruction on coping mechanisms after discharge. Refer patient/family to counseling/stress management programs when indicated. Provide emotional support to patient/family in the case of unsuccessful treatment outcomes, in reaching difficult decisions, and accepting inevitable outcomes.

- subjective report of decreased anxiety
- objective signs of decreased anxiety

Patient will begin acceptance process of long-term ventilator needs.

patient and family. Assess for appropriate level of anxiety and nervousness.

Allow flexible visitation to meet the needs of patient and family.

Help patient/family to identify and verbalize fears such as dying, being dependent on ventilator, losing control, being dependent on family, or being alone. Plan strategies to help alleviate and/or help patients process their fears.

Determine coping ability of patient/family and take appropriate measures to begin acceptance of long-term ventilator dependence. Provide frequent explanations to patient/family, allow patient to verbalize concerns, consult support services, and hold family conferences.

Administer sedatives and anxiolytics and monitor response.

Common emotional/psychological responses of ventilator-dependent patients include hopelessness, powerlessness, and loss of control. Incorporate the following strategies and others as appropriate into the patient's daily care to minimize these responses:

- provide daily progress reports for patient/family
- provide opportunities for patient to participate in care and decisions regarding health
- keep patient informed of condition, treatment, and results of tests

Address concerns patient and family may have on impact on quality of life.

Lung Cancer
Interdisciplinary Outcome Pathway

COORDINATION OF CARE

Diagnosis/Stabilization Phase		Acute Management Phase		Recovery Phase	
Outcome	Interventions	Outcome	Interventions	Outcome	Interventions
All appropriate team members and disciplines will be involved in the plan of care.	Obtain thorough patient and family history to include: • smoking history (active or passive) • environmental/occupational exposures such as aerosols, asbestos, hydrocarbons, nickel, uranium, radon, radiation, vinyl chloride, arsenic Develop the plan of care with the patient/family, surgeons, primary physician, oncologist, RN, advanced practice nurse, clinical pharmacist, RCP, PT, OT, social services, dietitian, SP, psychologist, and chaplain. Develop plan of care specific to type and stage of tumor: • surgical intervention (lobectomy or pneumonectomy) • radiation therapy • chemotherapy Develop plan of care specific to treatment goals: • curative • control • palliative	All appropriate team members will be involved in the plan of care.	Update the plan of care with all appropriate team members. Initiate consultations, if indicated (i.e., SP, case manager). Involve other disciplines as needed. Initiate discharge planning. Explain implications of staging, tumor type, and treatment recommendations to patient/family.	Patient/family will understand the discharge plan. Patient will achieve maximum functional capacity. Patient will understand how to maintain wellness and health.	Implement and update the plan of care with all appropriate team members. Develop discharge plan and make referrals to appropriate community services for ongoing health care needs: • American Cancer Society (I Can Cope) • National Cancer Institute Information Service • American Lung Association • Hospice/Respite (if applicable) • smoking cessation • pulmonary rehabilitation Patient/family will verbalize follow-up plan and supportive resources. Develop a systematic follow-up plan for long-term survivors. Develop a long-term follow-up plan to monitor disease recurrence and metastasis.

DIAGNOSTICS

Diagnosis/Stabilization Phase		Acute Management Phase		Recovery Phase	
Outcome	Interventions	Outcome	Interventions	Outcome	Interventions
Patient/family will understand the purpose of all diagnostic procedures: CXR, CT scan, MRI, bronchoscopy, biopsy.	Prepare patient for diagnostic procedures: CXR, CT scan of chest, bronchoscopy with rush or needle biopsy, MRI. Prepare patient for procedures to assess possible lymph node involvement: mediastinoscopy, scalene node biopsy, hilar tomography, CT scan. Explain all tests and procedures. Assess understanding. Be sensitive to patient and family's individualized needs for information.	Patient/family will understand all tests and procedures that must be completed (VS, lab work, chest tube removal, hemodynamic monitoring, x-rays, IS, cough and deep breathing).	Explain the purpose and results of labs to monitor hormone-like substances produced by tumor: ADH, ACTH. Explain the results of ongoing pulmonary evaluation: ABGs, pulmonary function studies, respiratory mechanics.	Patient/family will understand all diagnostic procedures in relation to continued health.	Prepare patient for procedures to monitor for metastasis: • liver and spleen scan • bone scan • brain CT • thoracentesis Review with patient/family before discharge the results of all tests and how patient's values compare to normal. Provide patient/family with guidelines concerning follow-up care.

FLUID BALANCE

Diagnosis/Stabilization Phase		Acute Management Phase		Recovery Phase	
Outcome	Interventions	Outcome	Interventions	Outcome	Interventions
Patient will achieve optimal hemodynamic status as evidenced by: • HR WNL • SBP > 90 mmHg • Hgb > 8 • MAP > 70 mmHg • free of dysrhythmias • normal hemodynamic parameters	Assess cardiac function: • heart sounds • rhythm • central peripheral pulses • presence or absence of edema • skin color and temperature Prepare patient for preop cardiovascular workup, if indicated. Anticipate the need for PA catheter, CVP, and arterial line for BP monitoring and to obtain lab specimens, intra- and postoperatively. Monitor and treat hemodynamic parameters: • BP • CO/CI • SV/SI • PA pressure • PCWP	Patient will maintain optimal hemodynamic status.	Obtain venous access for the following, if indicated: • fluid replacement if N & V present • preop fluids • chemotherapy administration If PA catheter and arterial line in place, VS, PAP, PCWP, CVP, q1h and PRN; SVR/PVR, CO/CI, SV/SI, q2–4h postop; progress to q4h until lines discontinued. I & O q1h postop; progressing to q8h. If chemotherapeutic agents toxic to bladder: • force fluids, if CV status does not contraindicate • encourage frequent voiding Weigh daily.	Patient will maintain optimal hemodynamic status.	Assess patient for the development of paraneoplastic syndromes and notify the physician: • Cushing's syndrome • hyponatremia • hypercalcemia • carcinoid syndrome • venous thrombosis Monitor patient for signs and symptoms of superior vena cava syndrome (SVCS) and notify physician: • facial swelling in a.m. • redness and edema of eyes • swelling of neck/arms • neck/thoracic vein distension • nonproductive cough • hoarseness/stridor • cyanosis

Lung Cancer Interdisciplinary Outcome Pathway (continued)

FLUID BALANCE (continued)

Diagnosis/Stabilization Phase		Acute Management Phase		Recovery Phase	
Outcome	Interventions	Outcome	Interventions	Outcome	Interventions
	• CVP • SvO_2 • O_2 delivery • O_2 consumption				Prepare patient for insertion of long-term central venous access device (CVAD). Include: • preop instructions • postop care Instruct patient/family on procedure for home care of CVAD: • catheter flushing • injection port cap changes • dressing changes Assess patient/family understanding of teaching. Reinforce as necessary.

NUTRITION

Diagnosis/Stabilization Phase		Acute Management Phase		Recovery Phase	
Outcome	Interventions	Outcome	Interventions	Outcome	Interventions
Patient will be adequately nourished as evidenced by: • stable weight • weight not >10% below or >20% above IBW • albumin >3.5 g/dL • total protein 6–8 g/dL • prealbumin >15 g/dL • total lymphocyte count 1,000–3,000	Consult dietitian to help determine and direct nutritional support. Assess nutritional status: weight, hydration status, signs of vitamin and mineral deficiencies. Monitor protein, prealbumin, and albumin. Assess for bowel sounds, abdominal distension, abdominal pain and tenderness q4h and PRN. Instruct patient/family on the adverse effects of chemotherapy (if applicable): • nausea • vomiting • diarrhea • malabsorption	Patient will be adequately nourished.	Estimate caloric and protein needs. Continue to monitor protein, albumin, prealbumin, and electrolytes. Place patient on a high calorie, high protein diet. Consider calorie count to assure patient is meeting caloric need. Consider nocturnal enteral feedings if patient's intake is not meeting caloric need. If GI tract is functional but patient unable to take oral feedings, initiate enteral nutrition. Start with low volumes and increase to estimated requirements.	Patient will maintain adequate nutritional status. Patient will be free from nausea.	Weigh weekly. Monitor for decrease in nutritional status and weight loss. Teach patient/family about dietary requirements: • increased calorie intake • caloric supplement, if needed • fluid restriction, if indicated • flexibility of mealtimes • small frequent meals, instead of three (3) large meals • healthy diet • vitamin/mineral supplements (especially antioxidants)

If patient at increased risk for N & V, administer antiemetics around the clock. Maintain naso/orogastric tube to suction, if intractable N & V. Keep NPO until extubated. If extubation is prolonged >24h, initiate alternative nutritional therapy.

Initiate parenteral nutrition via central circulation, if enteral route nonfunctional or if intractable N & V. Weigh daily.

MOBILITY

Diagnosis/Stabilization Phase		Acute Management Phase		Recovery Phase	
Outcome	Interventions	Outcome	Interventions	Outcome	Interventions
Patient will maintain normal ROM and muscle strength.	PT to assess physical limitations to ambulation mobility. OT to assess functional abilities for ADLs. PT/OT to help determine and direct activity goals. PT to assess muscle flexibility, strength, and tone. Initiate passive/active-assist ROM exercises. Institute progressive mobilization. If extubation prolonged >24h, initiate PT consult.	Patient will achieve optimal mobility.	Progress activity as tolerated. Monitor response to increased activity. Decrease if adverse effects occur (increased pain, tachycardia, dyspnea, ectopy, hypo/hypertension). Use assistive devices (pillows, splints, ambulation devices, etc.). Have patient demonstrate correct use of assistive devices. Schedule periods of rest between activities. Assess changes in sleep patterns. Consult inpatient pulmonary rehabilitation, if appropriate.	Patient will maintain optimal mobility.	Schedule long-term follow-up plan to monitor strength and activity level. Evaluate patient for dyspnea and modify therapy accordingly. Establish a home exercise program. Refer to outpatient pulmonary rehabilitation if feasible.

OXYGENATION/VENTILATION

Diagnosis/Stabilization Phase		Acute Management Phase		Recovery Phase	
Outcome	Interventions	Outcome	Interventions	Outcome	Interventions
Patient will have adequate gas exchange as evidenced by: • respiratory rate, depth, rhythm WNL • clear breath sounds	Assess respiratory functions: • breath sounds • respiratory muscle strength and movement • respiratory rate, depth, and quality • cough (acute/self-limiting or chronic/persistent)	Patient will have adequate gas exchange.	Assess chest drainage system (if applicable) q1–2h for: • fluctuation in waterseal chamber • amount and color of drainage • presence of clots or debris • dressing and connections remain secure	Patient will maintain adequate gas exchange.	Instruct patient in breathing exercises such as pursed-lip breathing. Have patient give return demonstration. Schedule patient for follow-up in pulmonary rehabilitation program, if applicable. Facilitate smoking cessation.

Lung Cancer Interdisciplinary Outcome Pathway (*continued*)

OXYGENATION/VENTILATION (continued)

	Diagnosis/Stabilization Phase		Acute Management Phase		Recovery Phase
Outcome	Interventions	Outcome	Interventions	Outcome	Interventions
• SaO_2 >90% • SpO_2 >92% • ABGs WNL • demonstrated ability to cough and clear secretions	• sputum production (character, color, odor, consistency, presence of blood, and microscopic exam) • CXR • SpO_2 • ABGs Assess patient for signs and symptoms of altered gas exchange: • dyspnea • wheezing • hoarseness • chest discomfort • restlessness • confusion • HA • clubbing • central cyanosis • pneumonia • pleural effusion Assist with placement and maintenance of artificial airway if needed. Be prepared for intubation and mechanical ventilation. Monitor ventilator settings and assess readiness to wean. Wean FIO_2 to keep SpO_2 >92%. Apply supplemental O_2 after extubation. Maintain adequate humidification. Optimize O_2 delivery by monitoring and treating CO, BP, HR, SaO_2, SvO_2, Hgb, and PaO_2. Assess for evidence of adequate tissue perfusion.		• air leak Assess for signs and symptoms of pneumothorax: • absent breath sounds • tracheal deviation • respiratory difficulty • subcutaneous emphysema If post/lobectomy/pneumonectomy, position patient to facilitate proper expansion into the lung space. Monitor patient for signs and symptoms of post-thoracotomy complications, if applicable: atelectasis, persistent air leak, failure of expansion of lung, pneumonia, pulmonary embolus. Monitor CXR. Provide pulmonary hygiene. Teach patient/family about IS. Have patient give return demonstration. Monitor oxygenation by continuous pulse oximetry and intermittent ABGs. If post/lobectomy/pneumonectomy, avoid deep suctioning. Assist with intrapleural infusion of antineoplastic agents, if indicated. Assess color and quantity of sputum. Administer high flow, humidified oxygen. Begin discussion of smoking cessation, if applicable.		Teach patient various cough techniques: cascade, huff. Have patient give return demonstration. Reevaluate pulmonary function 6–8 weeks upon completion of radiation therapy (if applicable).

COMFORT

Diagnosis/Stabilization Phase		Acute Management Phase		Recovery Phase	
Outcome	Interventions	Outcome	Interventions	Outcome	Interventions
Patient will be as comfortable and as pain free as possible, as evidenced by: • decreased incidence of pain • decreased severity of pain • normal VS	Obtain a thorough pain history: • previous or ongoing pain episodes • previous pain control methods • patient's attitude toward pain medication • any history of substance abuse Assess pain level through patient self-report: • description • location • intensity/severity, using a visual analogue scale • aggravating/relieving factors Assess pain level through direct observation for: • splinting or guarding • distorted posture • decreased mobility • anxiety Develop a proactive pain control plan. Education patient/family how to communicate unrelieved pain effectively. Administer analgesics and monitor response. Provide reassurance in a calm, caring, and competent manner. Keep HOB elevated to enhance breathing comfort. If intubated, establish effective communication techniques.	Patient will be as comfortable and as pain free as possible.	Reassess pain level: • routinely at scheduled intervals (at least q2–4h) • with each new report of pain • following pain medication administration Individualize route, dosage, and schedule for analgesics: • mild to moderate pain, use NSAIDs • moderate to severe pain, use opioid analgesics Offer PCA, if medically and psychologically indicated. Assess patient for referred pain. Provide uninterrupted periods of rest. Assess for complications that can cause discomfort: • pneumonia • pulmonary embolus • metastasis • DVT • fractured ribs from coughing Use complementary therapies such as imagery, humor, music, or touch therapy to enhance comfort. Provide analgesics as needed before painful procedures such as chest tube removal.	Patient will be as pain free as possible.	Instruct patient in the use of relaxation exercises, imagery, and distraction. Have patient give return demonstration. Assess effect of chronic pain on QOL. Instruct patient/family about long-term pain management to prevent unnecessary readmissions. Pain lasting > 6 months should be considered chronic pain. Refer to Chronic Pain Management Outcome Pathway as needed.

Lung Cancer Interdisciplinary Outcome Pathway (continued)

SKIN INTEGRITY

Diagnosis/Stabilization Phase		Acute Management Phase		Recovery Phase	
Outcome	Interventions	Outcome	Interventions	Outcome	Interventions
Patient will have intact skin without infection or pressure ulcers.	Obtain and document a complete baseline skin assessment. If patient to receive radiation therapy, teach patient/family the signs and symptoms of skin changes. Use preventive pressure-reducing devices if patient is at high risk for skin breakdown.	Patient will have intact skin without infection or pressure ulcers. Patient will have healing surgical wounds (if applicable). Patient will be free of skin breakdown secondary to radiation therapy, if applicable.	Continue as in Diagnosis/Stabilization Phase. Reassess skin daily and document size, location, and description of any breakdown. Treat any skin breakdown according to hospital protocol. Consider mattress overlay. Monitor areas of breakdown and incisions if applicable for signs and symptoms of infection. Maintain sterile technique with all dressing changes. If patient receiving radiation therapy: • assess irradiated skin for color, dryness, moisture, scaling, temperature, tenderness, desquamation, or itching • assess wet areas for signs of infection • apply water-based soothing ointments to dry areas • protect markings	Patient will have intact skin without abrasions or pressure ulcers. Patient will have healing wounds (surgical and traumatic) and be free of infection. Patient will be free of skin breakdown secondary to radiation therapy (if applicable).	Teach patient/family proper care of surgical incisions, signs and symptoms of infection, and when to call the physician. Teach patient/family proper techniques for dressing changes, if applicable. If patient receiving radiation therapy: • teach patient steps to prevent further skin irritation • avoid constrictive and rough clothing • avoid irritating substances such as perfumes, dyes, harsh soaps, and oil-based creams Reassess skin weekly.

PROTECTION/SAFETY

Diagnosis/Stabilization Phase		Acute Management Phase		Recovery Phase	
Outcome	Interventions	Outcome	Interventions	Outcome	Interventions

- activity limitations for after discharge
- signs and symptoms of infection
- when to call the physician

If patient receiving chemotherapy, obtain appropriate supplies/agents for treatment of extravasation and/or anaphylaxis.

Secure chest tube connections (if applicable) with tape.

Keep chest tubes free of kinks and monitor for air leaks.

Provide appropriate physical support as patient increases mobility.

OT consult for teaching of correct movement and appropriate functional skills to prevent joint stress, strain, or injury.

Initiate interventions to minimize patient/family/staff exposure to antineoplastic agents during preparation, administration, and disposal. Use sedatives as indicated and monitor response. Pay particular attention to possible respiratory depression.

PSYCHOSOCIAL/SELF-DETERMINATION

Diagnosis/Stabilization Phase		Acute Management Phase		Recovery Phase	
Outcome	Interventions	Outcome	Interventions	Outcome	Interventions
Patient/family utilize coping skills effectively to keep anxiety at a tolerable level. Patient will achieve psychophysiologic stability. Patient will begin acceptance of disease process.	Assess patient/family for current level of anxiety and fear. Recognize defensive coping mechanisms (repression, denial, regression, and projection). Introduce survivorship potential and phases of survival at time of diagnosis. Use calm, caring, reassuring approach with all interventions. Take measures to reduce sensory overload.	Patient/family will demonstrate effective coping skills. Patient will achieve psychophysiologic stability. Patient will begin acceptance of disease process.	Support patient through stages of loss and grieving. Assist patient with adaptation to altered body functions and body image. Reinforce and reward positive coping strategies by patient/family. Assess ineffective or maladaptive behaviors. Allow patient to participate in decision making. Identify and eliminate stressors. Teach patient in the use of diversion/relaxation techniques to overcome anxiety. Support patient through stages of loss and grieving. Allow flexible visitation to meet needs of patient and family.	Patient/family will maintain effective coping skills. Patient will achieve psychophysiologic stability. Patient will begin acceptance of disease process.	Assess patient for current stage of perception of illness and adaptation. Assist patient/family with identification and implementation of role changes. Monitor patient/family for changing psychological response. Assess for signs and symptoms of dysfunctional grief. Assess patient/family coping and resources throughout the survival process (American Lung Association, American Cancer Society, hospice). Address concerns patient may have about impact on daily life.

Lung Volume Reduction Surgery
Interdisciplinary Outcome Pathway

COORDINATION OF CARE

Diagnosis/Stabilization Phase		Acute Management Phase		Recovery Phase	
Outcome	Interventions	Outcome	Interventions	Outcome	Interventions
All appropriate team members and disciplines will be involved in the plan of care.	Develop the plan of care with patient/family, surgeon, primary physician, pulmonologist, RN, advanced practice nurse, RCP, PT, OT, social services, and dietitian. Refer to appropriate pulmonary rehabilitation program (inpatient or outpatient). Collate all diagnostic data. Assess need for housing while in rehabilitation program and during hospitalization. Make appropriate referrals to home medical supply company and home health agency.	All appropriate team members and disciplines will be involved in the plan of care.	Update the plan of care with the patient/family and team members including pulmonary rehabilitation staff and discharge planner. Instruct patient and family on all aspects of LVRS (presurgery, surgery, postsurgery, and rehabilitation). Anticipate changing team members (ICU nurse, medical-surgical staff nurses, and rehabilitation staff). Assess ability to manage at home. Initiate planning for anticipated discharge (home, SNF, pulmonary rehabilitation program, home health).	Patient/family will understand how to maintain optimal health at home.	Provide discharge teaching guidelines that discuss activity, wound care, and doctor visits. Refer to appropriate post discharge facility (SNF, pulmonary rehabilitation program, home health). Obtain necessary equipment for home care (oxygen, exercise equipment, walkers). Provide resource phone numbers.

DIAGNOSTICS

Diagnosis/Stabilization Phase		Acute Management Phase		Recovery Phase	
Outcome	Interventions	Outcome	Interventions	Outcome	Interventions
Rehabilitation/Presurgery Patient/family will understand any tests or procedures that must be completed during the rehabilitation and evaluation process for LVRS, including	Explain all tests and procedures. Arrange times for testing to meet patient/family needs. If out of town, arrange for housing for patient/family. Explain follow-up process postsurgery (3, 6, 9 months, and yearly).	Patient/family will understand any tests or procedures that must be completed post surgery (chest tube reinsertion, pleurodesis, 6 minute walk test).	Continue as in Diagnosis/Stabilization Phase.	Patient/family will understand meaning of diagnostic tests in relation to continued health care (follow-up evaluations).	Review with patient/family before discharge results of all pertinent lab tests, x-rays, exercise evaluation, and surgery. Discuss abnormal results and measures that can help patient return to normal. Review process of follow-up evaluations.

the repetition of all tests as follows:

- 6 minute walk test
- modified stress test
- pulmonary rehabilitation program
- ABGs
- complete PFT with body plethysmography and nitrogen washout
- bicore evaluation
- CXR
- quantitative perfusion scan
- lab work
- EKG
- dyspnea index
- dobutamine echocardiogram or dobutamine stress test as indicated
- questionnaires: stress profile, QOL, knowledge inventory, ADLs
- metabolic testing
- cardiac catheterization if indicated
- CT scans

Critical Care

Patient/family will understand any tests or procedures that must be completed post surgery (ABGs, CXR, bronchoscopy, lab work, intubation, daily weight, VS, SpO_2).

Establish effective communication technique with intubated patient.
Explain all tests and procedures.
Be sensitive to individual needs of patient/family for information.

Lung Volume Reduction Surgery Interdisciplinary Outcome Pathway *(continued)*

FLUID BALANCE

Diagnosis/Stabilization Phase		Acute Management Phase		Recovery Phase	
Outcome	Interventions	Outcome	Interventions	Outcome	Interventions
Rehabilitation/Presurgery Patient will maintain optimal hemodynamic status as evidenced by: • BP at baseline not > 150/90, nor < 90/40 • free from symptomatic dysrhythmias • UO > 0.5 mL/kg/hr • free from symptoms of heart failure (sudden weight gain, pedal edema, distended neck veins, S3, S4) • free from dehydration (concentrated urine, viscosity of secretions, poor skin turgor)	Monitor and treat all pulmonary and cardiac parameters: • HR • BP • concentrated urine • symptoms of CHF • dysrhythmias • viscous sputum • sudden weight gain of 2–3 pounds Obtain an order for additional cardiac diagnostic studies as needed (i.e., cardiac cath, 2D echocardiogram, transesophageal echocardiogram).	Patient will maintain optimal hemodynamic status. Patient will remain free of hemodynamic complications.	Monitor and treat all cardiac variables (HR, BP, symptomatic dysrhythmias). Maintain adequate hydration. Monitor daily weights, I & O. Monitor Hgb, Hct, PT, SMA-6/12, ABGs. Maintain SCD stockings until patient becomes ambulatory. Replace with antithrombolytic hose. Administer heparin 5,000 units q12h or as ordered. Maintain integrity of chest tubes. Record chest tube drainage systems separately. Chest tubes may be to gravity (water seal) or suction. Monitor and treat symptoms of heart failure (i.e., S3, S4, JVD, crackles). Administer vasopressors as indicated. Administer diuretics, normal saline fluid bolus as indicated.	Patient will maintain optimal hemodynamic status.	Continue as in Acute Management Phase. Instruct patient/family how to: • maintain optimal fluid balance • monitor for signs of dehydration and what to do if present (sudden weight loss, viscous sputum, concentrated urine)
Critical Care Patient will achieve optimal hemodynamic status as evidenced by: • HR 60–120 beats per minute • MAP > 70 mmHg or WNL for patient • UO > 0.5 mL/kg/hr	Monitor and treat the following: • HR • BP • I & O • LOC • peripheral pulses • dysrhythmias • chest tube drainage (sudden increase or decrease) • crackles				

- normothermic state
- absence of symptomatic dysrhythmias
- absence of crackles

Patient will remain free from bleeding.

Place sequential compression device (SCD) stockings on patient.
Maintain integrity of urinary catheter drainage.

NUTRITION

	Diagnosis/Stabilization Phase		Acute Management Phase		Recovery Phase	
	Outcome	Interventions	Outcome	Interventions	Outcome	Interventions
Rehabilitation/Presurgery	Patient will be adequately nourished or regain nutritional balance as evidenced by: • adequate weight • normal albumin, total protein, and prealbumin levels	Assess lab values (albumin, total protein, prealbumin). Assess nutritional status. Provide frequent, small meals throughout the day. Provide supplements 2–3 times a day. Provide vitamin supplements. Consult dietitian for weight gain or weight loss interventions. Anticipate possible tube feedings. Weigh daily. Assess/treat bloating (frequent meals, avoid gas-producing foods, use prescribed antacid medications or acid-blocking medications). Minimize alcohol intake to prevent poor nutrition intake and to avoid withdrawal at time of surgery.	Patient will be adequately nourished. Patient will be free from N & V. Patient will be free of bowel or elimination problems.	Advance to clear liquids and monitor response. If tolerated, advance to DAT and monitor response. Weigh daily. Estimate caloric needs and type of intake required. May need dietary consult. Administer laxative/stool softeners as needed. Administer antiemetics/H_2 blockers, antacids as indicated. Provide supplemental feedings as needed. May need to adjust carbohydrate intake if CO_2 retention is present.	Patient will be adequately nourished.	Continue as in Acute Management Phase. Reinforce nutritional education: • supplemental feedings • small frequent meals as guided by food pyramid • caloric reduction if needed • hydration • continue laxative/stool softener as needed • supplemental vitamins and minerals as needed. Assess patient/family understanding of diet and reinforce as necessary.
Critical Care	Patient will be adequately nourished.	Maintain NPO until extubation, intact swallowing mechanics, and/or no N & V. Monitor protein, albumin, and prealbumin levels. If extubation is delayed > 24h, anticipate need for alternative nutritional therapy.				

Lung Volume Reduction Surgery Interdisciplinary Outcome Pathway (continued)

MOBILITY

Diagnosis/Stabilization Phase		Acute Management Phase		Recovery Phase	
Outcome	Interventions	Outcome	Interventions	Outcome	Interventions
Rehabilitation/Presurgery					
Patient will achieve optimal functional capacity as evidenced by: • 30 minutes aerobic activity, preferably walking or treadmill at 1 mph or greater • 20% improvement in 6 minute walk test • 30–40 repetitions with weight tolerance 50% above baseline • completion of a pulmonary rehabilitation program • compliance with home maintenance program until surgical intervention	Inpatient or outpatient pulmonary rehabilitation program. Six minute walk evaluations and/or modified treadmill evaluation. Initiate exercise program: • calisthenics • arm and leg strengthening exercises • sit to stand maneuver at least 20 repetitions • stair climbing/stepping • bike ergometry • treadmill Progress exercise to RPE of 4–6 and Dyspnea Scale 4–6. If 6 minute walk test < 500 feet, begin bike ergometry and progress to endurance of 15 minutes with workload 50 rpm. Institute walking program (free walk at own pace). If 6 minute walk test > 500 feet, begin with treadmill and bike ergometry. Use assistive walk devices as needed. Discharge from pulmonary rehabilitation program with home maintenance program. Reinforce use of work simplification techniques, energy conservation, and pacing of activities.	Patient will achieve optimal mobility.	Continue as in Diagnosis/Stabilization Phase particularly if patient has not progressed. Progress LVRS Protocol: **Postop Day 3–4:** • pursed-lip breathing, IS • active ROM • sit to stand 5 times • march in place • treadmill (5–10 minutes) or walk (100–300 feet) or bike (5–10 minutes) TID • arm/leg exercises with or without weights **Postop Day 5:** • pursed-lip breathing, IS • arm/leg exercises with 1 pound weights • active ROM • sit to stand 5–20 times • treadmill (10–15 minutes) or walk (500+ feet) or bike (10–15 minutes) TID **Postop Day 6–7:** • pursed-lip breathing, IS • progress weights to 2 pounds • active ROM • sit to stand 20 times • treadmill (15 minutes +) or walk (1,000 feet) or bike (15–20 minutes) TID • if chest tubes are out, refer to pulmonary gym **Pulmonary Gym:** • pursed-lip breathing, IS • 6 minute walk test	Patient will achieve optimal functional capacity.	Reassess 6 minute walk test. Progress exercise protocol to maintenance level (20–30 minutes aerobic activity). Refer to inpatient, outpatient, or maintenance pulmonary rehabilitation program. Instruct patient/family on home maintenance program (include calisthenics, arm/leg strengthening, sit to stand, and aerobic activities such as bike or treadmill). Use oxygen as needed to keep SpO_2 > 90% with activity. Maximum lifting of 10 pounds, maximum exercise weights 2 pounds, until 6 week checkup. Refer to home health as needed for progression/maintenance of exercise therapy as indicated, especially if pulmonary rehabilitation program is not available.
Critical Care					
Patient will maintain normal ROM and muscle strength.	Consult pulmonary rehabilitation and physical therapy. Institute LVRS activity protocol:				

Postop Day 0 (while in ICU):
- passive to active ROM
- deep breaths, IS

Postop Day 1–2
- pursed-lip breathing, IS
- active ROM
- stand, march in place
- transfers (bed mobility, bed to chair)
- treadmill (1–5 minutes), walk (25–50 feet), or bike (2–5 minutes) three times a day

Assist patient to sit on side of bed, stand, and/or move into chair.

Monitor all activity with pulse oximetry. Titrate supplemental oxygen to maintain oxygen saturation greater than 90% with all activity.

Provide rest periods, pacing of activities, and simplify activities.

Turn and position q1–2h if patient is on bed rest for complications.

- increase aerobic activity to 30 minutes

Monitor response to exercise (HR, BP, oxygen saturation, RPE, dyspnea scale) and decrease if adverse events occur.

Medicate for pain as necessary prior to start of exercise therapy.

Use assistive walking devices as needed (pulmonary walker, rolling walkers).

Maintain suction on chest tubes as needed with portable suction device.

Use exercise bicycle in room if walking is not progressing.

Use portable treadmill as needed.

Refer to pulmonary rehabilitation gym for continued progressive exercise.

OXYGENATION/VENTILATION

Diagnosis/Stabilization Phase		Acute Management Phase		Recovery Phase	
Outcome	Interventions	Outcome	Interventions	Outcome	Interventions
Rehabilitation/Presurgery Patient will have adequate oxygenation and ventilation as evidenced by: • SpO_2 >90%–92% with or without supplemental O_2. • ABGs at baseline of pO_2 >60 mmHg with or without supplemental oxygen, pCO_2 <55 mmHg and pH 7.35–7.45	Monitor SpO_2 with activity and rest. Keep SpO_2 >90% at all times. Utilize supplemental oxygen as needed. Obtain baseline ABGs. Identify adequate oxygen system for home use, meeting portability needs. Identify adequate method of supplemental oxygenation at rest and with exercise (nasal cannula, oxymizer, transtracheal, nonrebreathing mask).	Patient will have adequate oxygenation and ventilation.	Continue as in Diagnosis/Stabilization Phase. Monitor and treat oxygenation/ventilation status per ABGs, respiratory assessment, SpO_2, CXR, tissue perfusion. Reintubate and ventilate as indicated. Titrate supplemental oxygen to patient's needs, particularly with activity. Monitor chest tubes. Assess for drainage and air leaks. If persistent air leak, anticipate pleurodesis with talc. Anticipate chest tube removal and prepare patient.	Patient will maintain adequate oxygenation and ventilation.	Instruct patient/family on home care: • pulmonary hygiene • home exercise • do's and don'ts with care • proper use of inhalers • proper breathing techniques • oxygen prescription with rest, activity, and exercise • medications • when to call physician Anticipate home needs and order as indicated (home health, oxygen).

Lung Volume Reduction Surgery Interdisciplinary Outcome Pathway (continued)

OXYGENATION/VENTILATION (continued)

Diagnosis/Stabilization Phase		Acute Management Phase		Recovery Phase	
Outcome	Interventions	Outcome	Interventions	Outcome	Interventions
• clear breath sounds • respiratory rate, depth, and rhythm WNL • CXR without acute processes • pursed-lip breathing, diaphragmatic breathing, inspiratory muscle training with resistive device • 25% improvement in negative inspiratory force (NIF) • effective airway clearance (huff, cascade, and augmented cough) • adequate use of IS, sustained maximum inhalation, breath stacking	Instruct patient on pursed-lip breathing, diaphragmatic breathing, inspiratory muscle training (starting at 30% of baseline with NIF goal, 15 minutes BID). Monitor for secretion problems. Institute pulmonary hygiene techniques (chest physiotherapy, flutter valve, breathing techniques, cough techniques, hydration). Maximize medication therapy (oral/inhaled bronchodilators short, long acting, steroid, and antibiotics). Instruct on proper inhaled medication techniques.		After chest tube removal, restart inspiratory muscle training with resistive device. Reinforce all pulmonary hygiene techniques. Assess response to bronchodilator therapy. Progress to . metered dose inhalers as indicated (patient must exhibit 30% of predicted vital capacity). Maintain exercise therapy protocol. Assess for adequacy of pain control but not to point of respiratory depression. Maintain/encourage upright position in bed as much as possible (HOB elevated, sit upright, or OOB in chair for eating). If nasal congestion is present, use saline nasal spray or commercially available nasal dilator.		

Critical Care

Patient will have adequate oxygenation and ventilation as evidenced by:
• extubation without respiratory distress within a few hours of surgery

Assess for airway adequacy, alertness, and orientation.
Assess respiratory functioning:
• breath sounds
• respiratory rate, depth, mechanics
• cough ability
• ABGs
• CXR
• SpO$_2$ with pulse oximetry

- SpO$_2$ >90–92% with supplemental O$_2$
- ABGs at baseline of pO$_2$ >60 mmHg, pCO$_2$ <60 mmHg, and pH 7.35–7.45
- normal Hgb
- clear breath sounds
- respiratory rate, depth, and rhythm WNL
- use of proper breathing techniques
- CXR with minimal pneumothoraces
- absence of subcutaneous emphysema
- minimal air leaks and adequate chest tube drainage with or without suction
- effective airway clearance

Reinforce use of pursed-lip breathing and diaphragmatic breathing.

Institute pulmonary hygiene techniques (IS, breath stacking, sustained maximal inspiration (SMI), chest physiotherapy, cough techniques, flutter valve, chest splint cough) q1–4h as indicated.

Suction as indicated.

Administer bronchodilator therapy via nebulizer and assess response.

Maintain adequate humidification.

Maintain integrity of chest tube drainage and assess for air leaks.

Administer oxygen therapy as needed.

COMFORT

Diagnosis/Stabilization Phase		Acute Management Phase		Recovery Phase	
Outcome	Interventions	Outcome	Interventions	Outcome	Interventions
Rehabilitation/Presurgery Patient will be comfortable and pain free as evidenced by: • no objective indicators of discomfort • no complaints of discomfort	Assess for discomfort especially of the musculoskeletal system. Evaluate and treat as indicated (cold, heat, ultrasound). Assess response to any treatments. Assess for signs of discomfort as related to exercise therapy, breathing discomfort, chest discomfort, and treat accordingly.	Patient will be as comfortable and pain free as possible.	Continue as in Diagnosis/Stabilization Phase. Anticipate need for analgesics. Provide as needed and assess response, particularly pre-exercise, pre–pulmonary hygiene, and pre–chest tube removal. Encourage comfortable positioning; tripod position leaning on bedside table.	Patient will be as comfortable and pain free as possible.	Instruct patient/family on use of pain medications and potential side effects. Reinforce relaxation therapy. Instruct patient/family on alternative therapies. Have patient/family give return demonstrations. Plan for rest periods and uninterrupted sleep in the home.

Lung Volume Reduction Surgery Interdisciplinary Outcome Pathway *(continued)*

COMFORT (continued)

Diagnosis/Stabilization Phase		Acute Management Phase		Recovery Phase	
Outcome	Interventions	Outcome	Interventions	Outcome	Interventions
	Instruct patient/family on comfort positions (tripod position, leaning on knees, or leaning on table). Encourage adequate rest. If interruptive sleep due to dyspnea exists, obtain appropriate medical therapy (long-acting bronchodilators, oxygen therapy as indicated by sleep oximetry). Instruct on relaxation techniques (progressive relaxation, music, imagery, breathing techniques).		Provide rest periods and uninterrupted sleep. Reinforce proper breathing techniques, particularly pursed-lip breathing. Reinforce relaxation therapy techniques. Anticipate removal of epidural analgesia and progress to oral medications. Assess response to oral analgesics. Support all tubing especially chest tubes when mobilizing patient. Use pulmonary walker to promote comfort when walking.		
Critical Care Patient will be as comfortable and pain free as possible as evidenced by: • no objective indications of discomfort • no complaints of discomfort	Provide reassurance in a calm, caring, and competent manner. Assess quantity and quality of pain and treat as indicated. Use a pain scale or visual analogue tool. Maintain integrity of epidural pain management. Assess constantly for respiratory depression and somnolence. Provide rest periods. Keep HOB elevated to enhance breathing comfort. Splint coughing maneuvers with huff cough technique.				

SKIN INTEGRITY

Diagnosis/Stabilization Phase		Acute Management Phase		Recovery Phase	
Outcome	Interventions	Outcome	Interventions	Outcome	Interventions
Rehabilitation/Presurgery		Patient will have intact skin without abrasions, pressure ulcers, or wound infections. Patient will have healing wounds.	Continue as in Diagnosis/Stabilization Phase. Assess all surgical wounds for drainage, erythema, and induration, and treat per hospital protocol or orders. Maintain adequate nutrition. Encourage/maintain patient mobility. Monitor temperature.	Patient will remain free of abrasions, pressure ulcers, or wound infections. Patient will have healing wounds.	Instruct patient/family on signs and symptoms of wound infections and measures to take should they occur. Reinforce adequate/sound nutritional intake. Instruct patient/family on proper skin care techniques to use at home. Have patient/family give return demonstration.
Patient will have intact skin without abrasions.	Assess skin for abrasions and healing ability, particularly patients on steroids. Assess nutritional status. Treat abrasions as indicated.				
Critical Care					
Patient will have intact skin without abrasions, pressure ulcers, or wound infections.	Preop shower/scrub with antibacterial soap. Prep chest with clippers morning of surgery. Administer antibiotics as ordered. Maintain integrity of all dressings. Use pressure-reducing devices when patient is at high risk for developing pressure ulcers. Reposition and turn patient q1–2h until patient is mobile. Assess skin and all bony prominences at least q4h and PRN. Treat all abrasions and skin breakdown per hospital protocol.				

PROTECTION/SAFETY

Diagnosis/Stabilization Phase		Acute Management Phase		Recovery Phase	
Outcome	Interventions	Outcome	Interventions	Outcome	Interventions
Rehabilitation/Presurgery		Patient will be protected from possible harm. Patient will be free of infection.	Continue as in Diagnosis/Stabilization Phase. Use assistive walking device (pulmonary walker) and gait belt as necessary. Provide support for all tubings when ambulating. Prevent kinking of chest tubes.	Patient will be protected from possible harm. Patient will be free of infection.	Reinforce use of any assistive device needed for ambulation. Instruct patient/family on proper use. Instruct patient/family about physical limitations:
Patient will be protected from possible harm. Patient will remain free of infection.	Instruct patient how to exercise safely. Instruct on how to use all exercise equipment safely. Assess for signs and symptoms of respiratory infections.				

Lung Volume Reduction Surgery Interdisciplinary Outcome Pathway (continued)

PROTECTION/SAFETY (continued)

Diagnosis/Stabilization Phase		Acute Management Phase		Recovery Phase	
Outcome	Interventions	Outcome	Interventions	Outcome	Interventions
	Instruct patient/family when to notify medical doctor.		Assess for signs and symptoms of pneumothorax after chest tube removal.		• no lifting or pushing objects > 10 pounds until 6 weeks postsurgery
Critical Care			Assess for signs and symptoms of respiratory decompensation (decreased SpO$_2$, change in ABGs, increase in respiratory rate, increased SOB, increased or colored secretions, infections, pneumonia).		• no exercises with > than 2 pound weights
Patient will be protected from possible harm.	Assess need for restraints if patient has decreased LOC or is agitated and restless. Follow hospital protocol.		Anticipate orders and administer antibiotics.		Review signs and symptoms of wound and respiratory infection and instruct patient to report these symptoms to physician.
Patient will be free of infection.	Provide sedatives sparingly. Be cognizant of the respiratory depressant effects.				Review signs and symptoms for which to notify physician (increasing SOB, infection, and unusual pain).
	Provide physical assistance for patient when dangling, standing, or beginning progressive exercises.				
	Assess for signs and symptoms of infection.				
	If chest tubes have air leak, do not clamp or kink tubing.				

PSYCHOSOCIAL/SELF-DETERMINATION

Diagnosis/Stabilization Phase		Acute Management Phase		Recovery Phase	
Outcome	Interventions	Outcome	Interventions	Outcome	Interventions
Rehabilitation/Presurgery		Patient will achieve psychophysiologic stability.	Continue as in Diagnosis/Stabilization Phase.	Patient will achieve psychophysiologic stability.	Reinforce positive coping behaviors.
Patient will achieve psychophysiologic stability.	Complete pulmonary rehabilitation program.	Patient will demonstrate minimal anxiety.	Include patient/family in all aspects of care and health care decisions.	Patient will demonstrate minimal anxiety.	Reinforce use of relaxation techniques in the home.
Patient will demonstrate a decrease in anxiety as evidenced by:	Conduct patient/family assessment and initiate measures to meet concerns.		Keep patient/family informed of condition, treatment, and test results.		Reinforce participation in support groups for patients with chronic lung disease.
• subjective reports of decreased anxiety	Instruct on measures to control anxiety: relaxation therapy; breathing techniques such as pursed-lip breathing, imagery, music.		Provide opportunity for discussion on outcomes of surgery and patient progress.		Address concerns patient may have about impact on daily life.
					Provide emotional support to patient/family in the case of unsuccessful outcomes with reaching decisions and accepting outcomes.

Refer to outside agencies as needed.

Provide all instructions in written format at time of discharge.

• objective signs of decreased anxiety (i.e., decreased HR, decreased respiratory rate, decreased SOB episodes, and controlled breathing pattern)

Patient will be compliant with pulmonary rehabilitation program.

Attend classes on psychology of breathing.

Assist patient/family on developing positive coping techniques.

Provide preop instruction on all aspects of LVRS. Reinforce realistic attitude toward surgery and postop expectations.

Coach patient through panic associated with SOB using pursed-lip breathing, gentle touch of hands on shoulders, staying with patient, talking in calm, soothing voice.

Use sedatives and antianxiety medications wisely and sparingly.

Assist patient/family in decisions regarding care.

Encourage participation in support groups.

Critical Care

Patient will achieve psychophysiologic stability.

Patient will demonstrate a decrease in anxiety.

Assess for stress and anxiety associated with critical care environment, surgery, and pain.

Provide sedatives wisely and sparingly, always noting the patient's response.

Use calm, caring, reassuring, and competent approach with patient and family.

Reinforce relaxation techniques.

Allow flexible visiting to meet needs of patient and family.

Provide explanations of all activities and status of patient.

Assist patient into best position to promote relaxation and improve breathing.

Provide rest periods and uninterrupted sleep.

Pneumonia
Interdisciplinary Outcome Pathway

COORDINATION OF CARE

Diagnosis/Stabilization Phase		Acute Management Phase		Recovery Phase	
Outcome	Interventions	Outcome	Interventions	Outcome	Interventions
All appropriate team members and disciplines will be involved in the plan of care.	Develop plan of care with patient, family, primary physician, pulmonologist, RN, advanced practice nurse, RCP, social services, chaplain, and outcome manager.	All appropriate team members and disciplines will be involved in the plan of care.	Update plan of care with patient, family, other staff members, PT, OT, pulmonary rehabilitation staff (if appropriate), dietitian, home health, medical equipment company (if home supplies necessary—e.g., home oxygen, nebulizer), and discharge planner. Assess social support systems. Initiate planning for anticipated discharge and arrange any equipment that may be needed at home. Assess ability to manage care at home. Begin home care teaching with patient/family.	Patient will understand how to maintain optimal health at home.	Instruct patient/family on any follow-up visits and/or pulmonary rehabilitation. Provide guidelines concerning care at home such as: • oxygen therapy • correct use of multidose inhalers and proper use of spacer, if used • medications (indication, dose and potential side effects) • breathing exercises • cough techniques • 6–8 glasses of water per day to keep secretions thin, white, watery (unless contraindicated due to other comorbidities, i.e., cardiovascular and/or renal disease) • energy conservation techniques to enhance ability and strengthening • when to call physician (change in secretions, fever, increased SOB) Coordinate home care with continuing care agency. Provide patient/family with phone number of resources available to answer questions and provide support. Remind patient/family that it takes at least a few months to recuperate from pneumonia and bodily defenses are typically still low. Patient may be very susceptible to further

					pulmonary/upper respiratory tract infections. Refer to outpatient pulmonary rehabilitation program if indicated. Assess risk factors for future episodes of pneumonia: elderly, smoking history, presence of other lung disease, AIDS, bedridden.

DIAGNOSTICS

Diagnosis/Stabilization Phase		Acute Management Phase		Recovery Phase	
Outcome	Interventions	Outcome	Interventions	Outcome	Interventions
Patient will understand any tests or procedures that must be completed (VS, I & O, CXR, intubation, mechanical ventilation, suctioning, lab work, ABGs, pulse oximetry, collection of sputum, blood, and/or urine culture, bronchoscopy, EKG, cardiac monitoring).	Explain all procedures and tests to patient and family. Be sensitive to individual needs of patient and family for information. Establish effective communication technique with patient if intubated.	Patient will understand any tests or procedures that must be completed (removal of ET, mechanical ventilation, ABGs, pulse oximetry, removal of urinary catheter, lab work, CXR).	Explain procedures and tests needed to assess respiratory ability and improvement in pneumonia such as respiratory mechanics, ABGs, and CXR.	Patient will understand any tests or procedures that must be completed (lab tests, CXR, follow-up ABGs).	Review with patient/family prior to discharge the results of significant tests (i.e., ABGs, SpO_2) and impact on continuing care. Make sure patient has a copy of tests that may be significant to continuing care. Provide patient with guidelines concerning follow-up care.

FLUID BALANCE

Diagnosis/Stabilization Phase		Acute Management Phase		Recovery Phase	
Outcome	Interventions	Outcome	Interventions	Outcome	Interventions
Patient will achieve optimal hemodynamic status as evidenced by: • MAP > 70 mmHg • normal hemodynamic parameters	Monitor and treat hemodynamic parameters: • BP • HR • dysrhythmias Monitor for fluid volume deficit related to fever and diaphoresis.	Patient will maintain optimal hemodynamic status.	Continue as in Diagnosis/Stabilization Phase. Monitor for complications that may occur such as hypoxemia, dysrhythmias, acute respiratory failure, pneumothorax, meningitis, endocarditis, empyema, or DIC.	Patient will maintain optimal hemodynamic status.	Teach patient and family: • optimal fluid balance and how to maintain it • signs/symptoms of fluid overload • importance of daily weight • importance of reporting changes in weight/fluid status to health care providers

Pneumonia Interdisciplinary Outcome Pathway (continued)

FLUID BALANCE (continued)

Diagnosis/Stabilization Phase		Acute Management Phase		Recovery Phase	
Outcome	Interventions	Outcome	Interventions	Outcome	Interventions
• free from dysrhythmias • optimal hydration • UO >0.5 mL/kg/hr • normothermia	Weigh daily. Monitor response to antibiotics. Determine hydration needs based on hemodynamics, I & O, viscosity of secretions, vital signs, CXR, breath sounds, SpO_2, and electrolytes. Monitor lab values: SMA-7, ABGs, CBC.		Maintain optimal hydration based on continued assessment.		

NUTRITION

Diagnosis/Stabilization Phase		Acute Management Phase		Recovery Phase	
Outcome	Interventions	Outcome	Interventions	Outcome	Interventions
Patient will be adequately nourished as evidenced by: • stable weight • weight not $>10\%$ below or $>20\%$ above IBW • albumin >3.5 g/dL • total protein 6–8 g/dL • prealbumin >15 • total lymphocyte count 1,000–3,000	Assess nutritional status. Assess gastric pH when possible. An elevated gastric pH may increase the risk of pneumonia. Monitor albumin, prealbumin, total protein, cholesterol, triglycerides, and lymphocytes.	Patient will be adequately nourished. Patient will be free of bowel and elimination problems.	Involve dietitian as needed: • if eating less than half of food on tray • for unanticipated weight loss • for albumin <3.0 • for instruction on general healthy nutrition and daily caloric requirements • safe weight-reducing or weight-gaining techniques if indicated Monitor patient's response to diet. Treat diarrhea, constipation, or ileus as indicated.	Patient will be adequately nourished.	Assess effectiveness of patient/family teaching. Reinforce as needed. Teach patient/family about: • food pyramid • suggested servings per day • daily caloric requirements • weight-reducing or weight-gaining techniques if needed • viatamin and mineral supplements (especially vitamins A, C)

MOBILITY

Diagnosis/Stabilization Phase		Acute Management Phase		Recovery Phase	
Outcome	Interventions	Outcome	Interventions	Outcome	Interventions
Patient will achieve optimal mobility.	Assess ambulation, mobility, muscle flexibility, strength, and tone. Allow frequent rest periods. Begin passive/active-assist ROM exercises.	Patient will maintain optimal mobility.	Develop individualized progressive activity program and advance as tolerated. Use oxygen if necessary to enhance exercise capability. Obtain PT consult for any limitation in mobility, flexibility, or limited strength or exercise capacity. OT consult if any functional limitations in ADLs. Teach energy conservation techniques to enhance activity ability and strengthening. Monitor response to increased activity. Decrease if adverse events occur (dyspnea, syncope, ectopy, tachycapnea, tachycardia, hypo/hypertension). Provide physical assistance or assistive devices as needed.	Patient will maintain optimal mobility.	Continue PT/OT in home if indicated. Assist patient in developing realistic goals for home exercise plan. Emphasize need for activity (even if only activity is getting up to chair daily). Refer to outpatient pulmonary rehabilitation program if applicable.

OXYGENATION/VENTILATION

Diagnosis/Stabilization Phase		Acute Management Phase		Recovery Phase	
Outcome	Interventions	Outcome	Interventions	Outcome	Interventions
Patient will have a patent airway and optimal ventilation/gas exchange as evidenced by: • normal CXR • respiratory rate, depth, and rhythm WNL for patient • clear breath sounds bilaterally	Monitor breath sounds, respiratory rate, SpO_2, and/or ABGs. Assess for increased tactile fremitus and pleural friction rub. Determine causative organism. (Obtain sputum sample for culture and gram stain. Analyze sensitive antibiotic coverage.) Be prepared for intubation and mechanical ventilation.	Patient will have optimal ventilation and gas exchange.	Continue as in Diagnosis/Stabilization Phase. Monitor sputum culture results closely and reaffirm proper antibiotic coverage. Assess for improvement in breath sounds, thin white secretions, and adequate cough reflexes. Assess readiness to wean from mechanical ventilation if intubated:	Patient will have optimal ventilation and gas exchange.	Teach patient/family home medications, oxygen therapy (if indicated), breathing exercises, relaxation exercises, energy conservation techniques, daily fluid intake requirements, cough techniques, signs/symptoms of respiratory infection, and symptoms to report to health care provider.

Pneumonia Interdisciplinary Outcome Pathway (continued)

OXYGENATION/VENTILATION (continued)

Diagnosis/Stabilization Phase		Acute Management Phase		Recovery Phase	
Outcome	Interventions	Outcome	Interventions	Outcome	Interventions
• SaO$_2$ >90% or SpO$_2$ >92% • ABGs, vital signs, mental status, and pulmonary function tests WNL for patient • demonstrated ability to cough and clear secretions • normal Hgb • normal degree of intrapulmonary shunting or WNL for patient • UO >0.5 mL/kg/hr • WBC returning to normal	Monitor and adjust ventilator settings to obtain appropriate level of assistance and minute ventilation. Maintain adequate humidification. Monitor quantity, color, and consistency of secretions. Observe sputum for rusty color or blood streaked. Monitor for signs/symptoms of respiratory distress: • weak ineffective cough • dyspnea; SOB • use of accessory muscles • adventitious breath sounds • alterations in level of consciousness • PCO$_2$ >50 mmHg or >normal limits for patient • SaO$_2$ <90% or SpO$_2$ <92% Administer antibiotics, bronchodilators, and corticosteroids as indicated. Monitor patient for signs/symptoms of altered gas exchange: • dyspnea • restlessness • confusion • headache • central cyanosis (not peripheral) • PaO$_2$ <50 mmHg on room air • PaO$_2$/PAO$_2$ ratio <60, PaO$_2$/FiO$_2$ <300 • PCO$_2$ >50 mmHg • SaO$_2$ <90% or SpO$_2$ <92% • use of accessory muscles • dysrhythmias		• measure respiratory mechanics; minute ventilation, negative inspiratory force, RR, tidal volume, and vital capacity • assess hemodynamic stability and factors that increase metabolic demand (fever, increased WBCs, hypo/hyperthyroid) • monitor electrolytes including calcium, magnesium, and phosphorous Monitor ventilatory and hemodynamic variables prior to, during, and after weaning from mechanical ventilation. Assist with extubation. Teach patient effective cough techniques such as cascade coughing, huff technique. Change medications to oral route and monitor response. Begin smoking cessation program if indicated. Determine motivation level of quitting (precontemplator, contemplator, or action) in order to provide appropriate support. Wean oxygen therapy as gas exchange improves. Measure SpO$_2$ with activity to assure oxygen level adequate with activity. Begin teaching patient/family on pulmonary system, current condition and treatment, expected clinical course, and future health implications.		Inform patient/family that energy may be low and susceptibility to other respiratory infections high for 2–3 months. Continue smoking cessation counseling if indicated. Refer to appropriate support group or agencies. Refer to pulmonary rehabilitation program if indicated.

- hypo/hypertension

Administer oxygen therapy as needed.

Assess for evidence of adequate tissue perfusion in all organ systems (normal BP, LOC, UO, and normal liver enzymes).

Monitor and treat complications such as hypoxemia, hypercapnea, acid-base disturbances, headache, restlessness, tachycardia, bronchospasm, hypo/hypertension, abscess, empyema, pleural effusion, or pneumothorax.

Be cognizant of fact that most pneumonias (bacterial and viral) occur when natural defenses are lowered by underlying illness. Those especially at risk are:

- elderly
- chronically ill
- critically ill
- immunosuppressed
- cancer patients
- receiving radiation
- hypoventilating (from alcohol, drugs, or head injury)
- those with significant smoking history
- AIDS patients

Assist patient to change position at least q2h to ventilate different components of lung and promote secretion clearance. Consider CLRT if significant degree of intrapulmonary shunting present (PaO_2/PAO_2 ratio is < 0.25, PaO_2/FIO_2 ratio is < 200, or QsQt > 30).

Pneumonia Interdisciplinary Outcome Pathway (continued)

COMFORT

Diagnosis/Stabilization Phase		Acute Management Phase		Recovery Phase	
Outcome	Interventions	Outcome	Interventions	Outcome	Interventions
Patient will be as comfortable and pain free as possible as evidenced by: • no objective indicators of discomfort • no complaints of discomfort	Plan interventions to provide optimal rest periods. Assess amount and degree of discomfort. Administer analgesics/sedatives cautiously when indicated considering effect on respiratory system. Use visual analogue scale or pain scale. Provide reassurance in a calm, caring, and competent manner. Keep HOB elevated to enhance breathing comfort. If intubated, establish effective communication methods. Observe for complications of pneumonia that can cause discomfort (dyspnea, SOB, bronchospasm).	Patient will be as comfortable as possible.	Continue as in Diagnosis/Stabilization Phase. Teach patient relaxation techniques. Use complementary therapies such as guided imagery, music, humor, or touch therapy to enhance patient's comfort. Involve family in strategies.	Patient will be as comfortable as possible.	Continue as in Acute Management Phase. Instruct patient/family on alternative methods to promote relaxation after discharge.

SKIN INTEGRITY

Diagnosis/Stabilization Phase		Acute Management Phase		Recovery Phase	
Outcome	Interventions	Outcome	Interventions	Outcome	Interventions
Patient will have intact skin without abrasions or pressure ulcers.	Assess all bony prominences q4h. Use preventative pressure-reducing devices when patients are at high risk for developing pressure ulcers. Treat pressure ulcers (if present) per hospital protocol.	Patient will have intact skin without abrasions or pressure ulcers.	Continue as in Diagnosis/Stabilization Phase.	Patient will have intact skin without abrasions or pressure ulcers.	Instruct patient/family on proper skin care postdischarge.

PROTECTION/SAFETY

Diagnosis/Stabilization Phase		Acute Management Phase		Recovery Phase	
Outcome	Interventions	Outcome	Interventions	Outcome	Interventions
Patient will be protected from possible harm.	Assess need for wrist restraints if patient is intubated. Balance the need to protect patient from dislodgment of ET with additional fear and anxiety that might be caused by restraints. Follow hospital protocol for use of restraints, if indicated. Assess response to restraints and check skin integrity/potential for impairment to circulation q1–2h. Explain need for restraints to family. Use sedatives as indicated (preferably short acting and/or those that have the least effect on respiratory drive). Allow family to remain with patient if they have calming influence and can promote rest and safety.	Patient will be protected from possible harm.	Support patient as indicated as mobility increases to avoid falls or injuries. Consider OT for teaching on correct movement and appropriate functional skills to prevent joint stress, strain, or injury. Determine need for oxygen with activity. Continue to allow family to stay with patient.	Patient will be protected from possible harm.	Review with patient/family any physical limitations in activity prior to discharge. Consult PT and/or OT for home follow-up if indicated.

PSYCHOSOCIAL/SELF-DETERMINATION

Diagnosis/Stabilization Phase		Acute Management Phase		Recovery Phase	
Outcome	Interventions	Outcome	Interventions	Outcome	Interventions
Patient will achieve psychophysiologic stability. Patient will demonstrate a decrease in anxiety as evidenced by: • vital signs WNL • subjective report of decreased anxiety • objective signs of decreased anxiety	Assess physiologic effect of environment on patient/family. Assess patient for appropriate level of stress. Observe patient's patterns of thinking and communicating. Use calm, competent, reassuring approach to all interventions. Take measures to reduce sensory overload such as providing uninterrupted periods of rest. Allow flexible visiting patterns to meet the psychosocial needs of patient and family.	Patient will achieve psychophysiologic stability. Patient will demonstrate a decrease in anxiety.	Same as in Diagnosis/Stabilization Phase. Provide adequate rest periods.	Patient will achieve psychophysiologic stability. Patient will demonstrate a decrease in anxiety.	Refer to outside agencies (Better Breathers Club, American Lung Association) or services as appropriate. Prepare patient for possible irreversible lung damage with some pneumonias. Address concerns patient may have about impact on daily life.

Pulmonary Embolism
Interdisciplinary Outcome Pathway

COORDINATION OF CARE

	Diagnosis/Stabilization Phase		Acute Management Phase		Recovery Phase	
	Outcome	**Interventions**	**Outcome**	**Interventions**	**Outcome**	**Interventions**
	All appropriate team members and disciplines will be involved in the plan of care.	Develop the plan of care with patient, family, primary physician, pulmonologist, RN, advanced practice nurse, RCP, social services, chaplain, and outcome manager.	All appropriate team members and disciplines will be involved in the plan of care.	Update plan of care with patient, family, other staff members, PT, OT, dietitian, home health, and discharge planner. Initiate planning for anticipated discharge and arrange any home health follow-up visits that may be necessary (such as PTT/PT tests if patient is on heparin or Coumadin). Begin home care teaching with patient and family.	Patient will understand how to maintain optimal health at home.	Instruct patient/family on any follow-up visits such as PT lab tests. Provide guidelines concerning care at home such as: • home anticoagulant therapy • when to call physician: SOB, pain, redness, or inflammation in lower extremities, bleeding tendencies and/or excessive bruising, excessive bleeding in gums, blood in stools (includes dark tarry stools), red or dark brown urine, vomiting blood or dark coffee ground material, excessive menstrual bleeding, and new or unexpected pain such as headache, stomach pain, or backache. • foods to limit and/or avoid that are high in vitamin K, which may alter PT levels:

High amount of vitamin K	Medium amount of vitamin K	
brussel sprouts	coffee	rolled oats
turnip greens	cabbage	
cauliflower	lettuce	
kale	cheddar	cheese
spinach	asparagus	
broccoli	chicken	
beef and pork	liver	
liver	bacon	
chick peas		
green tea		
(Chinese/Japanese)		
hummus (Middle Eastern food)		

- remind patients to inform their dentist if they are taking anticoagulants
- patients may want to wear a bracelet or carry a card indicating they are on anticoagulant therapy in case of accident
- remind patients not to take any new medications (prescription or nonprescription) without first checking with their health care provider

Provide patient/family with phone number of resources available to answer questions and provide support.

DIAGNOSTICS

Diagnosis/Stabilization Phase		Acute Management Phase		Recovery Phase	
Outcome	Interventions	Outcome	Interventions	Outcome	Interventions
Patient will understand any tests or procedures that must be completed (VS, I & O, CXR, hemodynamic monitoring, intubation, mechanical ventilation, suctioning, lab work, V/Q scan, pulmonary angiogram, EKG, cardiac monitoring).	Explain all procedures and tests to patient and family. Be sensitive to individual needs of patient and family for information. Establish effective communication technique with patient while intubated.	Patient will understand any tests or procedures that must be completed (removal of ET, mechanical ventilation, removal of urinary catheter, lab work, CXR).	Explain procedures and tests needed to assess respiratory ability such as respiratory mechanics and arterial blood gases. Explain any surgical interventions that may be needed.	Patient will understand any tests or procedures that must be completed (lab tests, CXR, ABGs).	Review with patient/family prior to discharge the results of significant tests and impact on continuing care (ABGs, PT if on Coumadin). Make sure patient has a copy of tests that may be significant to continuing care. Provide patient with guidelines concerning follow-up care.

Pulmonary Embolism Interdisciplinary Outcome Pathway (continued)

FLUID BALANCE (continued)

Diagnosis/Stabilization Phase		Acute Management Phase		Recovery Phase	
Outcome	Interventions	Outcome	Interventions	Outcome	Interventions
Patient will achieve optimal hemodynamic status as evidenced by: • MAP > 70 mmHg • normal hemodynamic parameters • free from dysrhythmias • free from dyspnea • UO > 0.5 mL/kg/hr	Monitor and treat hemodynamic parameters • BP • CO/CI • SV/SI • PA pressures • PCWP • CVP • SvO_2 • O_2T/O_2 consumption • I & O • LOC • evidence of tissue perfusion • dysrhythmias Monitor especially for hemodynamic consequences that may occur with pulmonary embolus such as pulmonary hypertension, right-sided heart failure, decreased SV, decreased CO/CI, tricuspid regurgitation/stenosis, distended neck veins, accentuated and/or split pulmonic sounds, and pulsus paradoxus. Monitor for signs/symptoms of pulmonary embolus such as sudden pleuritic pain, dyspnea, tachypnea, crackles, tachycardia, cough, hemoptysis, nonspecific EKG changes (especially T wave abnormalities/ST depression), and circulatory collapse with syncope and shock. Monitor for signs/symptoms of superficial thrombophlebitis (swelling, redness, rubor) in lower extremities. Monitor for positive Homan's sign (calf pain on dorsiflexion of foot).	Patient will maintain optimal hemodynamic status.	Continue as in Diagnosis/Stabilization Phase. Continue to monitor for complications that may be associated with pulmonary embolus such as atrial fibrillation, pulmonary hypertension, right-sided heart failure, acute respiratory failure, and hypoxemia. If receiving heparin therapy, try to convert to oral Coumadin or other anticoagulants. Monitor for appropriate lab values.	Patient will maintain optimal hemodynamic status.	Instruct patient/family on signs of bleeding. Instruct patient/family on follow-up lab tests that need to be checked.

Initiate and adjust heparin therapy (a bolus followed by continuous infusion) and/or thrombolytic therapy as ordered. Therapeutic anticoagulation is usually two to three times the control PTT value. May also monitor with ACT.

Try to avoid IM, IV, or skin punctures if receiving thrombolytic therapy (avoid IV or IM injections for 24h post thrombolytic therapy).

Check patient regularly for signs of bleeding (petecchiae, ecchymosis, gingival oozing, oozing from puncture sites). Monitor all emesis, nasogastric contents, stool, and urine for presence of fresh or occult blood. Monitor for nosebleeds, visual disturbances, joint swelling or pain.

Keep neutralizing agent on floor in case of acute bleeding emergencies (protamine for heparin therapy; Amicar or cryoprecipitate plasma for thrombolytic therapy). Monitor for complications of heparin therapy such as thrombocytopenia.

Weigh daily.

Monitor lab values: SMA-7, ABGs, CBC, PT/PTT, ACT.

NUTRITION

Diagnosis/Stabilization Phase		Acute Management Phase		Recovery Phase	
Outcome	Interventions	Outcome	Interventions	Outcome	Interventions
Patient will be adequately nourished as evidenced by: • stable weight • weight not >10% below or > 20% above IBW	Assess nutritional status. Monitor albumin, prealbumin, total protein, cholesterol, triglycerides, and lymphocytes	Patient will be adequately nourished. Patient will be free of bowel and elimination problems.	Involve dietitian as needed: • if eating less than half of food on tray • for unanticipated weight loss • for albumin <3.0 • for instruction on general healthy nutrition and daily caloric requirements	Patient will be adequately nourished.	Assess effectiveness of patient/family teaching. Reinforce as needed. If patient is on coumadin therapy, give list of foods to avoid with vitamin K.

Pulmonary Embolism Interdisciplinary Outcome Pathway (continued)

NUTRITION (continued)

Diagnosis/Stabilization Phase		Acute Management Phase		Recovery Phase	
Outcome	Interventions	Outcome	Interventions	Outcome	Interventions
• albumin > 3.5 g/dL • total protein 6–8 g/dL • prealbumin > 15 g/dL • total lymphocyte count 1,000–3,000			• safe weight-reducing or weight-gaining techniques if indicated Estimate patient's caloric need and type/amount of intake required. Monitor patient's response to diet. Begin teaching on foods to avoid or limit that have high amounts of vitamin K if Coumadin therapy is anticipated.		

MOBILITY

Diagnosis/Stabilization Phase		Acute Management Phase		Recovery Phase	
Outcome	Interventions	Outcome	Interventions	Outcome	Interventions
Patient will achieve optimal mobility.	Assess ambulation, mobility, muscle flexibility, strength, and tone. Begin passive/active-assist ROM exercises.	Patient will maintain optimal mobility.	Develop individualized progressive activity program and advance as tolerated. Obtain PT consult for any limitation in mobility, flexibility, or limited strength or exercise capacity. OT consult if any functional limitations in ADLS. Monitor response to increased activity. Activity may need to be limited due to anticoagulation therapy. Decrease if any adverse events occur (dyspnea, syncope, ectopy, tachycapnea, tachycardia, hypo/hypertension, excessive bruising or bleeding). Provide physical assistance or assistive devices as necessary.	Patient will maintain optimal mobility.	Continue PT/OT in home if indicated. Activity may have to be limited even on discharge due to anticoagulants and increased risk of excess bruising and/or bleeding tendencies with increased activity. Instruct family on activity limitations for the patient.

OXYGENATION/VENTILATION

Diagnosis/Stabilization Phase		Acute Management Phase		Recovery Phase	
Outcome	Interventions	Outcome	Interventions	Outcome	Interventions
Patient will exhibit optimal gas exchange, minimal V/Q mismatching, and normal tissue perfusion as evidenced by: • ABGs, VS, and mental status WNL for the patient • normal hemoglobin • normal degree of intrapulmonary shunting (V/Q mismatching) or WNL for patient • UO >0.5 mL/kg/hr • normal liver enzymes	Monitor breath sounds, respiratory pattern, SpO_2, and/or ABGs. Be prepared for intubation and mechanical ventilation. Monitor and adjust ventilator settings to obtain appropriate level of assistance and minute ventilation. Maintain adequate humidification. Monitor lung function closely especially for hypoxemia/VQ mismatch. Monitor PaO_2/PAO_2 ratio, PaO_2/FIO_2 ratio, or classical shunt equation as indicators of ventilation/perfusion mismatching. Monitor PCO_2 in relation to minute ventilation to determine if increased dead space (wasted ventilation) is present. For example, normal minute ventilation is 5–10 L/minute. Normal PCO_2 is 35–45. See the table below. Monitor for signs/symptoms of altered gas exchange: • dyspnea; SOB • SaO_2 <90% or SpO_2 <92% • PaO_2/PAO_2 ratio <60, PaO_2/FiO_2 <300 • alterations in LOC • adventitious breath sounds • pleuritic pain • restlessness, confusion, headache	Patient will exhibit optimal gas exchange, minimal V/Q mismatching, and normal tissue perfusion.	Continue as in Diagnosis/Stabilization Phase. Assess readiness to wean from mechanical ventilation. • measure respiratory mechanics; minute ventilation, negative inspiratory force, RR, tidal volume, and vital capacity • assess hemodynamic stability and factors that increase metabolic demand (fever, increased WBCs, hypo/hyperthyroid) • monitor electrolytes including calcium, magnesium, and phosphorous Monitor ventilatory and hemodynamic variables prior to, during, and after weaning from mechanical ventilation. Assist with extubation and continue oxygen therapy. Wean oxygen therapy as gas exchange improves. Anticipate further surgical treatment options if anticoagulation/thrombolytics are unsuccessful such as insertion of window/umbrella/filter in vena cava or pulmonary embolectomy. Begin teaching patient/family on pulmonary system, current condition, treatment, expected clinical course, and future health implications. Review risk factors for development of pulmonary embolus: • prolonged immobility/bed rest increasing venous stasis • obesity	Patient will have optimal ventilation and gas exchange.	Continue as in Acute Management Phase. Monitor oxygenation/gas exchange and treat as indicated. Reinforce teaching to patient/family.

Minute Ventilation	PCO_2	Alveolar Ventilation	Dead Space	Possible Cause
8 L/minute	42	normal	normal	normal ventilation
13 L/minute	44	increased	increased	pulmonary embolus
14 L/minute	32	increased	normal	hyperventilation
4 L/minute	50	decreased	normal	hypoventilation

Pulmonary Embolism Interdisciplinary Outcome Pathway *(continued)*

OXYGENATION/VENTILATION (continued)

Diagnosis/Stabilization Phase		Acute Management Phase		Recovery Phase	
Outcome	Interventions	Outcome	Interventions	Outcome	Interventions
	Assess for evidence of adequate tissue perfusion in all organ systems (normal BP, LOC, UO, and normal liver enzymes). Be prepared for V/Q scan and/or pulmonary angiography.		• hemorrhagic stroke • head or spinal trauma • hip, pelvis, or lower extremity trauma • orthopedic surgery • neurosurgery • obstetric/gynecologic surgery (especially pregnancy) • women who take oral contraceptives Begin teaching patient/family ways to prevent venous stasis and potentially further episodes of PE: • avoid prolonged sitting and standing positions • avoid constricting stockings or clothing • avoid crossing legs while sitting • perform regular exercise of legs • maintain adequate hydration Teach energy conservation techniques if indicated to increase activity capacity and strengthening.		

COMFORT

Diagnosis/Stabilization Phase		Acute Management Phase		Recovery Phase	
Outcome	Interventions	Outcome	Interventions	Outcome	Interventions
Patient will be as comfortable and pain free as possible as evidenced by:	Plan interventions to provide optimal rest periods. Assess amount and degree of discomfort.	Patient will be as comfortable as possible.	Continue as in Diagnosis/Stabilization Phase. Teach patient relaxation techniques. Have patient give return demonstration.	Patient will be as comfortable as possible.	Continue as in Acute Management Phase. Instruct patient/family on alternative methods to promote relaxation after discharge.

- no objective indicators of discomfort
- no complaints of discomfort

Administer analgesics/sedatives as needed considering effect on respiratory system.
Provide reassurance in a calm, caring, and competent manner.
Keep HOB elevated to enhance breathing comfort.
If intubated, establish effective communication methods.
Observe for complications of pulmonary embolism that can cause discomfort (dyspnea, SOB, chest pain).

Use complementary therapies such as guided imagery, music, humor, or touch therapy to enhance patient's comfort. Involve family in strategies.

SKIN INTEGRITY

Diagnosis/Stabilization Phase		Acute Management Phase		Recovery Phase	
Outcome	Interventions	Outcome	Interventions	Outcome	Interventions
Patient will have intact skin without abrasions or pressure ulcers.	Assess all bony prominences q4h. Use preventive pressure-reducing devices when patient is at high risk for developing pressure ulcers. Treat pressure ulcers (if present) per hospital protocol.	Patient will have intact skin without abrasions or pressure ulcers.	Continue as in Diagnosis/Stabilization Phase.	Patient will have intact skin without abrasions or pressure ulcers.	Instruct patient/family on proper skin care postdischarge.

PROTECTION/SAFETY

Diagnosis/Stabilization Phase		Acute Management Phase		Recovery Phase	
Outcome	Interventions	Outcome	Interventions	Outcome	Interventions
Patient will be protected from possible harm.	Assess need for wrist restraints if patient is intubated. Balance the need to protect patient from dislodgment of ET with additional fear and anxiety that might be caused by restraints. Follow hospital protocol for use of restraints. If indicated, assess response to	Patient will be protected from possible harm.	Support patient as indicated as mobility increases to avoid falls or injuries. Provide additional assistance if patient is on anticoagulants. Follow bleeding precautions if patient is on anticoagulants such as:	Patient will be protected from possible harm.	Review with patient/family any physical limitations in activity prior to discharge. Consult PT and/or OT for home follow-up if indicated.

Pulmonary Embolism Interdisciplinary Outcome Pathway (continued)

PROTECTION/SAFETY (continued)

Diagnosis/Stabilization Phase		Acute Management Phase		Recovery Phase	
Outcome	Interventions	Outcome	Interventions	Outcome	Interventions
	restraints. Check skin integrity and potential for impairment to circulation q1–2h. Explain need for restraints to family. Use sedatives as indicated (preferably short acting and/or those that have the least effect on respiratory drive). Allow family to remain with patient if they have calming influence and can promote rest and safety.		• limit venipunctures; if venipuncture is necessary, hold all sticks for 5 minutes • clean teeth with swabs or extra soft toothbrush • use only electric razor • avoid taking rectal temperature • avoid IM injections Continue to allow family to stay with patient.		

PSYCHOSOCIAL/SELF-DETERMINATION

Diagnosis/Stabilization Phase		Acute Management Phase		Recovery Phase	
Outcome	Interventions	Outcome	Interventions	Outcome	Interventions
Patient will achieve psychophysiologic stability. Patient will demonstrate a decrease in anxiety as evidenced by: • VS WNL • subjective report of decreased anxiety • objective signs of decreased anxiety	Assess physiologic effect of environment on patient/family. Assess patient for appropriate level of stress. Assess personal responses (affective, feelings) of patient regarding critical illness. Observe patient's patterns of thinking and communicating. Use calm, competent, reassuring approach to all interventions. Take measures to reduce sensory overload such as providing uninterrupted periods of rest. Allow flexible visiting patterns to meet the psychosocial needs of patient and family.	Patient will achieve psychophysiologic stability. Patient will demonstrate a decrease in anxiety.	Same as in Diagnosis/Stabilization Phase. Provide adequate rest periods. Include patient and family in all health care decisions. Continue to assess coping ability of patient and family and take measures as indicated.	Patient will achieve psychophysiologic stability. Patient will demonstrate a decrease in anxiety.	Continue to assess coping ability of patient and family. Provide information on coping mechanisms for use after discharge. Address concerns patient may have about impact on daily life.

Thoracic Surgery Interdisciplinary Outcome Pathway

COORDINATION OF CARE

Diagnosis/Stabilization Phase		Acute Management Phase		Recovery Phase	
Outcome	Interventions	Outcome	Interventions	Outcome	Interventions
All appropriate team members and disciplines will be involved.	Develop plan of care with the patient/family, primary care physician, thoracic surgeon, pulmonologist, anesthesiologist, RN, advanced practice nurse, RCP, social services, chaplain, and case manager.	All appropriate team members and disciplines will be involved in plan of care.	Update plan of care with patient/family and other team members including discharge planner and dietitian. Assess support systems at home. Initiate planning for anticipated discharge and call home health as indicated. Consult pulmonary rehabilitation if indicated. Begin teaching patient/family about care at home. Assess ability to manage at home versus extended care.	Patient will understand how to maintain optimal health at home.	Provide information concerning care at home and any follow-up visits. Provide patient/family with phone numbers of resources available to answer questions. Coordinate home care with appropriate home care agency as needed. Refer to pulmonary rehabilitation if feasible.

DIAGNOSTICS

Diagnosis/Stabilization Phase		Acute Management Phase		Recovery Phase	
Outcome	Interventions	Outcome	Interventions	Outcome	Interventions
Patient will understand any tests or procedures that must be completed (IVs, I & O, indwelling lines, ventilator, lab work, and chest tubes).	Explain all procedures and tests to patient/family. Be sensitive to individualized needs of patient/family for information. Establish effective communication technique with patient while intubated.	Patient will understand any tests or procedures that must be completed such as removal of chest tubes, indwelling line, lab work, CXR, IS.	Explain procedures and tests needed to assess recovery from surgery such as PFT, peak flow, and respiratory medicines.	Patient will understand meaning of diagnostic tests in relation to continued health (lab tests, increase in activity, coughing and deep breathing, IS).	Ensure that patient/family understand disease and surgery results. Discuss appropriate measures patient can take to help to return to normal. Provide patient with guidelines concerning follow-up care. Provide instruction on care at home after discharge (i.e., when to call the physician, care of incision, activity limitations, medications, and diet).

Thoracic Surgery Interdisciplinary Outcome Pathway (continued)

FLUID BALANCE

Diagnosis/Stabilization Phase		Acute Management Phase		Recovery Phase	
Outcome	Interventions	Outcome	Interventions	Outcome	Interventions
Patient will achieve optimal hemodynamic status as evidenced by: • MAP >70 mmHg • hemodynamic parameters WNL • UO >0.5 mL/kg/hr • free from dysrhythmias Patient will remain free from excessive bleeding.	Monitor and treat the following hemodynamic parameters: • HR • BP • CVP • I & O • LOC • peripheral pulses • dysrhythmias Assess for increase in chest tube drainage. Monitor lab values: Hgb, Hct, electrolytes, clotting studies. Monitor for complications: pneumonia, pulmonary embolus, MI, shock, bleeding.	Patient will maintain optimal hemodynamic status. Patient will remain free from dysrhythmias.	Monitor and treat cardiac variables. Assist with chest tube and indwelling line removal and monitor patient afterward. Monitor and treat dysrhythmias per protocol. Begin patient/family teaching on the disease process, current treatment, and expected clinical course. Monitor lab values: CBC, SMA-6, ABGs. Maintain optimal hydration based on assessment. Assess need for diuretics and/or K+ repletion, and blood products. Continue to monitor for complications.	Patient will maintain optimal hemodynamic status.	Continue assessment and interventions. Continue teaching and assess for understanding: • optimal fluid balance • signs and symptoms of fluid overload and dehydration • importance of daily weights

NUTRITION

Diagnosis/Stabilization Phase		Acute Management Phase		Recovery Phase	
Outcome	Interventions	Outcome	Interventions	Outcome	Interventions
Patient will be adequately nourished as evidenced by: • stable weight • weight not >10% below or >20% above IBW • albumin >3.5 g/dL • protein 6–8 g/dL • total lymphocyte count 1,000–3,000	Maintain patient NPO until extubation. If extubation is delayed >24h, assess need for alternative nutritional therapy. Monitor response to clear liquids once patient is extubated. Remove NG tube (if utilized), once extubated. Administer antiemetic, H2 blockers, and antacids if needed. Assess nutritional status.	Patient will be adequately nourished. Patient will remain free from nausea. Patient will demonstrate return of appetite.	Advance to heart healthy diet. Monitor response to diet. Assess bowel sounds. Administer laxatives/stool softeners as needed. Consult dietitian as needed for: • unanticipated weight loss • albumin <3.0 • eating less than half of food on tray Weigh daily.	Patient will be adequately nourished.	Estimate caloric need. Teach patient/family about need for adequate nutrition and need to follow heart healthy diet: • total fat intake <30% caloric intake • total saturated fat intake <10% of caloric intake • total cholesterol intake <300 mg daily intake • caloric restriction if needed • viatamin and mineral supplements • sodium restriction if needed Assess understanding.

MOBILITY

	Diagnosis/Stabilization Phase		Acute Management Phase		Recovery Phase
Outcome	**Interventions**	**Outcome**	**Interventions**	**Outcome**	**Interventions**
Patient will maintain normal ROM and muscle strength.	Begin passive/active-assist ROM exercises. Turn and position q2h (for pneumonectomy patients, affected side down only unless ordered otherwise). Dangle evening of surgery if possible. PT to assess ambulation, mobility, muscle flexibility, strength, and tone. OT to assess functional ability. PT/OT to help determine and direct activity goals.	Patient will achieve optimal mobility.	Progress exercise as tolerated: dangle, bathroom privileges, OOB for meals, and walking 50 feet. Monitor response to increased activity. Decrease if adverse events occur (tachycardia, chest discomfort, dyspnea, ectopy). Increase oxygen during exercise if needed based on SpO_2. Provide physical assistance or assistive devices as necessary. Begin patient/family teaching on principles of exercise program.	Patient will achieve optimal mobility.	Walk at least 200 to 300 feet TID to QID. Walk up and down one flight of stairs. Teach patient/family about home exercise program. Refer to outpatient pulmonary rehabilitation if feasible. Consider PT/OT in the home if necessary.

OXYGENATION/VENTILATION

	Diagnosis/Stabilization Phase		Acute Management Phase		Recovery Phase
Outcome	**Interventions**	**Outcome**	**Interventions**	**Outcome**	**Interventions**
Patient will have adequate gas exchange as evidenced by: • $SaO_2 2 > 90\%$ $SpO_2 > 92\%$ • ABGs WNL • clear breath sounds • respiratory rate, depth, and rhythm WNL • CXR clear • demonstrated ability to cough and clear secretions	Monitor ventilator settings and wakefulness and determine readiness to wean. Monitor hemodynamic variables before, during, and after weaning. Wean ventilator and monitor patient response: • wean FiO_2 to keep SpO_2 >92% • monitor effects of anesthesia and wean ventilator accordingly After extubation, apply supplemental oxygen. Monitor for signs and symptoms of respiratory distress as evidenced by: • use of accessory muscle	Patient will have adequate gas exchange.	Monitor and treat oxygenation/ventilatory status per ABGs, SpO_2, chest assessment, and CXR. Monitor and treat complications that may impair ventilation and oxygenation: pneumonia, atelectasis, pulmonary edema, ARDS, respiratory insufficiency, pneumothorax, MI, CHF, subcutaneous emphysema. Assess for improvement in breath sounds, thin white secretions, and adequate cough reflexes. Teach patient/family effective cough techniques (cascade, huff).	Patient will have optimal ventilation and gas exchange.	Obtain CXR before discharge. Teach patient/family about IS and the use of the chest splint pillow at home. Teach patient/family about medications when needed for underlying pulmonary disease. Teach patient/family signs and symptoms of respiratory infection and when to treat symptoms. Call physician for yellow or green sputum, fever, or cough.

Thoracic Surgery Interdisciplinary Outcome Pathway (continued)

OXYGENATION/VENTILATION (continued)

Diagnosis/Stabilization Phase		Acute Management Phase		Recovery Phase	
Outcome	Interventions	Outcome	Interventions	Outcome	Interventions
	• ineffective cough • dyspnea • adventitious breath sounds • alteration in LOC • abnormal ABGs Monitor pulse oximetry. Keep SpO$_2$ >92%. Reinforce use of SpO$_2$ q2h. IS when extubated. HOB elevated 30 degrees when possible. Maintain adequate humidification.		Support patient with oxygen therapy as indicated. Reinforce use of IS. Have patient give return demonstration. Provide chest splint pillow and instruct on proper use. Have patient give return demonstration. Monitor secretions and need for bronchodilator therapy.		

COMFORT

Diagnosis/Stabilization Phase		Acute Management Phase		Recovery Phase	
Outcome	Interventions	Outcome	Interventions	Outcome	Interventions
Patient will be as comfortable and pain free as possible as evidenced by: • no objective indicators of discomfort • no complaints of discomfort • normal VS	Anticipate need for analgesia and provide as needed. Use a pain scale or visual analogue tool. Assess response to analgesics and effects on ability to wean from ventilator when indicated. Use newer NSAID drugs with few side effects. Ensure safety and effectiveness of epidural catheter if used. Provide reassurance in a calm, caring, and competent manner.	Patient will be as comfortable and pain free as possible.	Anticipate need for analgesics and provide as needed; assess response. (Use sedation cautiously with COPD patients.) Provide chest splint pillow and instruct on proper use. Provide uninterrupted periods of rest. Assist patient with relaxation techniques and other therapies to promote relaxation such as music, touch therapy and imagery. Provide analgesics as needed before chest tube removal,	Patient will be relaxed and as comfortable as possible.	Progress analgesics to oral medications as needed; assess response. Teach patient/family regarding analgesic administration and potential side effects for postdischarge. Continue alternative methods to promote relaxation. Teach patient/family alternative methods to promote relaxation at home. Provide uninterrupted periods of rest.

Keep HOB elevated to increase breathing comfort. Establish effective communication with intubated patient.

ambulation, and any other procedures.
Observe for complications that may cause discomfort: pneumonia, pulmonary embolus, and bronchospasm.

SKIN INTEGRITY

Diagnosis/Stabilization Phase		Acute Management Phase		Recovery Phase	
Outcome	Interventions	Outcome	Interventions	Outcome	Interventions
Patient will have intact skin without abrasions or pressure ulcers. Patient will have healing surgical wound free of infection.	Assess all bony prominences at least q4h and treat if needed. Maintain integrity of all dressings. Use sterile technique with all dressing changes.	Patient will have intact skin without abrasions, pressure ulcers, or wound infections.	Use preventive pressure-reducing devices if patient is at high risk for developing pressure ulcers or has prolonged bed rest. Treat pressure ulcers according to hospital protocol. Assess chest incisions and chest tube sites for drainage, erythema, and induration. Observe for subcutaneous emphysema. Teach patient/family proper skin care at home; incision care.	Patient will have intact skin without abrasions, pressure ulcers, or wound infections.	Assess all wounds/incisions for signs/symptoms of infection. Culture if necessary. Reinforce importance of proper hygiene and wound care. Continue patient/family teaching on skin care at home. Assess need for home health care visits. Teach patient sterile dressing techniques if necessary.

PROTECTION/SAFETY

Diagnosis/Stabilization Phase		Acute Management Phase		Recovery Phase	
Outcome	Interventions	Outcome	Interventions	Outcome	Interventions
Patient will be protected from possible harm.	Assess need for wrist restraints while patient is intubated, has a decreased LOC, or is agitated and restless. Explain need for restraints to patient/family. Assess response to restraints and check q1–2h for skin integrity and impairment to circulation. Remove restraints as soon as patient is awake from anesthesia and able to follow instructions.	Patient will be protected from possible harm.	Provide physical assistance when dangling or getting OOB; monitor response. Support chest tubes when ambulating patient.	Patient will be protected from possible harm.	Provide support with ambulation and climbing stairs. Teach patient/family about physical limitations postdischarge. Review signs and symptoms to report to physician. Continue PT/OT in the home if necessary. Refer to outpatient pulmonary rehabilitation if feasible.

Thoracic Surgery Interdisciplinary Outcome Pathway (continued)

PROTECTION/SAFETY (continued)

Diagnosis/Stabilization Phase		Acute Management Phase		Recovery Phase	
Outcome	Interventions	Outcome	Interventions	Outcome	Interventions
	Follow hospital protocol for use of restraints. Provide sedatives/anxiolytic agents as needed. Be mindful of effect on respiratory status.				

PSYCHOSOCIAL/SELF-DETERMINATION

Diagnosis/Stabilization Phase		Acute Management Phase		Recovery Phase	
Outcome	Interventions	Outcome	Interventions	Outcome	Interventions
Patient will achieve psychophysiologic stability. Patient will demonstrate a decrease in anxiety as evidenced by stable VS and subjective reports. Patient will begin acceptance of disease process.	Assess psychologic effects of critical care. Provide sedatives as indicated. Play close attention to effect on respiratory status. Take measures to reduce sensory overload such as uninterrupted periods of rest. Develop effective interventions to communicate with patient while intubated. Allow flexible visiting to meet family/patient needs. Determine emotional impact and coping ability of patient and take appropriate measures to meet needs. Diagnosis may be cancer. Conduct a family needs assessment and employ measures to meet identified concerns.	Patient will achieve psychophysiologic stability. Patient will demonstrate a decrease in anxiety. Patient will continue acceptance of disease process.	Take measures to decrease sensory overload. Provide adequate rest periods. Provide sedatives as needed; monitor respiratory status. Continue to assess coping ability of patient/family and take measures as indicated. Involve patient/family in health care decisions.	Patient will achieve psychophysiologic stability. Patient will demonstrate a decrease in anxiety. Patient will continue acceptance of disease process.	Provide adequate periods of rest. Continue to assess coping ability of patient and family. Provide information on coping mechanisms for use after discharge. Refer to outside services or agencies as appropriate (chaplain, social services, or home health). Include patient/family in decisions concerning care. Continue to use alternative therapies to promote relaxation. Address concerns patient may have about impact on daily life.

CHAPTER 3

Gastrointestinal Pathways

Cirrhosis and Portal Hypertension Interdisciplinary Outcome Pathway

COORDINATION OF CARE

Diagnosis/Stabilization Phase		Acute Management Phase		Recovery Phase	
Outcome	Interventions	Outcome	Interventions	Outcome	Interventions
All appropriate team members and disciplines will be involved in the plan of care.	Develop the plan of care with the patient/family, primary physician(s), gastroenterologist, RN, advanced practice nurse, transplant team, RCP, and other specialists as needed.	All appropriate team members and disciplines will be involved in the plan of care.	Update the plan of care with all team members, dietitian, chaplain, social worker, and PT. Initiate planning for anticipated discharge. Involve home health care and home equipment supply company if necessary. Begin teaching patient/family about home care. Involve transplant team as necessary.	Patient/family will understand how to maintain optimal health at home.	Teach patient/family about any follow-up visits. Coordinate home care with continuing care agency. Arrange for any equipment needed at home. Provide guidelines concerning follow-up care to patient/family: • medications • dietary restrictions • activity limitations • when to call the physician Provide patient/family with phone number of resources available to answer questions. Confer as needed with outpatient care team members.

DIAGNOSTICS

Diagnosis/Stabilization Phase		Acute Management Phase		Recovery Phase	
Outcome	Interventions	Outcome	Interventions	Outcome	Interventions
Patient/family will understand any tests or procedures that must be completed (lab tests, endoscopy, x-rays, CT scan, biopsies, surgical procedures, transplant workup, and angiography).	Explain all procedures and tests to patient/family. Be sensitive to patient and family's individual needs for information. Be prepared to repeat information frequently in easy to understand terminology.	Patient/family will understand tests and procedures that are necessary (monitoring, critical care, further diagnostic testing).	Explain procedures and tests needed to assess progress and prognosis of liver dysfunction. Anticipate need for further diagnostic tests and interventions. Continue to involve transplant team as needed.	Patient/family will understand tests and procedures that are needed in course of liver dysfunction.	Review with patient and family before discharge the results of significant tests and how the patient's baseline values compare to normal. Discuss any measures patient will need to take to deal with abnormal findings (i.e., hypercholesterolemia). Provide patient/family with guidelines concerning care at home: • when to call the physician

- when to call other health care providers
- medications
- physical limitations
- dietary restrictions
- skin care
- follow-up care

FLUID BALANCE

Diagnosis/Stabilization Phase		Acute Management Phase		Recovery Phase	
Outcome	Interventions	Outcome	Interventions	Outcome	Interventions
Patient will achieve optimal hemodynamic status as evidenced by: • MAP > 70 mmHg • hemodynamic parameters WNL • UO >0.5 mL/kg/hr • no bleeding • absence of cardiac dysrhythmias	Monitor and treat: • hemodynamic parameters • BP • SvO_2 • CO/CI • SV/SI Assess for alterations in LOC. Monitor evidence of tissue perfusion (pain, pulses, color, temperature, altered LOC, ileus, decreased UO). Monitor lab values: bilirubin, albumin, aspartate aminotransferase, alanine aminotransferase, ABGs, PT, PTT, CBC, ammonia level, creatinine, gamma-glutamyl transferase, lactate dehydrogenase, alkaline phosphatase, cholesterol. Monitor and treat potentially life-threatening cardiac dysrhythmias. Observe for signs of obvious or insidious bleeding and administer blood products as needed. Assess response. Anticipate need for vasopressor agents; assess response and titrate according to BP, HR, and evidence of tissue perfusion. Assess for peripheral edema and ascites. Be prepared for paracentesis.	Patient will maintain optimal hemodynamic status.	Continue as in Diagnosis/Stabilization Phase. Weigh daily. Administer diuretics if required and monitor UO. Begin patient/family teaching on liver dysfunction, current treatment, and expected clinical course. Monitor for signs of decreased tissue perfusion (decreased UO, MI, altered LOC, ARDS, ileus).	Patient will maintain optimal hemodynamic status.	Continue to monitor for signs of decreased tissue perfusion. Teach patient/family: • signs of complications (jaundice, bleeding tendencies, neurologic changes) • when to seek medical attention • fluid management • signs of fluid overload/deficit and actions to take • daily weight

Cirrhosis and Portal Hypertension Interdisciplinary Outcome Pathway (continued)

FLUID BALANCE (continued)

Diagnosis/Stabilization Phase		Acute Management Phase		Recovery Phase	
Outcome	Interventions	Outcome	Interventions	Outcome	Interventions
	Monitor for possible complications associated with liver dysfunction and treat accordingly (coagulopathies, pleural effusion, renal insufficiency, upper GI bleed, bacteremia, bleeding varices, altered LOC, infection, cardiac problems, ascites). Assess need for referral for liver transplantation evaluation. Monitor EKG continuously. Administer IV Pitressin as ordered. Monitor for side effects (coronary vasoconstriction, dysrhythmias, MI, bradycardia, decreased CO, hypertension, abdominal cramps, and tissue sloughing).				

NUTRITION

Diagnosis/Stabilization Phase		Acute Management Phase		Recovery Phase	
Outcome	Interventions	Outcome	Interventions	Outcome	Interventions
Patient will be adequately nourished as evidenced by: • correction of nutritional deficiencies including carbohydrates, fat, protein stores, vitamin and trace elements • albumin at least 3.0–3.5 g/dL	Assess nutritional status. If intubated, initiate alternative nutritional therapy. Consult dietitian or nutritional support team to determine/direct nutritional support. Initiate recommended diet and monitor response. Restrict sodium and/or protein if appropriate. Assess bowel sounds, abdominal distension, and ascites.	Patient will be adequately nourished as evidenced by continued correction of nutritional deficiencies, liver enzymes returning to normal, and no evidence of fluid retention.	Continue recommended diet and monitor response. Progress to DAT and monitor response. Monitor serum protein and albumin levels. Weigh daily. Be cognizant that fluid shifts may occur resulting in ascites or edema. Thus loss of lean body mass may occur with no change in weight.	Patient will be adequately nourished.	Teach patient/family: • daily caloric requirements • low fat, low sodium, low protein diet restrictions as recommended for patient • no alcohol Teach patient/family to monitor for sudden weight gain and actions to take should such weight gain occur. Recommend services to assist with alcohol dependence if necessary.

- total protein at least 6.0 g/dL
- total lymphocyte count 1,000–3,000

Monitor albumin, prealbumin, total protein, cholesterol, triglycerides, and lymphocyte count.

Consider calorie count to determine if intake meeting nutritional goals.

MOBILITY

Diagnosis/Stabilization Phase		Acute Management Phase		Recovery Phase	
Outcome	Interventions	Outcome	Interventions	Outcome	Interventions
Patient will maintain normal muscle strength and tone.	PT to assess ambulation, mobility, muscle strength, flexibility, and tone. OT to assess functional ability. PT/OT to help determine and direct activity goals. Begin passive/active-assist ROM exercises.	Patient will achieve optimal mobility.	Continue as in Diagnosis/Stabilization Phase. Monitor response to increased activity and decrease if adverse events occur (tachycardia, dysrhythmias, dyspnea, syncope). Monitor SpO$_2$ with increased activity. Apply supplemental oxygen to keep SpO$_2$ > 92%. Provide physical assistance or assistive devices with activity as necessary. Space activities to allow for adequate rest periods. Allow patient to assist in ADLs as tolerated.	Patient will achieve optimal mobility.	Instruct patient/family about activity limitations. Instruct patient/family about progressive activity program.

OXYGENATION/VENTILATION

Diagnosis/Stabilization Phase		Acute Management Phase		Recovery Phase	
Outcome	Interventions	Outcome	Interventions	Outcome	Interventions
Patient will have adequate gas exchange as evidenced by: • normal CXR • respiratory rate, depth, and rhythm WNL • clear breath sounds bilaterally • SaO$_2$ > 90 • ABGs WNL	Monitor respiratory pattern, SaO$_2$, breath sounds, muscle strength, coughing ability, ABGs, Hgb, SpO$_2$, and CXR. Be prepared for intubation and mechanical ventilation. Monitor ventilator settings and hemodynamic variables before, during, and after weaning. Apply supplemental oxygen and monitor with pulse oximetry to keep SpO$_2$ > 92%.	Patient will have adequate gas exchange.	Monitor oxygenation disturbances with ABGs, SaO$_2$, and SpO$_2$. Treat as needed. Monitor ventilation disturbances with CXR, chest assessments, ABGs, and breath sounds. Treat as needed. Observe for complications of liver dysfunction that may impair oxygenation/ventilation status: ascites, pleural effusion, infection, pneumonia, pulmonary embolus.	Patient will have optimal ventilation and gas exchange.	Teach patient/family about home medications. Teach patient/family signs and symptoms of respiratory infection and when to report symptoms. Refer to outpatient pulmonary rehabilitation program if indicated. Refer to smoking cessation program if needed. Recommend support groups or organizations to provide assistance with smoking cessation.

Cirrhosis and Portal Hypertension Interdisciplinary Outcome Pathway (continued)

OXYGENATION/VENTILATION (continued)

Diagnosis/Stabilization Phase		Acute Management Phase		Recovery Phase	
Outcome	Interventions	Outcome	Interventions	Outcome	Interventions
• absence of dyspnea, cyanosis, and secretions • VS WNL • CO WNL • SpO_2 > 92%	Assess effects of ascites on respiratory status. If patient can tolerate, elevate HOB.		Wean from oxygen therapy or mechanical ventilation as condition improves. Monitor SpO_2. Encourage coughing and deep breathing at least q2h. Use humidification to thin secretions if indicated. Assess effects of increased activity on respiratory status. Monitor with pulse oximetry. Use supplemental oxygen to keep SpO_2 > 92%. Initiate discussion on smoking cessation if applicable.		

COMFORT

Diagnosis/Stabilization Phase		Acute Management Phase		Recovery Phase	
Outcome	Interventions	Outcome	Interventions	Outcome	Interventions
Patient will be as comfortable and pain free as possible as evidenced by: • no objective indicators of discomfort • no complaints of discomfort • normal VS	Assess absence of, or quantity and quality of, discomfort. Use visual analogue scale or other pain scale. Administer analgesics when indicated and assess response. Monitor effect of analgesics on respiratory status and liver function. Provide reassurance in a calm, caring, and competent manner. In intubated patients, establish effective communication method so patient can communicate discomfort.	Patient will be as comfortable and pain free as possible.	Continue as in Diagnosis/Stabilization Phase. Observe for complications of liver dysfunction that may cause discomfort: ascites, bleeding, pleural effusion. Teach patient/family relaxation techniques and have them give return demonstration. Use complementary therapies such as guided imagery, music, humor, or touch therapy to promote relaxation.	Patient will be as comfortable and pain free as possible.	Teach patient/family alternative methods to promote relaxation and comfort after discharge. Teach patient/family proper use of analgesics, both prescribed and OTC.

SKIN INTEGRITY

Diagnosis/Stabilization Phase		Acute Management Phase		Recovery Phase	
Outcome	Interventions	Outcome	Interventions	Outcome	Interventions
Patient will have intact skin without abrasions or pressure ulcers.	Assess for jaundice, erythema, dry skin, and other skin disorders associated with liver dysfunction. Assess all body prominences q4h and treat if needed. Use preventive pressure-reducing devices when patient is at high risk for developing pressure ulcers. Follow hospital protocol for treatment of pressure ulcers. Maintain meticulous oral hygiene.	Patient will have intact skin without abrasions or pressure ulcers.	Continue as in Diagnosis/Stabilization Phase.	Patient will have intact skin without abrasions or pressure ulcers.	Instruct patient/family about interventions to continue at home for proper skin care. Instruct patient/family to inspect skin at least daily and to report lesions and nonhealing wounds to physician.

PROTECTION/SAFETY

Diagnosis/Stabilization Phase		Acute Management Phase		Recovery Phase	
Outcome	Interventions	Outcome	Interventions	Outcome	Interventions
Patient will be protected from possible harm.	Assess need for wrist restraints if patient is intubated, restless, agitated, or has altered LOC. Explain need for restraints to patient/family. Follow hospital protocol for use of restraints. If restraints are used, check for skin integrity and impairment to circulation q1–2h. Remove restraints as soon as possible. Assess need for assistance with activities and provide physical support as needed. Monitor for hepatic encephalopathy. Allow family to remain with patient if they have calming influence.	Patient will be protected from possible harm.	Give appropriate physical assistance as patient increases mobility to prevent falls or injury. Continue to monitor for hepatic encephalopathy. Allow family to remain with patient if they have calming influence.	Patient will be protected from possible harm.	Review with patient/family any physical limitations in activity before discharge.

Cirrhosis and Portal Hypertension Interdisciplinary Outcome Pathway (continued)

PSYCHOSOCIAL/SELF-DETERMINATION

Diagnosis/Stabilization Phase		Acute Management Phase		Recovery Phase	
Outcome	Interventions	Outcome	Interventions	Outcome	Interventions
Patient will achieve psychophysiologic stability. Patient will demonstrate a decreased level of anxiety as evidenced by: • normal VS • normal mental status for patient • patient reports feeling less anxious Patient will begin acceptance process of liver disease.	Assess physiologic effect of environment on patient (hemodynamic variables, psychological status, signs of increased sympathetic response). Assess patient for appropriate level of stress. Assess personal responses of patient regarding critical illness. Determine coping ability of patient/family and take appropriate measures (provide explanations, allow patient/family to verbalize feelings and concerns, consult support services, allow flexible visiting to meet patient/family needs, have family conferences). Begin discussion of possible liver transplantation if indicated. Observe patient's patterns of thinking and communicating. Use calm, caring, competent, and reassuring approach with all interventions. Take measures to reduce sensory overload such as providing uninterrupted periods of rest. Arrange for flexible visitation to meet needs of patient and family.	Patient will achieve psychophysiologic stability. Patient will continue acceptance process of liver disease.	Continue as in Diagnosis/Stabilization Phase. Continue psychological and emotional support of patient and family. Assist patient in identifying quality of life issues important to him or her. Assist patient in identifying positive coping mechanisms. Allow patient/family to verbalize feelings. Involve transplant team as needed.	Patient will achieve psychophysiologic stability. Patient will continue acceptance process of liver disease.	Continue to assess patient for psychophysiologic stability. Include patient/family in decisions regarding care. Provide support and instruct on coping mechanisms for chronic illness. Refer to outpatient counseling as needed. Involve transplant team as necessary. Address concerns patient may have about impact on daily life.

Gastrointestinal Bleeding Interdisciplinary Outcome Pathway

COORDINATION OF CARE

Diagnosis/Stabilization Phase		Acute Management Phase		Recovery Phase	
Outcome	Interventions	Outcome	Interventions	Outcome	Interventions
All appropriate team members and disciplines will be involved in the plan of care.	Develop the plan of care with patient/family, primary nurse(s), primary physician(s), gastroenterologist, other specialists as needed, RN, advanced practice nurse, RCP, chaplain, and social services. The patient's history may be obtained from the family if the patient is unable to give it.	All appropriate disciplines will be consulted.	Update the plan of care with patient/family, other team members, dietitian, discharge planner, case manager, home health agency, PT (if indicated). Initiate planning for anticipated discharge. Begin teaching patient/family about home care: • medications • dietary restrictions • signs/symptoms of bleeding • fluid volume deficit	Patient/family will understand how to maintain optimal health at home.	Provide guidelines concerning follow-up care to patient/family. Provide patient/family with phone numbers of resources available to answer questions. Assist patient/family with identification of risk factors for further bleeding. Teach patient/family measures to take to prevent further bleeding. Refer to support group, if applicable.

DIAGNOSTICS

Diagnosis/Stabilization Phase		Acute Management Phase		Recovery Phase	
Outcome	Interventions	Outcome	Interventions	Outcome	Interventions
Patient/family will understand any tests or procedures that need to be completed: VS, I & O, hemodynamic monitoring, x-rays, CT scan, MRI, lab work, GI tubes, endoscopy, sclerotherapy, arteriography, barium radiographs, ABGs, EKG, pulse oximetry, IV lines, blood therapy, endoscope electrocoagulation, transcatheter embolization, photocoagulation.	Explain all tests and procedures to patient/family. Be sensitive to patient/family individualized needs for information.	Patient/family will understand any tests or procedures that need to be completed. Patient/family will understand any surgical interventions that may be required.	Anticipate need for and prepare patient/family for further treatment such as surgery, endoscopy, and photocoagulation. Explain surgical interventions to patient/family.	Patient/family will understand meaning of diagnostic tests in relation to continued health.	Review with patient/family results of tests before discharge. Discuss abnormal findings and appropriate measures patient/family can take to return to prehospital condition. Provide guidelines concerning: • when to call physician • physical restrictions • dietary restrictions • skin care • medications • care of incision • follow-up appointments

Gastrointestinal Bleeding Interdisciplinary Outcome Pathway (continued)

FLUID BALANCE

Diagnosis/Stabilization Phase		Acute Management Phase		Recovery Phase	
Outcome	Interventions	Outcome	Interventions	Outcome	Interventions
Patient will achieve optimal hemodynamic status as evidenced by: • MAP > 70 mmHg • VS WNL for the patient • hemodynamic parameters WNL • no bleeding • UO > 0.5mL/kg/hr • LOC WNL Patient will achieve good tissue perfusion as evidenced by: • warm, dry skin • good pulses • no pallor	Monitor and treat hemodynamic parameters: • BP • CO/CI • SV • PA pressures • CVP • PCWP • SVR/PVR • SvO_2 • temperature • pulse pressure • cardiac rhythm Monitor VS q1h and PRN until stable. Monitor for orthostatic changes in blood pressure and narrowing pulse pressure. Assess I & O q1h. Measure and record gastric drainage every shift or as indicated during acute bleed. Use a large-bore NG tube. Monitor lab values: CBC, electrolytes, sodium, coagulation studies, BUN, platelets, creatinine, reticulocyte count. If acute upper GI bleed continues, use room temperature saline and lavage stomach until clear. Monitor patient for abdominal pain and rebound tenderness. Monitor for signs and symptoms of fluid volume deficit: • sluggish skin turgor • dry mouth • skin and mucous membranes • sunken eyes • weight loss	Patient will maintain optimal hemodynamic status. Patient will maintain good tissue perfusion.	Continue as in Diagnosis/Stabilization Phase. Monitor and treat hemodynamic parameters, VS, I & O, and fluid volume status q2–4h and PRN. Monitor lab values: CBC, electrolytes, coagulation studies, platelets, BUN, and creatinine. Begin teaching patient/family about GI system, current problems, treatment plans, and expected clinical course. Administer antacids as ordered and monitor for side effects.	Patient will maintain optimal hemodynamic status. Patient will maintain good tissue perfusion.	Continue as in Diagnosis/Stabilization and Acute Management phases. Monitor and treat hemodynamic parameters, VS, I & O, and fluid volume status q4h and PRN. Teach patient/family risk factors that increase gastric acidity, thus increasing the chance of bleeding: • smoking • alcohol abuse • NSAIDs • reserpine • caffeine • aspirin • corticosteroids • oral contraceptives Instruct patient on purpose, dose, schedule, and side effects of antacids, H_2 receptor antagonists, prostaglandins, and any other antiulcer medications as prescribed. Teach patient also about OTC medications now available. Monitor Hgb for several weeks. Teach patient/family signs and symptoms of recurrent bleeding and fluid volume deficit.

Administer normal saline, lactated Ringer's, crystalloids, colloidal agents, and blood products as ordered.

Monitor for signs and symptoms of fluid overload: dyspnea, JVD, edema, crackles.

Assess gastric pH and check GI aspirate for blood q1–4h and administer antacids or sucralfate as ordered.

Administer H_2 receptor antagonists as ordered and monitor for side effects.

Guiac all stools. Stools may be guiaic positive up to 12 days after the bleed.

Monitor for complications that can occur from GI bleed:
- hypovolemic shock
- acute tubular necrosis
- hepatic failure
- metabolic acidosis
- loss of consciousness
- neurologic insult
- dysrhythmias
- cardiac ischemia
- DIC
- sepsis

If massive blood transfusion is necessary, monitor for complications of massive blood therapy:
- hyperkalemia
- hypocalcemia
- hypothermia
- metabolic acidosis
- infection
- coagulopathies
- DIC
- ARDS
- hypervolemia
- circulatory overload
- febrile transfusions

Monitor UO q1h.

Monitor for hematemesis, melena, and/or hematochezia.

Gastrointestinal Bleeding Interdisciplinary Outcome Pathway (continued)

FLUID BALANCE (continued)

Diagnosis/Stabilization Phase		Acute Management Phase		Recovery Phase	
Outcome	Interventions	Outcome	Interventions	Outcome	Interventions
	Assist with endoscopic or angiographic procedures to assess and treat bleeding. Prepare patient/family for surgery if indicated. Assess evidence of tissue perfusion (pain, pulses, color, temperature, sign of decreased perfusion such as decreased VO_2, altered LOC, and ileus). Administer vasopressin infusion and observe for side effects (angina, dysrhythmias, MI, edema, HA, N & V, pulmonary edema). Vasodilators may be used concomitantly. Assess bowel sounds q2h and PRN.				

NUTRITION

Diagnosis/Stabilization Phase		Acute Management Phase		Recovery Phase	
Outcome	Interventions	Outcome	Interventions	Outcome	Interventions
Patient will be adequately nourished as evidenced by: • stable weight not >10% below or >20% above IBW • albumin >3.5 g/dL • total protein 6–8 g/dL • total lymphocyte count 1,000–3,000	NPO if acutely bleeding. Assess total protein, albumin, prealbumin, and lymphocyte count. Begin alternative nutrition such as total parenteral nutrition if bleeding precludes enteral route. Assess bowel sounds q4h (hyperactive in upper GI bleed, hypoactive/normal in lower GI bleed). Weigh daily. Monitor electrolytes.	Patient will be adequately nourished.	Begin clear liquids and monitor patient's response. Consult dietitian to help determine and direct nutritional support. Consider need for caloric count. Continue to monitor weight and nutritional parameters daily. Consult dietitian if: • albumin <3.0 • eating less than half of food on tray • for dietary counseling	Patient will be adequately nourished.	Teach patient/family necessary dietary changes: restrictions on coffee, tea, chocolate, spicy foods, high roughage, alcohol, and milk products Products just listed may contribute to mucosal irritation, acid secretions, or varices irritation.

MOBILITY

Diagnosis/Stabilization Phase		Acute Management Phase		Recovery Phase	
Outcome	Interventions	Outcome	Interventions	Outcome	Interventions
Patient will achieve optimal mobility.	Assess degree of mobility and muscle strength. Begin passive/active-assist ROM exercises.	Patient will achieve optimal mobility.	Continue as in Diagnosis/Stabilization Phase. PT to assess ambulation, mobility, ROM, muscle strength and tone. OT to assess functional ability. Monitor response to increased activity. Decrease activity if adverse events occur (tachycardia, discomfort, dyspnea, ectopy, or hypotension). PT/OT to help determine and direct activity goals. Allow patient to assist in ADLs as tolerated. Monitor for orthostatic hypotension and treat accordingly. Provide physical assistance or assistive devices as necessary.	Patient will achieve optimal mobility.	Instruct patient/family about exercise program. Teach patient/family proper use of assistive devices. Have patient/family give return demonstration.

OXYGENATION/VENTILATION

Diagnosis/Stabilization Phase		Acute Management Phase		Recovery Phase	
Outcome	Interventions	Outcome	Interventions	Outcome	Interventions
Patient will have adequate gas exchange and tissue perfusion as evidenced by: • SaO_2 >90% • SpO_2 >92% • ABGs WNL for the patient • SvO_2 60–80% • UO >0.5mL/kg/hr • alert and oriented	Monitor respiratory status: rate, rhythm, and depth of breathing; CXR; ABGs; pulse oximetry; and SvO_2. Be prepared for intubation and mechanical ventilation. If necessary, assist with monitoring or adjusting of ventilator settings to maintain appropriate level of assistance and minute ventilation. Involve RCP. Monitor Hgb and Hct q2–4h until stable.	Patient will have adequate gas exchange and tissue perfusion.	Continue as in Diagnosis/Stabilization Phase. Monitor Hgb and Hct q12–24h. Monitor and treat oxygenation/ventilation disturbances as per ABGs or SaO_2/SvO_2. Wean oxygen therapy/mechanical ventilation as indicated. Involve RCP as necessary. Teach patient/family about oxygenation needs and treatments provided. Assess effects of increased activity on oxygenation status.	Patient will have adequate gas exchange and tissue perfusion.	Continue as in Acute Management Phase. Teach patient/family about home care O_2 needs if applicable. Monitor Hgb for several weeks after bleed.

Gastrointestinal Bleeding Interdisciplinary Outcome Pathway (continued)

OXYGENATION/VENTILATION (continued)

Diagnosis/Stabilization Phase		Acute Management Phase		Recovery Phase	
Outcome	Interventions	Outcome	Interventions	Outcome	Interventions
• respiratory rate, depth, and rhythm WNL • absence of dyspnea, cyanosis, and secretions • hemodynamic parameters WNL for the patient • Hgb WNL	Monitor ABGs or SpO_2/SvO_2 closely. Apply supplemental oxygen if indicated and monitor response. Monitor for hyperventilation. Monitor for signs of adequate tissue perfusion: • alert and oriented • BP and pulse WNL for patient • SvO_2 60–80% • UO > 0.5 mL/kg/hr • normal skin color and temperature Reduce tissue oxygen demands through bed rest and comfort measures. Reduce fever if present. Assess for lactic acidosis.		If patient has surgery, monitor effects of anesthesia on respiratory system. Also, supply abdominal pillow splint to assist with coughing and deep breathing. Have patient give return demonstration.		

COMFORT

Diagnosis/Stabilization Phase		Acute Management Phase		Recovery Phase	
Outcome	Interventions	Outcome	Interventions	Outcome	Interventions
Patient will be as comfortable and pain free as possible as evidenced by: • no objective indicators of pain • no complaints of discomfort	Assess discomfort: • time discomfort started • location • radiation • quantity • quality • factors that relieve • factors that aggravate Administer analgesics and monitor response. Monitor effect on respiratory status and BP. Provide mouth care frequently, especially if patient is NPO to	Patient will be as comfortable as possible.	Continue as in Diagnosis/Stabilization Phase. Instruct patient on relaxation techniques. Use complementary therapies such as touch therapy, music therapy, humor, and imagery to promote relaxation. Involve family members in strategies. Observe for complications of GI bleed that may cause discomfort: bleeding, abdominal distension, and infection.	Patient will be as comfortable as possible.	Instruct patient/family on alternative methods to promote relaxation after discharge. Refer to outpatient clinic or stress management program. Instruct patient/family on stress management techniques. Refer to support group if applicable.

minimize oral discomfort. Avoid the use of lemon and glycerin swabs, which can be drying to the mucosa. Provide reassurance in a calm, caring, and competent manner. Keep lights dimmed and environment as quiet as possible to keep physical and verbal stimulation at a minimum. Allow flexible visitation if family has calming effect on patient.

Assess any postop discomfort and treat accordingly. If surgical discomfort, use an abdominal splint pillow to assist with coughing and deep breathing. Ask patient to give a return demonstration.

SKIN INTEGRITY

Diagnosis/Stabilization Phase		Acute Management Phase		Recovery Phase	
Outcome	Interventions	Outcome	Interventions	Outcome	Interventions
Patient will have intact skin without abrasions or pressure ulcers.	Assess all bony prominences at least q4h and treat if needed. Turn q2h as hemodynamic status allows. Use preventive pressure-reducing devices if patient is at high risk for developing pressure ulcers. Treat pressure ulcers according to hospital protocol. Use superfatted or lanolin-based soap for bathing and apply emollients for dry skin.	Patient will have intact skin without abrasions or pressure ulcers.	Continue as in Diagnosis/Stabilization Phase. If surgical procedure is done, monitor incision site closely. Take measures to keep skin clean and dry. Monitor for signs and symptoms of infection at incision site.	Patient will be as comfortable as possible.	Continue as in Acute Management Phase. Teach patient/family proper skin care after discharge. If surgical procedure is done, instruct patient/family on care of incision.

PROTECTION/SAFETY

Diagnosis/Stabilization Phase		Acute Management Phase		Recovery Phase	
Outcome	Interventions	Outcome	Interventions	Outcome	Interventions
Patient will be protected from possible harm.	Assess need for wrist restraints and institute if needed. If used, check skin integrity and circulation q1h. Explain need for restraints to patient/family. Follow hospital protocol for use of restraints.	Patient will be protected from possible harm.	Continue as in Diagnosis/Stabilization Phase. If surgical procedure is done, use aseptic technique with dressing changes. Monitor incision for signs of infection.	Patient will be protected from possible harm.	Teach patient/family about any physical limitations in activity after discharge. Teach patient/family about any risk factors that can aggravate or cause another GI bleed.

Gastrointestinal Bleeding Interdisciplinary Outcome Pathway (*continued*)

PROTECTION/SAFETY (continued)

	Diagnosis/Stabilization Phase		Acute Management Phase		Recovery Phase	
Outcome	Interventions	Outcome	Interventions	Outcome	Interventions	
	Assess need for assistance with activities. Provide physical support as needed. Maintain NG suction at low level to avoid further trauma to gastric mucosa. Take measures to prevent infection.					

PSYCHOSOCIAL/SELF-DETERMINATION

	Diagnosis/Stabilization Phase		Acute Management Phase		Recovery Phase	
Outcome	Interventions	Outcome	Interventions	Outcome	Interventions	
Patient will achieve psychophysiologic stability. Patient will demonstrate a decrease in anxiety as evidenced by: • VS WNL for the patient • subjective report of decreased anxiety • objective signs of decreased anxiety Patient will begin acceptance process of GI bleed.	Assess physiologic effects of critical care environment on patient (hemodynamic variables, psychological status, signs of increased sympathetic response). If intubated, find alternative techniques with which to communicate with patient. Administer sedatives and antianxiety agents and monitor response. Use calm, caring, competent, and reassuring approach with patient/family. Allow flexible visitation to meet patient/family needs. Determine coping ability of patient/family and take appropriate measures (provide frequent explanations, allow patient to verbalize concerns, consult support services, allow family to visit often, and have family conferences). Encourage patient to verbalize feelings about condition.	Patient will achieve psychophysiologic stability. Patient will demonstrate a decrease in anxiety. Patient will continue acceptance of GI bleed.	Continue as in Diagnosis/Stabilization Phase. Allow patient to verbalize any feelings.	Patient will achieve psychophysiologic stability. Patient will demonstrate a decrease in anxiety. Patient will continue acceptance of GI bleed.	Continue as in Acute Management Phase. Provide support to patient/family in the case of unsuccessful treatment outcomes in reaching difficult decisions and accepting inevitable consequences. Address concerns about possible effects on sexual function, activities, return to work. When patient is discharged, refer to outpatient counseling, stress management program, and/or support groups.	

Pancreatitis Interdisciplinary Outcome Pathway

COORDINATION OF CARE

Diagnosis/Stabilization Phase		Acute Management Phase		Recovery Phase	
Outcome	Interventions	Outcome	Interventions	Outcome	Interventions
All appropriate team members and disciplines will be involved in the plan of care.	Develop the plan of care with patient/family, primary physician, gastroenterologist, RN, advanced practice nurse, RCP, chaplain, social services, and outcome manager.	All appropriate disciplines will be consulted.	Update the plan of care with patient, family, other team members, dietitian, discharge planner, home health agency, PT. Initiate planning for anticipated discharge. Begin teaching patient/family about home care: • medications • dietary restrictions • signs and symptoms of recurrence • activity limitations	Patient/family will understand how to maintain optimal health at home.	Provide guidelines concerning follow-up care to patient and family. Provide patient/family with phone numbers of resources available to answer questions concerning postdischarge medications and dietary regimens. Provide information about appropriate support groups.

DIAGNOSTICS

Diagnosis/Stabilization Phase		Acute Management Phase		Recovery Phase	
Outcome	Interventions	Outcome	Interventions	Outcome	Interventions
Patient/family will understand any tests or procedures that need to be completed (VS, I & O, hemodynamic monitoring, x-rays, CT scan, MRI, lab work, GI tubes, cardiac monitoring, glucose monitoring, EKG, ABGs, pulse oximetry, IV lines, blood therapy, endoscopic examinations, ultrasounds).	Explain all tests and procedures to patient/family. Be sensitive to individualized needs for information.	Patient/family will understand any tests or procedures that need to be completed.	Anticipate need for and prepare patient/family for further treatment such as surgery, intubation, long hospitalization, fluid replacement, pain control, glucose monitoring, and dietary management.	Patient/family will understand meaning of diagnostic tests in relation to continued health.	Review with patient/family results of tests before discharge. Discuss abnormal findings and appropriate measures patient/family can take to return to prehospital condition. Provide guidelines concerning follow-up care: • when to call physician • physical restrictions • dietary restrictions • skin care • medications

Pancreatitis Interdisciplinary Outcome Pathway *(continued)*

FLUID BALANCE

Diagnosis/Stabilization Phase		Acute Management Phase		Recovery Phase	
Outcome	Interventions	Outcome	Interventions	Outcome	Interventions
Patient will achieve optimal hemodynamic status as evidenced by: • MAP >70 mm Hg • PCWP WNL • CVP WNL • hemodynamic parameters WNL • stable Hgb and Hct • serum electrolytes WNL • coagulation studies WNL • blood glucose WNL	Monitor and treat hemodynamic parameters: • BP • CO/CI • SV/SI • PA pressures • CVP • SVR/PVR • SvO₂ Monitor closely q1h for signs of: • pulmonary complications (hypoxemia, atelectasis, ARDS) • cardiovascular complications (hypotension, decreased cardiac output, increased SVR) • electrolyte problems (hypokalemia, hypocalcemia) • sepsis • coagulation problems If necessary, infuse FFP, albumin, colloids, and electrolyte solutions. Administer fluids to prevent dehydration. Administer vasopressors as necessary and titrate according to response. Record temperature q4h and PRN. Monitor closely for renal failure. Administer analgesics (meperidine) as needed and monitor response. Morphine and other opiates are usually avoided because they cause spasms of sphincter of Oddi.	Patient will maintain optimal hemodynamic status. Patient's weight will return to baseline with a positive nitrogen balance.	Continue as in Diagnosis/Stabilization Phase. Decrease monitoring time to q2h and PRN. Monitor albumin, glucose, amylase, and lipase levels. Monitor for ascites, jaundice, and rebound tenderness. Institute nutritional supplements as needed through enteral or parenteral access. Weigh daily. Measure abdominal girth. Administer colloids, albumin, and FFP as needed. Administer vasopressors as needed and monitor response. Monitor hemodynamic parameters q2–4h. Administer pancreatic enzyme replacement immediately after meals and assess response. Do not mix pancreatic enzyme preparations with foods containing protein. Use fruit juice or applesauce. Wipe patient's lips after ingestion, since residual enzymes can cause irritation and skin breakdown. Institute peritoneal dialysis as needed.	Patient will maintain optimal hemodynamic status.	Monitor and treat hemodynamic parameters. Monitor and treat fluid and electrolytes imbalances. Begin teaching patient and family about postdischarge measures to monitor fluid balance and medications for glucose metabolism.

Be prepared to administer vitamin K, insulin, and calcium gluconate as needed.
Monitor for Cullen's sign (discoloration or bruising around umbilicus) or Grey Turners sign (discoloration or bruising of the flank). These are usually secondary to hemorrhagic pancreatitis.
Assess for causes of pancreatitis: biliary disease, trauma, surgery, alcohol, tumors, medications, infection.

NUTRITION

Diagnosis/Stabilization Phase		Acute Management Phase		Recovery Phase	
Outcome	Interventions	Outcome	Interventions	Outcome	Interventions
Patient will be adequately nourished as evidenced by: • positive nitrogen balance • serum amylase WNL • total protein WNL • electrolytes (especially glucose) WNL	Remain NPO until: • abdominal pain relieved • no ileus is present • serum amylase is returning to normal Consult dietitian or nutritional support team to coordinate/direct nutritional support. Patient may need total parenteral nutrition. Assess response. May feed enterally with long duodenal feeding tube using elemental, low fat formula tube feedings. NG tube to low wall suction. Monitor for N & V. Administer antiemetics as needed and monitor response. Replace pancreatic enzymes as needed. Peritoneal lavage if needed. Assess total protein, albumin, prealbumin, and lymphocyte count. Assess bowel sounds q4h.	Patient will be adequately nourished. Patient will return to baseline weight without evidence of fluid retention.	Monitor amylase, lipase, and glucose levels daily. Advance DAT starting with clear liquids and monitor response. Consider calorie count to determine if patient's intake meeting nutritional goals. Supplement diet as needed. Monitor for hyperglycemia (polydypsia, polyuria, polyphagia, weakness). Assess need for lipids. If given, monitor triglyceride levels. Weigh daily. Begin teaching patient/family about any dietary restrictions.	Patient will be adequately nourished. Patient will maintain normal nutritional and metabolic metabolism. Patient will have sufficient information to comply with discharge dietary regimen.	Teach patient/family: • use of insulin and pancreatic enzymes • avoidance of alcohol, fat, or spicy foods • increase carbohydrate intake • vitamin/mineral supplements Provide phone number of dietitian.

Pancreatitis Interdisciplinary Outcome Pathway (*continued*)

MOBILITY

Diagnosis/Stabilization Phase		Acute Management Phase		Recovery Phase	
Outcome	Interventions	Outcome	Interventions	Outcome	Interventions
Patient will achieve optimal mobility.	PT to assess degree of ambulation, mobility, muscle strength, tone, and flexibility. OT to assess functional ability. PT/OT to help determine and direct activity goals. Begin passive/active-assist ROM exercises.	Patient will achieve optimal mobility.	Continue as in Diagnosis/Stabilization Phase. Monitor response to increased activity. Decrease activity if adverse events occur (tachycardia, discomfort, dyspnea, or hypotension). Allow patient to assist in ADLs as tolerated.	Patient will achieve optimal mobility.	Instruct patient/family about exercise program.

OXYGENATION/VENTILATION

Diagnosis/Stabilization Phase		Acute Management Phase		Recovery Phase	
Outcome	Interventions	Outcome	Interventions	Outcome	Interventions
Patient will have adequate gas exchange and tissue perfusion as evidenced by: • SaO_2 > 90% • SpO_2 > 92% • ABGs WNL for patient • SvO_2 60–80% • UO > 0.5mL/kg/hr • alert and oriented × 3 • respiratory rate, depth, and rhythm WNL • absence of dyspnea, cyanosis, and secretions • hemodynamic parameters WNL for patient	Monitor respiratory status—rate, rhythm, and depth of breathing, CXR, ABGs, pulse oximetry, and SvO_2. Be prepared for intubation and mechanical ventilation. If necessary, assist with monitoring or adjusting of ventilator settings to maintain appropriate level of assistance and minute ventilation. Monitor ABGs or SpO_2/SvO_2 closely. Apply supplemental oxygen if indicated and monitor response. Monitor for signs of adequate tissue perfusion: alert and oriented, BP and pulse WNL for patient, SvO_2 60–80%, SpO_2 > 90%, UO > 0.5 mL/kg/hr, normal skin color and temperature. Reduce tissue oxygen demands through bed rest and comfort measures.	Patient will have adequate gas exchange and tissue perfusion.	Continue as in Diagnosis/Stabilization Phase. Monitor and treat oxygenation/ventilation disturbances as per ABGs or SaO_2/SvO_2. Wean oxygen therapy/mechanical ventilation as indicated. Teach patient/family about oxygenation needs and treatments provided. Assess effects of increased activity on oxygenation status.	Patient will have adequate gas exchange and tissue perfusion.	Continue as in Acute Management Phase. Teach patient/family about home care oxygen needs if applicable. Continue instruction on IS, use of splint pillow, and coughing and deep breathing.

- absence of effusions or areas of consolidation
- no use of accessory muscles of respiration
- absence of ARDS

Reduce fever if present. Instruct patient to cough and deep breathe. Instruct on use of IS. Have patient give return demonstration. Instruct patient on use of pillow to splint abdomen. Have patient give return demonstration. Monitor for suspected microemboli. Monitor for complications of pancreatitis that may impair oxygenation/ventilation: pleural effusion, infiltrates, pleuritis, ARDS.

COMFORT

Diagnosis/Stabilization Phase		Acute Management Phase		Recovery Phase	
Outcome	Interventions	Outcome	Interventions	Outcome	Interventions
Patient will be as comfortable and pain free as possible as evidenced by: • no objective indicators of discomfort • no complaints of discomfort	Assess quantity and quality of pain. The pain may fluctuate. Use pain scale to evaluate objectively. Assess location of discomfort (usually in the epigastric area but may radiate to the back). Administer analgesics (meperidine) and monitor response. Monitor effect on respiratory status and blood pressure. Teach patient use of PCA pump if used. Provide frequent oral care, especially if patient is NPO, to minimize oral discomfort. Avoid the use of lemon and glycerin swabs, which can be drying to the mucosa. Provide reassurance in a calm, caring, and competent manner. Keep lights dimmed and environment as quiet as possible to keep physical and verbal stimulation at a minimum. Position knee to chest for optimal comfort. Assess for any accompanying symptoms: N & V, fever, jaundice.	Patient will be as comfortable as possible.	Continue as in Diagnosis/Stabilization Phase. Instruct patient on relaxation techniques. Have patient give return demonstration. Use complementary therapies such as touch therapy, music therapy, humor, and imagery to promote relaxation. Involve family members in strategies. Observe for complications of pancreatitis that may cause discomfort: bleeding, abdominal distension, infection. Assist to most comfortable position, usually knee to chest, to decrease intensity of the discomfort.	Patient will be as comfortable as possible.	Instruct patient/family on alternative methods to promote relaxation after discharge. Teach patient appropriate use of analgesics.

Pancreatitis Interdisciplinary Outcome Pathway (*continued*)

SKIN INTEGRITY

Diagnosis/Stabilization Phase		Acute Management Phase		Recovery Phase	
Outcome	Interventions	Outcome	Interventions	Outcome	Interventions
Patient will have intact skin without abrasions or pressure ulcers.	Assess all bony prominences at least q4h and treat if needed. Use preventive pressure-reducing devices if patient is at high risk for developing pressure ulcers. Treat pressure ulcers according to hospital protocol. Use superfatted or lanolin-based soap for bathing and apply emollients for dry skin.	Patient will have intact skin without abrasions or pressure ulcers.	Continue as in Diagnosis/Stabilization Phase.	Patient will have intact skin without abrasions or pressure ulcers.	Continue as in Acute Management Phase. Teach patient/family proper skin care after discharge.

PROTECTION/SAFETY

Diagnosis/Stabilization Phase		Acute Management Phase		Recovery Phase	
Outcome	Interventions	Outcome	Interventions	Outcome	Interventions
Patient will be protected from possible harm.	Assess need for restraints and institute if needed. If used, check skin integrity and circulation q1h. Explain need for restraints to patient/family. Follow hospital protocol for use of restraints. Assess need for assistance with activities. Provide physical assistance as needed. Maintain NG suction at low level to avoid trauma to gastric mucosa.	Patient will be protected from possible harm.	Continue as in Diagnosis/Stabilization Phase.	Patient will be protected from possible harm.	Teach patient/family about any physical limitations in activity after discharge.

PSYCHOSOCIAL/SELF-DETERMINATION

Diagnosis/Stabilization Phase		Acute Management Phase		Recovery Phase	
Outcome	Interventions	Outcome	Interventions	Outcome	Interventions
Patient will achieve psychophysiologic stability. Patient will demonstrate a decrease in anxiety as evidenced by: • VS WNL for patient • subjective report of decreased anxiety • objective signs of decreased anxiety Patient will begin acceptance process of possible long-term or chronic disorder.	Assess physiologic effects of critical care environment on patient (hemodynamic variables, psychological status, signs of increased sympathetic response). Administer sedatives and antianxiolytics and monitor response. Use calm, caring, competent, and reassuring approach with patient and family. Allow flexible visitation to meet patient/family needs. Determine coping ability of patient/family and take appropriate measures (provide frequent condition reports, provide frequent explanations, allow patient to verbalize concerns, consult support services, allow family to visit often, and have family conferences). Allow patient/family to verbalize concerns about possibility of long-term or chronic illness.	Patient will achieve psychophysiologic stability. Patient will demonstrate a decrease in anxiety. Patient will continue acceptance process of possible long-term or chronic illness.	Continue as in Diagnosis/Stabilization Phase. Continue to allow patient/family to verbalize concerns about condition. Consult support services (chaplain, counselor) as needed.	Patient will achieve psychophysiologic stability. Patient will demonstrate a decrease in anxiety. Patient will continue acceptance of possible long-term or chronic illness.	Provide emotional support to patient/family. Refer to outpatient counseling or stress management programs if needed, such as diabetic counseling and/or alcohol abstinence. Address concerns patient may have about impact on daily life.

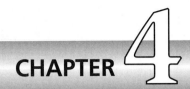

CHAPTER 4

Neurologic Pathways

Acute Head Injury
Interdisciplinary Outcome Pathway

COORDINATION OF CARE

Diagnosis/Stabilization Phase		Acute Management Phase		Recovery Phase	
Outcome	Interventions	Outcome	Interventions	Outcome	Interventions
All appropriate team members and disciplines will be involved in the plan of care.	Develop the plan of care with patient/family, primary physician(s), neurologist, neurosurgeon, RN, advanced practice nurse, RCP, chaplain, and other specialists as needed.	All appropriate team members and disciplines will be involved in the plan of care.	Update the plan of care with patient/family, other team members, dietitian, PT, recreational therapist, OT, speech and language pathologist. Initiate planning for anticipated discharge. Begin teaching patient/family about care at home if discharge to home is anticipated. Involve home health agency if needed.	Patient/family will understand how to maintain optimal health at home, extended care facility, or physical rehabilitation facility.	Provide guidelines concerning follow-up care to patient/family especially in regard to patient/family progressive activity toward independent living and energy conservation techniques. Provide patient/family with phone number of resources available to answer questions. Continue to involve PT and physical rehabilitation consults. Prepare for discharge to extended care facility, physical rehabilitation facility, or home. If discharged to home, provide instructions on care at home: • when to call the physician • physical restrictions • exercise program • diet • medications

DIAGNOSTICS

Diagnosis/Stabilization Phase		Acute Management Phase		Recovery Phase	
Outcome	Interventions	Outcome	Interventions	Outcome	Interventions
Patient/family will describe any tests or procedures that need to be completed (hemodynamic monitoring, ICP monitoring, x-rays, CT scan, MRI, angiography, lab work, EKG, LP).	Explain all procedures and tests to patient/family. Be sensitive to individualized needs of patient/family for information. Assess patient's ability to understand procedures. If patient is unresponsive, use tactile and verbal methods to communicate. Establish effective communication technique with intubated patient.	Patient/family will describe any tests or procedures that need to be completed (hemodynamic monitoring, ICP monitoring, lab tests, CT scan, MRI, x-rays, test to determine physical functioning, EEG).	Explain procedures and tests to assess recovery from head injury to patient/family. Assess individualized needs of patient/family for information. Anticipate need for further diagnostic tests such as EMG, EEG, CT scan, and any interventions that may result.	Patient/family will describe or discuss the meaning of diagnostic tests in relation to continued health (MRI, CT scan, EMG, further testing to assess potential for healing/mobility).	Review with patient/family before discharge results of all tests. Discuss abnormal findings and appropriate measures patient/family can take to return to normal or to regain as much physical and mental functioning as possible. Stress this is a long-term process.

FLUID BALANCE

Diagnosis/Stabilization Phase		Acute Management Phase		Recovery Phase	
Outcome	Interventions	Outcome	Interventions	Outcome	Interventions
Patient will achieve optimal hemodynamic status as evidenced by: • VS WNL • ICP WNL • hemodynamic parameters WNL • adequate LOC • clear lung sounds • normothermia Patient will maintain optimal neurologic status as evidenced by cerebral perfusion pressure (CPP) > 50 mmHg.	Monitor and treat hemodynamic parameters: • SvO₂ • BP • ICP • I & O • LOC • evidence of tissue perfusion (pain, pulses, temperature, color, altered LOC, decreased UO) • CPP Monitor lab values: electrolytes, SMA-18, CK, CK-BB. Assess for fluid overload or deficit and treat accordingly. Anticipate need for vasopressor agents and assess response. Titrate accordingly. Assess neurologic status q1h and PRN. If used, assess ICP q1h and PRN. Anticipate need for diuretics. Monitor for signs of increased ICP and treat accordingly. Monitor temperature and watch for signs of shivering. Use hypo/hyperthermia unit if necessary. Avoid rapid cooling. Raise HOB 30–45 degrees. Monitor CPP. Attempt to keep CPP > 50 mmHg. (CPP = mean arterial pressure – ICP). A low CPP could indicate edema, mass, or hyperemia. Assess for other conditions that may affect LOC: alcoholism, seizures, age, cardiac disease, pulmonary disease, coagulation defects. If ICP changes with activity, space activities. Determine baseline ICP before any activity.	Patient will maintain optimal hemodynamic status. Patient will maintain optimal neurologic status. Patient will remain normothermic.	Continue to monitor and treat hemodynamic parameters as needed. Assess for fluid overload or deficit and treat accordingly. Anticipate need for diuresis. Continue to monitor CPP. Include diaphoretic episodes in estimation of I & O. Assess neurologic status q2–4h and PRN. If used, assess ICP q2–4h and PRN. Assess temperature and signs of shivering. Maintain normal temperature with hypo/hyperthermia unit or other measures. Avoid rapid cooling. Monitor for complications associated with head injury and treat accordingly: • pneumonia • muscle atrophy • infection • embolus • thrombus formation • renal failure • diabetes insipidus • hematoma formation • increased ICP • hypo/hyperglycemia • leukocytosis • uremic encephalopathy • hepatic encephalopathy Monitor urine specific gravity and osmolality. Monitor blood osmolality.	Patient will maintain optimal hemodynamic status. Patient will maintain optimal neurologic status. Patient will remain normothermic.	Maintain strict I & O. Assess neurologic status q4–8h and PRN. Continue to monitor for complications. Teach patient/family fluid management for after discharge.

Acute Head Injury Interdisciplinary Outcome Pathway (continued)

NUTRITION

Diagnosis/Stabilization Phase		Acute Management Phase		Recovery Phase	
Outcome	Interventions	Outcome	Interventions	Outcome	Interventions
Patient will be adequately nourished as evidenced by: • stable weight within 20% of IBW • albumin 3.5–4.0 g/dL • total protein 6–8 g/dL • absolute lymphocyte count 1,000–3,000	Consult dietitian to coordinate/direct nutritional support. NPO until able to swallow fluids. If needed, initiate total parenteral or enteral nutrition as soon as possible and monitor response. Assess bowel sounds, abdominal distension, abdominal pain and tenderness q4h and PRN. If intubated, initiate alternative nutritional therapy.	Patient will be adequately nourished.	Continue as in Diagnosis/Stabilization Phase. If able, advance to DAT and monitor response. Consult SP to assess gag reflex and swallowing ability. Dietary consult as needed if: • albumin <3.0 • caloric intake less than needed Speech and language therapy consult as needed. OT consult for physical inabilities of feeding when indicated. OT to determine special equipment needed when eating such as lightweight utensils or specially built-up handles. Monitor protein and albumin lab values.	Patient will be adequately nourished.	Teach patient/family about diet: • type (regular, soft, liquid) • restrictions • supplements as needed Consider need for outpatient dietitian follow-up.

MOBILITY

Diagnosis/Stabilization Phase		Acute Management Phase		Recovery Phase	
Outcome	Interventions	Outcome	Interventions	Outcome	Interventions
Patient will maintain normal muscle strength and tone. Patient will be free of joint contractures.	Assess degree of mobility, strength, muscle tone, and sensation. Consult PT/OT to help establish mobility, functional ability, and activity goals. Keep HOB elevated 30 degrees. Begin passive/active-assist ROM exercises as tolerated.	Patient will achieve optimal mobility. Patient will maintain normal muscle strength and tone. Patient will be free of joint contractures.	Continue as in Diagnosis/Stabilization Phase. Continue passive/active-assist ROM exercises. Obtain PT/physical rehabilitation consult. OT consult for ADLs. Monitor response to increased activity. Decrease if adverse events occur (dyspnea, increased intracranial pressure, syncope, tachycardia, hypo/hypertension). Monitor effects of increased activity on	Patient will achieve optimal mobility. Patient will maintain normal muscle strength and tone. Patient will be free of joint contractures.	Prepare for transfer to SNF, home, or physical rehabilitation facility. Include family in all plans of continuing care. Teach patient/family about exercise program. OT to teach progressive increase in ADLs and IADLs. Teach patient/family proper use of assistive devices or orthotics. Have patient/family give return demonstration of proper use.

respiratory status. Use pulse oximetry as needed. Apply supplemental oxygen to keep SpO2 >92%.
Provide physical support as necessary.
Provide physical assistive devices as necessary.
Take measures to prevent joint contractures (may need orthotic devices).
Begin discussion with patient/family about potential physical limitations and required resources after discharge.

OXYGENATION/VENTILATION

Diagnosis/Stabilization Phase		Acute Management Phase		Recovery Phase	
Outcome	Interventions	Outcome	Interventions	Outcome	Interventions
Patient will have adequate gas exchange as evidenced by: • SaO2 >90% • SpO2 >92% • ABGs WNL • PaCO2 27-33 mm Hg • clear breath sounds • respiratory rate, depth, and rhythm WNL • CXR WNL • absence of dyspnea, cyanosis, secretions	Monitor ventilator settings and hemodynamic variables before, during, and after weaning (if applicable). Anticipate need for hyperventilation and hyperoxygenation, particularly before suctioning. Wean ventilator when appropriate and monitor patient response: • wean FIO2 to keep SpO2 >92% • use humidification to keep secretions thin Involve RCP. Assess respiratory functioning including lung sounds, respiratory muscle strength, respiratory rate and depth, coughing ability, ABGs, and CXR. If not intubated, apply supplemental oxygen. Monitor with pulse oximetry. Keep SpO2 >92%.	Patient will have adequate gas exchange.	Monitor and treat oxygenation/ventilation disturbances as per ABGs, SaO2, SpO2, chest assessment, adventitious breath sounds, and CXR. Wean oxygen therapy and/or mechanical ventilation as tolerated. Continue to involve RCP in care. Begin teaching patient/family about mechanical ventilation if home care is expected. Assess effects of increased activity on respiratory status. Monitor with pulse oximetry. Observe for complications of head injury that may impair oxygenation/ventilation: • embolus • increased ICP • thrombus formation • seizures • fever • neurogenic shock	Patient will have adequate gas exchange.	Assess respiratory functioning and intervene as indicated. Provide instruction to patient/family on mechanical ventilation as needed (see "Chronic Ventilator-Dependent Patient Pathway"): • caring for tracheostomy tube • suctioning • use of ambu bag • emergency measures Continue to assess for complications of head injury that may impair oxygenation/ventilation (i.e., pneumonia, infection, embolus, thrombus formation). Assess patient/family understanding of home care needs. Reinforce knowledge and skills as needed.

Acute Head Injury Interdisciplinary Outcome Pathway (continued)

OXYGENATION/VENTILATION (continued)

Diagnosis/Stabilization Phase		Acute Management Phase		Recovery Phase	
Outcome	Interventions	Outcome	Interventions	Outcome	Interventions
	Assess evidence of tissue perfusion (pain, pulses, temperature, color, decreased UO, altered LOC). Monitor lab values: ABGs, CO_2, Hgb.		Assess need for long-term mechanical ventilation. If indicated, initiate plans to place in SNF, physical rehabilitation facility, or in the home. If going home, involve home health agency and home medical equipment company early in process.		

COMFORT

Diagnosis/Stabilization Phase		Acute Management Phase		Recovery Phase	
Outcome	Interventions	Outcome	Interventions	Outcome	Interventions
Patient will be as comfortable and pain free as possible as evidenced by: • no objective indicators of discomfort • no complaints of discomfort	Assess absence of, or quantity and quality of, pain. Administer analgesics and monitor for response. Administer sedatives cautiously. Monitor effect on LOC. Assess response to all analgesics and effects on ability to wean from ventilator if applicable. If patient is intubated, establish effective communication technique with which patient can communicate discomfort. Provide reassurance in a calm, caring, and competent manner. Keep HOB elevated at least 30 degrees to decrease cerebral edema. Plan interventions to provide optimal rest periods.	Patient will be relaxed and as comfortable as possible.	Continue as in Diagnosis/Stabilization Phase. Teach patient relaxation techniques. Have patient give return demonstration. Use touch therapy humor, music therapy, and imagery to promote relaxation. Involve family in strategies. Observe for complications of head injury that may cause discomfort such as increased ICP, HA, seizures, restlessness, or irritability.	Patient will be relaxed and as comfortable as possible.	Progress analgesics to oral medications as needed. Assess response. Teach patient/family alternative methods to promote relaxation after discharge. Have patient/family give return demonstration.

SKIN INTEGRITY

Diagnosis/Stabilization Phase		Acute Management Phase		Recovery Phase	
Outcome	Interventions	Outcome	Interventions	Outcome	Interventions
Patient will have intact skin without abrasions or pressure ulcers.	Assess all bony prominences at least q4h and treat if needed. Use preventive pressure-reducing devices if patient is at high risk for developing pressure ulcers. Treat pressure ulcers according to hospital protocol. Initiate passive/active-assist ROM exercises.	Patient will have intact skin without abrasions or pressure ulcers. Patient will have healing wounds.	Continue as in Diagnosis/Stabilization Phase. Use sterile technique with all dressing changes. Assess wounds for healing, signs of infection, erythema.	Patient will have intact skin without abrasions or pressure ulcers. Patient will have healing wounds.	Teach patient/family: • proper skin care • care of incision • signs and symptoms of infection • when to call the physician

PROTECTION/SAFETY

Diagnosis/Stabilization Phase		Acute Management Phase		Recovery Phase	
Outcome	Interventions	Outcome	Interventions	Outcome	Interventions
Patient will be protected from possible harm.	Seizure precautions. Assess need for restraints. If indicated, assess response to restraints. Follow hospital protocol for use of restraints. Check q1–2h for skin integrity and impairment to circulation. Explain need for restraints to patient/family. Remove restraints when patient is able to follow instructions. Administer sedatives and anxiolytics cautiously and monitor neurologic effect. Allow family to remain with patient if they have calming influence and can promote rest and safety. OT consult for splinting to prevent joint deformities and monitor joint integrity when indicated.	Patient will be protected from possible harm.	Continue as in Diagnosis/Stabilization Phase. When activity is increased, provide any necessary support. Use assistive devices as needed. Continue to allow family to remain with patient.	Patient will be protected from possible harm.	Teach patient/family about any physical limitations in activity after discharge and proper use of any assistive devices. Have patient/family give return demonstration. Consult PT/OT for home follow-up if indicated.

Acute Head Injury Interdisciplinary Outcome Pathway (continued)

PSYCHOSOCIAL/SELF-DETERMINATION

Diagnosis/Stabilization Phase		Acute Management Phase		Recovery Phase	
Outcome	Interventions	Outcome	Interventions	Outcome	Interventions
Patient will achieve psychophysiologic stability. Patient will demonstrate a decrease in anxiety as evidenced by: • VS WNL • subjective report of anxiety level • objective signs of anxiety level Patient/family will begin acceptance process for head injury and possible effects.	Assess physiologic effect of critical care environment on patient (hemodynamic variables, psychological status, signs of increased sympathetic response). Develop effective interventions to communicate with intubated patient. If patient is unresponsive, maintain verbal and tactile contact with patient. Use calm, caring, competent, and reassuring approach with patient and family. Arrange for flexible visitation to meet patient and family needs. Determine coping ability of patient/family and take appropriate measures to meet their needs (i.e., explain condition, explain equipment, provide frequent condition reports, use easy to understand terminology, repeat information as needed, allow family to visit, answer all questions). Provide counseling and support for family to help process the acute head injury event as well as subsequent events.	Patient will achieve psychophysiologic stability. Patient will demonstrate a decrease in anxiety. Patient/family will continue acceptance process of head injury and any possible effects.	Continue as in Diagnosis/Stabilization Phase. Provide adequate rest periods. Continue to assess coping ability of patient/family and take measures as indicated (i.e., help patient/family verbalize feelings, initiate family conferences, use support services, counseling). Help patient/family identify past positive coping mechanisms. Obtain psychological consult if needed. Initiate discharge planning to either SNF, physical rehabilitation facility, or home. Include patient/family in decisions concerning care. Refer family to support programs.	Patient will achieve psychophysiologic stability. Patient will demonstrate a decrease in anxiety. Patient/family will continue acceptance process for head injury and possible effects.	Continue to assess coping ability of patient/family. OT to continue progression of ADLs and IADLs to increase independence and self-esteem. Provide patient/family with detailed information regarding transfer to rehabilitation facility, SNF, or home. Provide detailed information regarding continued care to decrease anxiety and increase confidence. Provide patient and family information about support groups. Reinforce positive coping mechanisms. Discourage use of inappropriate coping mechanisms. Address concerns patient may have about impact on daily life.

Acute Ischemic Stroke Interdisciplinary Outcome Pathway

COORDINATION OF CARE

Diagnosis/Stabilization Phase		Acute Management Phase		Recovery Phase	
Outcome	Interventions	Outcome	Interventions	Outcome	Interventions
All appropriate team members and disciplines will be involved in the plan of care.	Develop plan of care with patient/family, Emergency Department (ED) physician, primary care physician, neurologist, RN, advanced practice nurse, and other specialists as needed.	All appropriate team members and disciplines will implement the plan of care.	Consult physiatrist for rehabilitation evaluation. Consult SP, PT, and OT based on assessments and physiatrist's recommendations. Begin teaching patient/family about stroke, poststroke care, and rehabilitation. Initiate planning for anticipated discharge. Update the plan of care.	Patient/family will understand how to maintain optimal health postdischarge.	Provide individualized education on risk factors for stroke and recurrent stroke: • smoking • hypertension • hyperlipidemia • atrial fibrillation • diabetes • obesity Ensure that patient/family can recognize signs/symptoms of stroke and take appropriate action. These signs and symptoms may include: • weakness, numbness, or paralysis, particularly on one side • blurred or decreased vision • problems understanding or speaking • dizziness or loss of balance • sudden severe or unexplained headache Provide guidelines regarding follow-up care. Inform patient/family of post discharge health information, resources in community, stroke support groups, national organizations, and so on. Involve home health as necessary.

Acute Ischemic Stroke Interdisciplinary Outcome Pathway (continued)

DIAGNOSTICS

Diagnosis/Stabilization Phase		Acute Management Phase		Recovery Phase	
Outcome	Interventions	Outcome	Interventions	Outcome	Interventions
Patient/family will describe any tests or procedures that need to be completed (VS, I & O, hemodynamic monitoring, x-rays, CT, MRI, labwork, EKG, GCS, NIH Stroke Scale, and other assessment tools).	Explain all procedures and tests to patient/family. Be sensitive to individualized needs of patient/family for information. Assess patient's ability to understand explanations and procedures.	Patient/family will describe any tests/procedures that need to be completed (VS, hemodynamic monitoring, labwork, CT, MRI, angiography, x-rays, EEG, 2D and transesophageal echocardiography, and carotid Doppler/ultrasonography).	Explain all procedures and tests to assess type and severity of stroke, level of functioning, and stroke etiology to patient/family. Assess individualized needs of patient/family for information. Anticipate need for further diagnostic tests, and any intervention that might result from testing.	Patient/family will describe or discuss the meaning of tests in relation to continued health (follow-up CT or MRI, labwork, and assessment tools).	Review with patient/family discharge results of all tests. Discuss abnormal findings and appropriate measures for patient/family to take to return to normal or to regain as much function as possible. Review with patient/family tests ordered as part of postdischarge care, associated with postdischarge treatment regimen.

FLUID BALANCE

Diagnosis/Stabilization Phase		Acute Management Phase		Recovery Phase	
Outcome	Interventions	Outcome	Interventions	Outcome	Interventions
Patient will achieve optimal hemodynamic status as evidenced by: • HR 60–120 • systolic BP 90–180 • diastolic BP 50–100 • adequate LOC • UO >0.5 mL/kg/hr • stable neurologic status • normothermia	Monitor and treat hemodynamic parameters: • HR <60 or >120 • SBP <90 or >180 • DBP <50 or >100 • I & O Monitor neurologic status for: • decreased LOC • seizure activity • changes from baseline neurological assessment and notify physician promptly of changes Monitor for cardiac dysrhythmias and treat as indicated.	Patient will maintain optimal hemodynamic status.	Continue as in Diagnosis/Stabilization Phase. Monitor and treat hemodynamic parameters. Assure adequate hydration if patient unable to handle oral fluids due to LOC or swallowing difficulties; infuse ½ NS at 50–75 mL/hr.	Patient will maintain optimal hemodynamic status.	Educate patient/family regarding hydration, medications affecting fluid balance, and potential bleeding. Assess for understanding and reinforce as needed. Assure adequate hydration and route for medication administration postdischarge.

Monitor temperature; treat fever >101°F with antipyretics; investigate cause.

If thrombolytic or anticoagulant therapy given, monitor hemodynamic parameters as listed earlier, *plus* coagulation studies and signs and symptoms of systemic and intracranial bleeding.

Institute seizure precautions.

NUTRITION

Diagnosis/Stabilization Phase		Acute Management Phase		Recovery Phase	
Outcome	Interventions	Outcome	Interventions	Outcome	Interventions
Patient will be adequately nourished as evidenced by: • stable weight • not >10% below or >20% above IBW • albumin 3.5–4.0 g/dL • total protein 6–8 g/dL • prealbumin >15 • total lymphocyte count 1,000–3,000	Consult SP to assess swallowing ability and gag reflex (complete bedside swallow evaluation recommended). Consult dietitian or nutritional support team to coordinate/direct nutritional support. If swallow is adequate without choking or aspiration, initiate oral medications and heart healthy diet: • total fat <30% of daily intake • total saturated fat <10% of daily intake • total daily cholesterol intake <300 mg • caloric reduction if indicated If choking or aspiration noted, make patient NPO, alert physician and other team members, order video swallow, and begin enteral or parenteral feedings.	Patient will be adequately nourished.	Continue as in Diagnosis/Stabilization Phase. Monitor daily weight, prealbumin, albumin, total protein, and lymphocyte count. Consider calorie count to determine if intake is meeting nutritional goals. Utilize SP for oral motor exercises. Monitor for signs of aspiration. If video swallow shows signs of aspiration/penetration, change diet accordingly. Consider surgeon consult for gastrostomy tube in case of severe dysphasia. OT consult for feeding issues if functional ability to feed self is impaired. OT to determine special equipment needs when eating such as built-up handles or light-weight utensils.	Patient will be adequately nourished. Patient will take meals safely.	Monitor response to nutrition given. Educate patient/family regarding swallowing safety and individualized diet modifications to reduce risk of recurrent stroke. Teach patient/family about heart healthy diet.

Acute Ischemic Stroke Interdisciplinary Outcome Pathway (continued)

MOBILITY

Diagnosis/Stabilization Phase		Acute Management Phase		Recovery Phase	
Outcome	Interventions	Outcome	Interventions	Outcome	Interventions
Patient will achieve optimal mobility.	Assess for degree of ataxia and weakness. Promote safety measures for patient's level of mobility (i.e., bed rails raised if patient on complete bed rest). Teach patient/family active and active-assist ROM if hemiparesis present.	Patient will achieve optimal mobility.	Continue as in Diagnosis/Stabilization Phase. Consult PT and OT to establish ambulation, mobility, functional ability, muscle strength, tone, flexibility, and activity goals. Goals should encourage independence with ADLs as quickly as possible. Monitor response to increased activity, and advise care team if adverse effects occur, such as changes in neurologic status, severe fatigue, or dyspnea. Provide physical assistance and assistive devices as needed. Discuss potential physical limitations with patient/family in regard to discharge. Initiate stroke rehabilitation program if feasible.	Patient will achieve optimal mobility. Patient will be free of joint contractures.	Continue as in Diagnosis/Stabilization and Acute Management Phases. Prepare for transfer to appropriate level of care: home, home with home health or outpatient therapies, inpatient acute or subacute rehabilitation facility, or SNF. Educate patient/family regarding progressive exercise and activity plan.

OXYGENATION/VENTILATION

Diagnosis/Stabilization Phase		Acute Management Phase		Recovery Phase	
Outcome	Interventions	Outcome	Interventions	Outcome	Interventions
Patient will have adequate gas exchange as evidenced by: • SpO_2 > 92% • clear breath sounds • respiratory depth and rate WNL • ABGs WNL (only drawn if necessary) • CXR WNL	Monitor respiratory status continually. Assure that patient is NPO unless swallow evaluated as adequate. Observe patient for signs/symptoms of increased ICP: decreased LOC, widening pulse pressure, Cheyne-Stokes respirations, and notify primary physician or neurologist immediately.	Patient will have adequate gas exchange.	Monitor and treat oxygenation status per SpO_2 and ABGs. Monitor and treat ventilation status per respiratory assessment, ABGs, adventitious breath sounds, CXR. Assess effects of progressing activity on respiratory status. Observe for signs/symptoms of respiratory complications such as pneumonia/aspiration pneumonitis, pulmonary embolus.	Patient will have adequate gas exchange. Patient will perform pulmonary toilet measures as needed postdischarge.	Teach patient/family methods to reduce aspiration: • increase HOB for feedings and 30 minutes postfeedings • use appropriate medication routes • use appropriate diet consistency • perform oral motor exercises and swallow pocketing and aspiration

Assess patient for evidence of tissue perfusion.
Monitor ventilator settings and wakefulness, and determine readiness to wean, if applicable.

COMFORT

Diagnosis/Stabilization Phase		Acute Management Phase		Recovery Phase	
Outcome	Interventions	Outcome	Interventions	Outcome	Interventions
Patient will be as comfortable and pain free as possible, as evidenced by: • no objective indicators of pain/discomfort • no complaints of pain/discomfort	Assess for presence of pain, quality and quantity of pain if present (utilize pain scale). Administer non-narcotic analgesics and monitor response. Avoid sedatives and narcotic analgesics; administer cautiously if needed for continued or severe pain. Monitor response on LOC and neurologic status. Provide reassurance in a calm, caring, and competent manner.	Patient will be as relaxed and comfortable as possible.	Continue as in Diagnosis/Stabilization Phase. Provide uninterrupted rest periods in a quiet environment. Teach patient relaxation techniques (i.e., imagery, music therapy, deep breathing). Use touch therapy and relaxation methods as described to promote relaxation. Involve family in relaxation strategies.	Patient will be as relaxed and comfortable as possible.	Continue as in Diagnosis/Stabilization and Acute Management phases. Teach patient/family alternative methods used to promote relaxation, for use after discharge. Have patient/family give return demonstration. Teach patient/family regarding smoking as general and stroke-specific health hazard. Teach patient about smoking cessation.

SKIN INTEGRITY

Diagnosis/Stabilization Phase		Acute Management Phase		Recovery Phase	
Outcome	Interventions	Outcome	Interventions	Outcome	Interventions
Patient's skin will be intact without breaks, abrasions, or hematoma.	Assess patient's level of mobility; if independent mobility decreased, institute measures to minimize pressure on bony prominences. Assess patient's skin at least q4h and treat as needed. Use hospital prevention and skin care treatment protocols as needed. If thrombolytic therapy given, assess puncture sites, skin, and mucous membranes qh ×24h post-thrombolytic; hold manual pressure ×5–10 minutes post IV and lab punctures until coagulation studies WNL.	Patient's skin will be intact without breaks, abrasions, or hematoma.	Continue as in Diagnosis/Stabilization Phase. If antiembolic compression stockings or sequential/pneumatic compression device in use for DVT prophylaxis, remove and inspect skin at least q8h.	Patient's skin will be intact without breaks, abrasions, or hematoma.	Develop discharge plan to appropriate facility: home, home with home health or outpatient therapy, inpatient acute or subacute rehabilitation facility, or SNF. Teach patient/family to care for skin properly postdischarge. Assess understanding and reinforce as needed.

Acute Ischemic Stroke Interdisciplinary Outcome Pathway (continued)

PROTECTION/SAFETY

Diagnosis/Stabilization Phase		Acute Management Phase		Recovery Phase	
Outcome	Interventions	Outcome	Interventions	Outcome	Interventions
Patient will be protected from possible harm. Patient will demonstrate a decrease in anxiety as evidenced by: • VS WNL • subjective report of decreased anxiety	Assess for decreased LOC, presence of confusion; if present, restrain patient per hospital policy. Explain restraints and patient safety to patient/family. If restraints used, check patient response, skin integrity, and neurovascular status q1h. Remove restraints when patient alert and not confused, and continue to monitor neurologic status. Administer sedatives cautiously, and only for severe agitation/confusion. Sedatives should be avoided if at all possible, so as not to mask changes in neurologic status.	Patient will be protected from possible harm.	Continue as in Diagnosis/Stabilization Phase. Assess need for assistance with activities. Provide physical support as needed. OT to teach correct movement and appropriate functional skills to prevent joint stress, strain, or injury. Splinting to prevent joint deformities and maintain joint integrity when indicated. Assess for signs of progressing stroke (changes in VS, LOC, baseline neurologic deficits, or physical mobility or function) and notify primary physician or neurologist promptly of any changes.	Patient will be protected from physical harm.	Educate patient/family regarding measures to promote safety postdischarge. Ensure that patient/family are prepared to deal with patient's physical limitations postdischarge: • assistive devices provided as appropriate • patient/family trained in proper use and care of assistive devices • home environment is adequately prepared Assess patient/family understanding of protection/safety measures.

PSYCHOSOCIAL/SELF-DETERMINATION

Diagnosis/Stabilization Phase		Acute Management Phase		Recovery Phase	
Outcome	Interventions	Outcome	Interventions	Outcome	Interventions
Patient will achieve psychophysiologic stability. Patient will demonstrate a decrease in anxiety as evidenced by: • VS WNL • subjective report of decreased anxiety	Assess physiologic effects of care environment on patient (hemodynamic variables, psychosocial status, signs of increased sympathetic response). Avoid sedatives and other medications that might mask changing neurologic status. Take measures to reduce sensory overload.	Patient will achieve psychophysiologic stability. Patient will demonstrate decreased anxiety. Patient will demonstrate decreased fear. Patient will continue acceptance process of stroke.	Continue as in Diagnosis/Stabilization Phase. Encourage family to visit with patient and to participate in therapies. Assure rest periods are given and that patient is not overstimulated. Allow patient to verbalize feelings of anxiety, fear, and loss of control. Include family in all aspects of care. Initiate discharge planning process to include patient/family.	Patient will achieve psychophysiologic stability. Patient will continue acceptance process of stroke.	Continue to assess coping ability of patient/family and take appropriate measures to promote positive coping mechanisms (psychology consultation, social services, chaplain services). Explain process of stroke recovery. Offer sources of stroke information postdischarge such as community health informa-

- objective signs of decreased, or absence of, anxiety

Patient will begin acceptance process of stroke.

Calmly reassure patient regarding condition and care provided.

Allow flexible visiting to meet needs of patient/family.

Determine coping ability of patient/family and take measures to meet their needs (i.e., explain condition, equipment, and medications, provide frequent condition reports, use lay terminology, and repeat information as needed).

Teach other measures to promote relaxation (i.e., imagery, deep breathing, music therapy, touch therapy).

OT to teach progressive increase in ADLs and IADL skills to increase independence and self-esteem.

tion centers, national stroke organizations, stroke support groups, and caregiver support groups.

Address concerns patient may have about impact on daily life.

Guillain-Barré Syndrome Interdisciplinary Outcome Pathway

COORDINATION OF CARE

Diagnosis/Stabilization Phase		Acute Management Phase		Recovery Phase	
Outcome	Interventions	Outcome	Interventions	Outcome	Interventions
All appropriate disciplines will be consulted and involved in the development of the plan of care.	Consult the following as needed: neurologist, primary physician, other specialists as needed, RN, advanced practice nurse, RCP, OT, PT, and chaplain.	All appropriate disciplines and team members will be involved in the plan of care.	Review/revise plan of care with patient/family and all team members, dietitian, physical rehabilitation specialist, and social worker. Initiate planning for anticipated discharge. If applicable, arrange for home health care and home equipment needs. Begin teaching patient/family about care at home if discharge to home is anticipated.	Patient/family will understand how to maintain optimal health at home, SNF, or physical rehabilitation facility.	Provide guidelines concerning follow-up care to patient/family: • medications • dietary restrictions • exercise program • activity limitations • use of assistive devices • follow-up visits Provide patient/family with phone number of resources available to answer questions. Inform patient/family that full recovery may take years and some permanent neurologic deficit may be present. Refer to a support group if appropriate. Arrange visits with Guillain-Barré syndrome (GBS) survivor.

DIAGNOSTICS

Diagnosis/Stabilization Phase		Acute Management Phase		Recovery Phase	
Outcome	Interventions	Outcome	Interventions	Outcome	Interventions
Patient/family will understand any tests or procedures that need to be completed (hemodynamic monitoring, x-rays, CT scan, MRI, EMG, lab work, EKG, EEG, LP).	Explain all procedures and tests to patient/family. Be sensitive to individualized needs of patient/family for information. Establish effective communication technique with intubated patient.	Patient/family will understand any tests or procedures that need to be completed (hemodynamic monitoring, lab work, x-rays, EEG, and tests to determine physical functioning).	Explain procedures and tests to assess progress and recovery from GBS to patient/family. Assess individualized needs of patient/family for information. Anticipate need for further diagnostic tests such as EMG, EEG, CT scan, and any interventions that may result.	Patient/family will understand meaning of diagnostic tests in relation to continued health (MRI, CT scan, PFT, EMG, further testing to assess potential for healing/mobility).	Review with patient/family before discharge results of all tests. Discuss abnormal findings and appropriate measures patient/family can take to return to normal or to regain as much physical functioning as possible (i.e., exercise program).

Patient/family will understand tests needed to rule out other pathology.

Provide patient/family with guidelines concerning follow-up care.

Prepare for discharge to SNF, physical rehabilitation facility, or home.

Continue to involve PT and OT. Obtain physical rehabilitation consult.

If discharged to home, provide instruction on care at home:
- when to call physician
- physical restrictions
- exercise
- care of mechanical ventilator/tracheostomy, if needed
- diet
- medications

FLUID BALANCE

Diagnosis/Stabilization Phase		Acute Management Phase		Recovery Phase	
Outcome	Interventions	Outcome	Interventions	Outcome	Interventions
Patient will achieve optimal hemodynamic status as evidenced by: • MAP >70 mmHg • hemodynamic parameters WNL • adequate LOC • adequate respiratory functioning • neurologic status WNL	Monitor and treat hemodynamic parameters such as BP, CO, SvO_2. Assess evidence of tissue perfusion (pain, pulses, color, temperature, signs of decreased perfusion such as decreased UO, ileus, and altered LOC). Constantly monitor level of muscle functioning, paralysis, and paresthesia. Assess neurologic status with GCS q1–2h and PRN. Constantly monitor respiratory functioning and anticipate respiratory complications. Be prepared for intubation and mechanical ventilation. Monitor I & O. Remember insensible fluid loss. Anticipate need for vasopressor therapy.	Patient will maintain optimal hemodynamic status.	Continuously monitor muscle functioning, paralysis, and paresthesias. Monitor and treat hemodynamic parameters. Assess neurologic status q2–4h and PRN with GCS. Continue to monitor for possible complications and treat accordingly. Weigh daily. Continue cardiac monitoring. Monitor serum sodium osmolality.	Patient will maintain optimal hemodynamic status.	Assess neurologic status q4–8h and PRN. Teach patient/family proper fluid management after discharge. Weigh daily.

Guillain-Barré Syndrome Interdisciplinary Outcome Pathway (continued)

FLUID BALANCE (continued)

Diagnosis/Stabilization Phase		Acute Management Phase		Recovery Phase	
Outcome	Interventions	Outcome	Interventions	Outcome	Interventions
	Cardiac monitoring. Treat potentially life-threatening dysrhythmias. Monitor for possible complications associated with GBS and treat accordingly: • respiratory deterioration • autonomic dysfunction • pharyngeal paralysis • dysphagia • aspiration • muscle cramps • hyperesthesia • orthostatic hypotension • respiratory infection • pneumonia • contractures Monitor UO with indwelling catheter q1–2h. Maintain UO at least 0.5 mL/kg/hr.				

NUTRITION

Diagnosis/Stabilization Phase		Acute Management Phase		Recovery Phase	
Outcome	Interventions	Outcome	Interventions	Outcome	Interventions
Patient will be adequately nourished as evidenced by: • stable weight not > 10% below or > 20% above IBW • albumin 3.5–4 g/dL • total protein 6–8 g/dL	Consult SP to assess swallowing and gag reflexes. If present, initiate DAT. Monitor response to diet. If swallowing and gag reflexes are not present, initiate enteral or parenteral feeding. Assess bowel sounds, abdominal distension, abdominal pain and tenderness q4h and PRN. Consult dietitian to coordinate/direct nutritional support.	Patient will be adequately nourished.	Continue as in Diagnosis/Stabilization Phase. Weigh daily. Monitor protein, albumin, and total lymphocyte counts. Involve dietitian in plan of care as necessary. Assess response to diet and progress as tolerated. Teach patient/family oral motor exercises. Consult SP as needed.	Patient will be adequately nourished.	Monitor response to nutrition given. Instruct patient/family on type of diet at home (i.e., soft, liquid, supplements, heart healthy). Allow family to bring in patient's favorite foods. Arrange for speech therapist in the home as needed. Have patient demonstrate oral motor exercises.

• total lymphocyte count 1,000–3,000	Begin oral motor exercises if indicated. Keep HOB 60–90 elevated degrees if not contraindicated.	If receiving enteral feeding, assess for excessive gastric residual, diarrhea, or constipation. Initiate calorie count when solid foods are started to make certain nutritional needs are met. OT consult for feeding self if able to do so. OT to determine special equipment needs when eating such as built-up handles or lightweight utensils.

MOBILITY

Diagnosis/Stabilization Phase		Acute Management Phase		Recovery Phase	
Outcome	Interventions	Outcome	Interventions	Outcome	Interventions
Patient will maintain muscle strength and tone. Patient will be free of joint contractures.	Assess degree of mobility, muscle strength, paresthesia, and paralysis. This may worsen during the first phase of the illness so frequent assessment is essential, at least q8h. Utilize the Medical Research Council Scale. PT to assess ambulation, mobility, ROM, muscle strength, tone, and flexibility. Institute other types of bed therapy as indicated (i.e., kinetic bed). OT to assess functional ability. Begin passive/active-assist ROM exercises. PT/OT to help determine and direct activity goals.	Patient will achieve optimal mobility. Patient will maintain muscle strength and tone. Patient will be free of joint contractures.	Continue as in Diagnosis/Stabilization Phase. Obtain physical rehabilitation consult. Monitor response to increased activity; decrease activity if adverse events occur (tachycardia, dyspnea, hypotension, ectopy, syncope). Monitor respiratory response to increased activity with pulse oximetry. Use supplemental oxygen to keep $SpO_2 > 92\%$. Provide physical support as necessary. Provide assistive devices as necessary. Begin discussion with family about potential residual physical limitations and required home resources. Continue to assess the degree of mobility. This should stabilize and start to improve in the second stage of the illness. Assess for complications that may be a result of immobility: infection, DVT, pulmonary embolus. Initiate isometric and isotonic exercises. Continue to assess return of function.	Patient will achieve optimal mobility. Patient will be free of joint contractures. Patient will maintain muscle strength and tone.	Prepare for transfer to SNF, home, or physical rehabilitation facility. Arrange for home health visits and equipment. Have patient demonstrate proper use of assistive devices. Include family in all transfer plans. Teach patient/family about progressive exercise program. Have patient/family demonstrate exercises. Monitor patient for return of function. Prepare patient/family for long-term recovery period. Teach patient progressive increase to ADLs as able.

Guillain-Barré Syndrome Interdisciplinary Outcome Pathway (continued)

OXYGENATION/VENTILATION

Diagnosis/Stabilization Phase		Acute Management Phase		Recovery Phase	
Outcome	Interventions	Outcome	Interventions	Outcome	Interventions
Patient will have adequate gas exchange as evidenced by: • SaO$_2$ >90% • ABGs WNL • clear breath sounds • respiratory rate, depth, and rhythm WNL • CXR WNL • absence of dyspnea, cyanosis, and secretions • effective cough • VC >1 L or >30% of predicted value	Constantly monitor respiratory status: functioning, respiratory muscle strength, pulse oximetry, rate, rhythm, depth of respirations, lung sounds, coughing ability, ABGs, and CXR. Be prepared for intubation and mechanical ventilation. Encourage coughing and deep breathing at least q2h. If patient is on ventilator, monitor settings and hemodynamic variables before, during, and after weaning. If patient is not intubated, apply supplemental oxygen. Monitor with pulse oximetry. Keep SpO$_2$ >92%. Assess evidence of tissue perfusion (pain, color, temperature, pulses, signs of decreased perfusion such as altered LOC, decreased UO, ileus). Monitor lab values: ABGs, Hgb.	Patient will have adequate gas exchange.	Monitor and treat oxygenation status per ABGs and/or SpO$_2$. Monitor and treat ventilation status per chest assessment, ABGs, adventitious breath sounds, and CXR. Support patient with oxygen therapy and/or mechanical ventilation as indicated. Use humidification to keep secretions thin. Monitor lab values: ABGs, HGB. Assess effects of increased activity on respiratory status. Monitor with pulse oximetry. Apply supplemental oxygen to keep SpO$_2$ >92%. Observe for complications of GBS that may impair oxygenation/ventilation: respiratory arrest, pneumonia, infection, thrombus, embolus, atelectasis, aspiration. If necessary, prepare patient/family for long-term mechanical ventilation and need for tracheostomy. If so, monitor ventilator settings as described. If long-term mechanical ventilation is indicated, initiate plans to place in SNF, physical rehabilitation facility, or in the home. If going home, involve home health personnel as soon as possible as well as home oxygen supply company. Wean from mechanical ventilation when: • respiratory muscle strength returns	Patient will have adequate gas exchange.	Obtain CXR before discharge. Encourage coughing and deep breathing at least q2h. Begin to teach patient/family about mechanical ventilation and/or tracheostomy care if needed. Involve RCP as necessary. Continue to assess for complications of GBS that may impair oxygenation/ventilation. Teach patient/family about potential complications of GBS and when to call the physician. Assess patient/family understanding of home care. Reinforce knowledge and skills as needed. Arrange RCP follow-up after discharge as needed. Continue respiratory muscle training. Have patient demonstrate various techniques.

- VC >30% of predicted
- NIF >20 cm H_2O

Begin respiratory muscle training. Involve RCP.

Assess autonomic disturbances that can be seen in patients with respiratory muscle paralysis (sinus tachycardia, orthostatic hypotension, asystole, heart blocks, and SIADH).

COMFORT

Diagnosis/Stabilization Phase		Acute Management Phase		Recovery Phase	
Outcome	Interventions	Outcome	Interventions	Outcome	Interventions
Patient will be as comfortable and pain free as possible as evidenced by: • no objective indicators of discomfort • no complaints of discomfort • absence of dyspnea	Assess absence of, or quantity and quality of, pain. Use a pain scale or visual analogue tool. Administer analgesics (narcotic and non-narcotic) and monitor response, particularly respiratory system. Administer sedatives cautiously and monitor effects on respiratory status. Reposition extremities frequently. If patient is intubated or unable to speak, establish effective communication technique with which patient can communicate discomfort. Provide reassurance in a calm, caring, and competent manner. Assess for other symptoms: paresthesias, aches, and hyperesthesias.	Patient will be as relaxed and comfortable as possible.	Continue as in Diagnosis/Stabilization Phase. Provide uninterrupted rest periods in a quiet environment. Instruct patient on relaxation techniques. Use touch therapy, humor, music therapy, and imagery to promote relaxation. Involve family in strategies. Consider alternative methods to control discomfort (i.e., cutaneous stimulation or TENS, ice/heat). Consult PT/OT for splinting as appropriate. Observe for complications of GBS that may cause discomfort: contractures, pulmonary embolus, infection. Repositioning may help alleviate discomfort. Passive ROM exercises may help promote comfort.	Patient will be as relaxed and comfortable as possible.	Continue as in Acute Management Phase. Progress analgesics to oral medications if patient is able to swallow; assess effect on respiratory system. Teach patient/family proper use of analgesics, both prescribed and OTC. Teach patient/family alternative methods to promote relaxation after discharge. Have them give return demonstration.

Guillain-Barré Syndrome Interdisciplinary Outcome Pathway (continued)

SKIN INTEGRITY

Diagnosis/Stabilization Phase		Acute Management Phase		Recovery Phase	
Outcome	Interventions	Outcome	Interventions	Outcome	Interventions
Patient will have intact skin without abrasions or pressure ulcers.	Assess muscle strength, movement, paresthesia, and paralysis at least q4-8h. Consult OT/PT. OT/PT to help determine/direct activity goals. Assess all bony prominences at least q4h and treat if needed. Use preventive pressure-reducing devices if patient is at high risk for developing pressure ulcers. These patients are at high risk of pressure necrosis. Treat pressure ulcers according to hospital protocol.	Patient will have intact skin without abrasions or pressure ulcers.	Continue as in Diagnosis/Stabilization Phase. Establish a turning schedule. Teach family the proper way to turn and allow them to assist with care if they so desire. OT/PT will assess need for splints and assistive devices.	Patient will have intact skin without abrasions or pressure ulcers.	Begin plans for transfer to SNF, physical rehabilitation facility, or home. Teach patient/family about proper skin care after discharge: • turning schedule • massage bony prominences • application of lotion • keep skin dry • gel pad in chair • assistive devices • splints

PROTECTION/SAFETY

Diagnosis/Stabilization Phase		Acute Management Phase		Recovery Phase	
Outcome	Interventions	Outcome	Interventions	Outcome	Interventions
Patient will be protected from possible harm.	Assess need for assistance with activities. Provide physical support as needed. Continue to enlist assistance of PT/OT. Start passive/active-assist ROM exercises at least q4h to prevent joint contractures.	Patient will be protected from possible harm.	Assess need for assistance with activities. Provide physical support as needed. Teach patient/family about ROM exercises. Have patient/family demonstrate these exercises. Keep schedule posted. Position joints in neutral position when possible. When patient is getting OOB, consider possibility of orthostatic hypotension and/or autonomic dysreflexia. Monitor all VS with any activity and decrease activity if adverse events occur. Elevate HOB slowly or use tilt table or Stryker frame.	Patient will be protected from possible harm.	Teach patient/family about any physical limitations in activity after discharge/transfer. Teach patient/family proper use of assistive devices as needed. Have them give return demonstration.

Consider antithrombotic hose. If used, remove at least q8h and inspect skin.
Continue exercise program as discussed under Mobility.

PSYCHOSOCIAL/SELF-DETERMINATION

Diagnosis/Stabilization Phase		Acute Management Phase		Recovery Phase	
Outcome	Interventions	Outcome	Interventions	Outcome	Interventions
Patient will achieve psychophysiologic stability. Patient will demonstrate a decrease in anxiety as evidenced by: • VS WNL • subjective report of decreased anxiety • objective signs of decreased anxiety Patient will begin acceptance of GBS.	Assess physiologic effects of critical care environment on patient (hemodynamic variables, psychological status, signs of increased sympathetic response). Administer sedatives or hypnotics cautiously and monitor respiratory effects. Take measures to reduce sensory overload. If patient is intubated or unable to speak, develop effective interventions to communicate with patient. Alternative techniques include magic slates, talk trach, picture board, elective artificial larynx, and/or clicking pressure-sensitive call devices. Determine coping ability of patient/family and take appropriate measures to meet their needs (i.e., explain condition, explain equipment, provide frequent condition reports, use easy to understand terminology, repeat information as needed, answer all questions, allow verbalization of fears and concerns). Begin explanation of process of GBS and required treatment to patient and family. If patient is unresponsive, maintain verbal and tactile contact with patient.	Patient will achieve psychophysiologic stability. Patient will demonstrate a decrease in anxiety. Patient will demonstrate a decrease in fear. Patient will continue acceptance process of GBS.	Continue as in Diagnosis/Stabilization Phase. Provide adequate rest periods. Allow patient to verbalize/communicate feelings of anxiety and fear. Continue to include family in all aspects of care. Continue to assess coping ability of patient/family and take measures as indicated. Initiate discharge planning: SNF, physical rehabilitation facility, or home. Include patient/family in all decisions concerning care. Continue explanation of GBS.	Patient will achieve psychophysiologic stability. Patient will demonstrate a decrease in anxiety. Patient will demonstrate a decrease in fear. Patient will continue acceptance process of GBS.	Encourage uninterrupted rest periods. Continue to assess coping ability of patient/family and take measures as appropriate (psychological consult, social services, home health agency, chaplain). Refer to outside agencies as needed. Explain process of GBS and any anticipated future effects of illness including potential effects on sexual functioning, returning to work, recreation. Arrange visit from GBS survivor, if possible.

Subarachnoid Hemorrhage
Interdisciplinary Outcome Pathway

COORDINATION OF CARE

Diagnosis/Stabilization Phase		Acute Management Phase		Recovery Phase	
Outcome	Interventions	Outcome	Interventions	Outcome	Interventions
All appropriate disciplines will be involved in the plan of care.	Develop the plan of care with the patient, family, neurologist, neurosurgeon, primary physician, pulmonologist, other specialists as needed, RN, advanced practice nurse, RCP, dietitian, PT, OT, social services, and chaplain.	All appropriate disciplines and team members will be involved in the plan of care.	Develop and update plan of care with the patient/family, other team members, case manager, speech pathologist, and discharge planner. Initiate patient/family/interdisciplinary conferences during hospitalization to reevaluate plan of care, implement new interventions, and anticipate discharge plans.	Patient/family will understand how to maintain optimal health at home, rehabilitation facility, or extended care facility.	Continue planning for anticipated discharge: obtain family social/environmental history, contact home health agency/rehabilitation facility/extended care facility. Begin teaching patient/family about home care if discharge to home is anticipated. Initiate patient/family/interdisciplinary conference to finalize discharge care plan. Provide guidelines concerning follow-up care to patient/family. Provide patient/family with list of resources and phone numbers available for contact to answer questions and for support.

DIAGNOSTICS

Diagnosis/Stabilization Phase		Acute Management Phase		Recovery Phase	
Outcome	Interventions	Outcome	Interventions	Outcome	Interventions
Patient/family will understand tests or procedures that need to be completed (VS, invasive/noninvasive monitoring, assessments, x-rays, CT scans, LP, EKG, EEG, laboratory work, ABGs,	Assess cognitive level of patient and establish effective communication techniques if intubated. Explain all procedures and tests to patient/family and evaluate perceptions/understanding; reeducate as necessary to meet individual needs. Prepare for surgery if indicated.	Patient/family will understand tests or procedures that need to be completed.	Assess patient/family needs for information. Plan and coordinate patient/family/professional conferences as needed to meet identified needs. Explain all procedures and tests, diagnosis and prognosis, plans and interventions. Anticipate further diagnostic tests/procedures and interven-	Patient/family will express understanding of diagnostic tests and procedures in relation to continued health maintenance, rehabilitation, and discharge home (to include MRI, CT scan,	Plan and coordinate patient/family/professional conference to discuss results of diagnostic tests and prognosis, further interventions, and transfer/discharge plans. Provide guidelines for follow-up care. Prepare patient/family for transfer to extended care facility if needed.

(continued from previous page)

Diagnosis/Stabilization Phase		Acute Management Phase		Recovery Phase	
Outcome	Interventions	Outcome	Interventions	Outcome	Interventions
	angiography, transcranial Doppler studies, I & O, fluid restrictions, and environmental restrictions).		tions that may be needed and provide education and emotional support to patient/family.	repeat angiography, laboratory testing, EKG, EEG).	Provide information regarding support groups and educational resources for patient/family for home discharge to maintain optimal physical/neurologic function and psychological emotional balance.

FLUID BALANCE

Diagnosis/Stabilization Phase		Acute Management Phase		Recovery Phase	
Outcome	Interventions	Outcome	Interventions	Outcome	Interventions
Patient will achieve optimal hemodynamic status as evidenced by: • MAP > 70 mm Hg • BP controlled to achieve adequate cerebral blood flow (CBF), CPP of 50–80 mmHg and ICP < 15 mmHg • hemodynamic parameters WNL • absence of cardiac dysrhythmias • normal LOC and neurologic function	Monitor and treat increased ICP, rebleeding, and/or vasospasm including: • stimuli-controlled environment • bed rest • HOB elevated 30 degrees (contraindicated in posterior fossa surgical treatment approaches) • medications for seizure, anxiety, pain, or nausea; may need paralysis and sedation • calcium channel blockers for vasospasm if ordered • colloidal agents, crystalloids, diuretics, or vasoactive drugs as indicated to maintain normal CPP and MAP • anticonvulsant agents if seizure activity present • fluid restriction (usually 500 cc/8 hours including oral and intravenous) Monitor and treat abnormal hemodynamic parameters: • BP • CO/CI • SV/SI • PA pressures, CVP, PCWP • SvO$_2$	Patient will maintain optimal hemodynamic status/cardiovascular and neurologic function. Patient will maintain normal cerebral and tissue perfusion as evidenced by: • SvO$_2$ • LOC • CPP • UO > 0.5 mL/kg/hr • stable cognitive skills, motor function, muscle tone, position, and reflexes. Patient will maintain normal electrolyte balance.	Continue as in Diagnosis/Stabilization Phase. Monitor cardiopulmonary and neurologic parameters closely. Any deterioration warrants *immediate action.* Weigh daily. Monitor and treat electrolyte disturbances such as diabetes insipidus or SIADH. Monitor for complications of infection such as sepsis, pneumonia, interstitial pneumonitis, or meningitis by monitoring WBC, fever, and CXR abnormalities. Monitor and treat signs of inadequate tissue perfusion such as decreased LOC, < 0.5 mL/kg/hr of urine, faint or absent peripheral pulses, pupillary changes. Wean intravenous sedation, therapeutic paralysis, diuretics, vasoactive drugs, and mechanical ventilation as patient improves.	Patient will maintain optimal cardiovascular/hemodynamic/neurologic status.	Monitor effects of all discontinued medications, treatments, and therapies on cardiovascular, hemodynamic, pulmonary, and neurologic function. Monitor I & O and daily weight until transfer/discharge. Provide information to patient/family regarding signs and symptoms of neurologic deficits to report to physician such as confusion, lethargy, or seizure activity.

Subarachnoid Hemorrhage Interdisciplinary Outcome Pathway (*continued*)

FLUID BALANCE (continued)

Diagnosis/Stabilization Phase		Acute Management Phase		Recovery Phase	
Outcome	Interventions	Outcome	Interventions	Outcome	Interventions
	Monitor I & O. Assess and monitor neurologic status q2h including: • GCS • LOC • cognitive and motor function deficits • abnormal muscle tone/posture • abnormal reflexes (Bruzinski and Kernig's signs) • cranial nerve deficits • pupillary size/response changes				

NUTRITION

Diagnosis/Stabilization Phase		Acute Management Phase		Recovery Phase	
Outcome	Interventions	Outcome	Interventions	Outcome	Interventions
Patient will be adequately nourished as evidenced by: • stable weight • weight not >10% below or >20% above IBW • albumin >3.5 g/dL • prealbumin >15 g/dL • total protein 6–8 g/dL • total lymphocyte count 1,000–3,000	Consult dietitian to help determine and direct nutritional support. Monitor albumin, prealbumin, total protein. Assess for and institute measures to control N & V. Assess bowel function for potential complications such as an ileus, GI bleed.	Patient will be adequately nourished.	Consult SP to assess swallowing and gag reflexes: if present, initiate diet as tolerated; if not, initiate enteral or parenteral feeding based on laboratory data and nutritional/metabolic needs assessment by interdisciplinary team. Assess and teach oral/motor exercises as they relate to adequate food intake and chewing such as small bites, chewing completely, and double swallowing. Monitor for signs of aspiration.	Patient will be adequately nourished.	Reevaluate nutritional goals and alter treatment appropriately. Instruct patient/family regarding nutritional goals and diet at home. Provide phone number of outpatient dietitian.

Consider calorie count when patient is on oral feedings to assure patient is meeting nutritional goals.

Involve dietitian if:
- patient eating less than half of food of tray
- albumin <3.5 g/dL

Monitor serum albumin level, serum protein levels, and total lymphocyte counts.

Monitor for signs of negative nitrogen balance such as edema in feet, ankles, or trunk, decreased protein, albumin count.

Monitor and treat patient with abnormal GI function such as diarrhea.

Consult OT for any problems with feeding self. OT to obtain any specific equipment needed for eating such as built-up handles or light-weight utensils.

MOBILITY

Diagnosis/Stabilization Phase		Acute Management Phase		Recovery Phase	
Outcome	Interventions	Outcome	Interventions	Outcome	Interventions
Patient will maintain optimal motor function. Patient will be free of joint contractures.	PT to assess ambulation, mobility, muscle flexibility, strength, and tone. OT to assess functional activity. PT/OT to determine and direct activity goals. Begin progressive activity program such as passive/active-assist ROM, bed transfers, ambulation. Monitor response to activity.	Patient's neurologic function will improve or remain stable. Patient will maintain joint integrity and be free of joint contractures. Patient will be free of immobility complications such as: • pneumonia • atelectasis • deep vein thrombosis • pressure ulcers	Continue as in Diagnosis/Stabilization Phase. OT to teach correct positioning to maintain joint integrity and prevent joint stress, strain, or injury. Provide physical assistance or assistive devices as indicated. Assess for negative effects of immobility and initiate preventative measures to prevent: • deep vein thrombosis • peripheral edema • muscle wasting • atelectasis, pneumonia, increased intrapulmonary shunting	Patient will have optimal mobility.	Rehabilitative or physiatry consult if indicated. Develop home exercise plan. Consult PT/OT for home care if needed.

Subarachnoid Hemorrhage Interdisciplinary Outcome Pathway (continued)

MOBILITY (continued)

Diagnosis/Stabilization Phase		Acute Management Phase		Recovery Phase	
Outcome	Interventions	Outcome	Interventions	Outcome	Interventions
			gastrointestinal complications such as ileus, nausea, constipation. Initiate antiembolic hose and SCD devices as preventative therapeutic measures.		

OXYGENATION/VENTILATION

Diagnosis/Stabilization Phase		Acute Management Phase		Recovery Phase	
Outcome	Interventions	Outcome	Interventions	Outcome	Interventions
Patient will have adequate airway and gas exchange as evidenced by: • $SaO_2 > 90\%$, SpO_2 saturation $> 92\%$ • ABGs WNL; $PaO_2 > 90$, $PaCO_2$ 25–35 mmHg • respiratory rate, depth, and pattern WNL • clear breath sounds • CXR WNL • absence of dyspnea, cyanosis, and secretions • effective cough • ventilation to maintain moderate hyperventilation (PCO_2 25–35) for first 24–48 hours.	Monitor respiratory status: strength, rate, depth, pattern, ability to cough, secretions, lung sounds, ABGs, SpO_2, and pulmonary parameters. Monitor CXR reports. Prepare client/family for impending intubation and mechanical ventilation if applicable. Initiate and maintain sedation/paralysis as prescribed if indicated.	Patient will have adequate ventilation and gas exchange as evidenced by $SaO_2 > 90\%$ and ABGs within normal limits.	Support client with O_2 therapy and/or mechanical ventilation as indicated. Monitor and treat oxygenation status per SaO_2/ABG results. Monitor and treat ventilation status per chest assessments (at least q2–4h), ABG results, adventitious breath sounds, and CXR results. Assess the relationship of increased ICP and respiration/ventilation. Observe and report complications such as pneumothorax, atelectasis, pulmonary edema/congestive heart failure, pneumonia, and pulmonary embolus. Turn and position to prevent aspiration of emesis or oral secretions. Deep breathe q2h and discourage forceful coughing.	Patient will have adequate airway management, ventilation, and gas exchange.	Obtain CXR before transfer/discharge to ensure absence of complications. Plan and coordinate patient/family/professional conference to provide information/education regarding airway/oxygenation maintenance after transfer/discharge. Consult with interdisciplinary team to provide necessary equipment and teaching regarding use of equipment for patient/family/other upon discharge as needed (may need to consult home health agency for assistance with care). Assess patient/family for comprehension of care and use of equipment/skills, plan of care, and guidelines for prevention of complications; provide necessary teaching and reinforcement.

Provide continuous lateral rotational therapy (CLRT) as indicated by patient identification systems; consider a-A ratio and/or other indicator of intrapulmonary shunting. CLRT may also be helpful in preventing pneumonia and/or lower respiratory tract infections as long as CLRT is not contraindicated by placement of ventricular drains.

Assess patient perceptions and psychological/emotional coping responses to mechanical ventilation; provide education and support through identified means of communication; sedation as prescribed.

Assess readiness and initiate weaning of mechanical ventilation/oxygen therapy as patient tolerates (normal respiratory parameters and SpO_2 >92%).

Assess need for long-term mechanical ventilation; if indicated, begin contact with social services and/or discharge planner to long-term care discharge planning.

COMFORT

Diagnosis/Stabilization Phase		Acute Management Phase		Recovery Phase	
Outcome	Interventions	Outcome	Interventions	Outcome	Interventions
Patient will show clinical signs of comfort, rest, and relaxation. Patient will express comfort and freedom from pain if capable of verbal communication.	Assess objective signs and symptoms of pain, comfort, rest, and relaxation. Assess verbalized quantity and quality of pain as well as causes/relief. Use pain scale or visual analogue scale to evaluate patient's pain.	Patient will be as relaxed and comfortable as possible.	Continue as in Diagnosis/Stabilization Phase. Plan and provide uninterrupted periods of rest/sleep. Observe for complications of head injury that may prolong discomfort. Assess psychological impact of pain perception.	Patient will be as relaxed and comfortable as possible.	Continue as in Diagnosis/Stabilization and Acute Management phases. Progress analgesics to oral medications and assess responses; wean from medication as indicated. Teach patient/family alternative methods to promote relaxation and comfort after discharge such as guided imagery, touch therapy, humor, and music therapy.

Subarachnoid Hemorrhage Interdisciplinary Outcome Pathway (continued)

COMFORT (continued)

Diagnosis/Stabilization Phase		Acute Management Phase		Recovery Phase	
Outcome	Interventions	Outcome	Interventions	Outcome	Interventions
	Administer analgesics/sedatives and monitor responses (in particular, monitor level of consciousness and neurologic status). Assess psychological perceptions of pain/emotional responses; provide education and information as well as support/reassurance as indicated.		Teach patient relaxation techniques. Suggest alternative therapies (i.e., touch therapy, humor, music, and imagery) to promote relaxation. Involve family in strategies. Observe for and institute measures to control pain and nausea (increased or recurrent pain or N & V may indicate increased ICP).		

SKIN INTEGRITY

Diagnosis/Stabilization Phase		Acute Management Phase		Recovery Phase	
Outcome	Interventions	Outcome	Interventions	Outcome	Interventions
Patient will have intact skin without abrasions or pressure ulcers.	Assess color, temperature of skin, sensation, presence of edema, capillary refill, vascularity, and pulses of all extremities and bony prominences. Use protective pressure-reducing devices if patient is at risk for development of breakdown.	Patient will have intact skin without abrasions or pressure ulcers.	Same as in Diagnosis/Stabilization Phase. Treat pressure ulcers according to hospital policy. May need to obtain pressure-reducing mattress or specialty bed.	Patient will have intact skin without abrasions or pressure ulcers.	Teach patient/family proper skin care maintenance before discharge. Teach patient/family all aspects of pressure relief in preventing alterations in skin integrity.

PROTECTION/SAFETY

Diagnosis/Stabilization Phase		Acute Management Phase		Recovery Phase	
Outcome	Interventions	Outcome	Interventions	Outcome	Interventions
Patient will be protected from possible harm.	Monitor and treat for seizure activity. Assess need for assistance with activities. Provide physical assistance as needed. Assess need for wrist restraints if patient is intubated, has a decreased LOC, or is agitated	Patient will be protected from possible harm.	Continue as in Diagnosis/Stabilization Phase. Provide appropriate physical assistance as patient increases mobility to prevent falls or injury. Pad side rails to prevent injury if patient is prone to or having seizures.	Patient will be protected from possible harm.	Review with patient/family any physical limitations in activity before discharge. Consult PT/OT for home follow-up if limitations are present.

or restless. Explain need for restraints to patient/family. Assess response to restraints when used and check q1h for skin integrity and impairment to circulation. Follow hospital protocol for use of restraints. Promote adequate sleep patterns with reduced activity, stimuli, and lighting in room.

PSYCHOSOCIAL/SELF-DETERMINATION

Diagnosis/Stabilization Phase		Acute Management Phase		Recovery Phase	
Outcome	Interventions	Outcome	Interventions	Outcome	Interventions
Patient will achieve psychophysiologic stability. Patient will demonstrate a decrease in anxiety as evidenced by: • VS WNL • expressed decrease in anxiety • overt behavioral evidence of calmness	Assess physiologic effects of critical situation/knowledge deficit on patient (hemodynamic variables, psychological status, signs of increased sympathetic response). Assess need for patient/family conference to allow expression of needs, desires, fears, concerns, and to voice questions regarding physical and neurologic outcome.	Patient will achieve psychophysiologic stability. Patient will demonstrate a decrease in anxiety as evidenced by: • VS WNL • expressed decrease in anxiety	Continue as in Diagnosis/Stabilization Phase. Provide adequate sleep/rest periods for patient. Encourage patient to progress in ADLs and IADLs to become as independent as possible to enhance self-esteem. Encourage discussion with patient/family regarding feelings of anxiety and fear about diagnosis, prognosis, and treatment plans. Encourage discussion regarding self-perception of change in physical attributes secondary to surgery, paralysis, or other complications. Consult chaplain, psychologist, and/or psychiatrist as needed for psychological and emotional support.	Patient will achieve psychophysiologic stability.	Continue as in Acute Management Phase. Encourage family to allow patient to be as independent as possible but still maintain safety and protection. Assess and provide information regarding health maintenance after discharge. Continue to assess patient/family coping abilities and provide information on appropriate support groups/resources. Provide list of resources with phone numbers. Address concerns patient may have about impact on daily life.

CHAPTER 5

Renal Pathways

Acute Renal Failure
Interdisciplinary Outcome Pathway

COORDINATION OF CARE

	Diagnosis/Stabilization Phase		Acute Management Phase		Recovery Phase	
	Outcome	Interventions	Outcome	Interventions	Outcome	Interventions
	All appropriate team members and disciplines will be involved in the plan of care.	Develop the plan of care with the patient, family, primary physician, nephrologist, cardiologist, pulmonologist, hematologist, RN, advanced practice nurse, PT, OT, chaplain, and dialysis staff.	All appropriate team members and disciplines will be involved in the plan of care.	Update the plan of care with patient/family, other team members, nephrologist, social services, dietitian, and discharge planner. Initiate planning for anticipated discharge. Begin teaching patient/family about home care (i.e., hemodialysis, peritoneal dialysis) if indicated.	All appropriate disciplines will be consulted.	Provide instructions for dialysis and/or follow-up care. Provide patient/family with phone numbers of resources available.

DIAGNOSTICS

	Diagnosis/Stabilization Phase		Acute Management Phase		Recovery Phase	
	Outcome	Interventions	Outcome	Interventions	Outcome	Interventions
	Patient will understand any tests or procedures that must be completed (serum labs, urine electrolytes, urine osmolality, specific gravity, x-rays, ABGs, IV urography studies, renal biopsy, and ultrasounds). Patient will understand dialysis process.	Explain procedures and tests to patient/family. Be sensitive to patient/family's individualized need for information. Explain dialysis process.	Patient will understand any tests or procedures that must be completed. Patient will understand the dialysis process.	Continue as in Diagnosis/Stabilization Phase.	Patient will understand meaning of diagnostic tests in relation to continued care.	Review with patient family: • discharge results of lab tests • renal function • what to expect in renal function/health Assist with making appointments and travel arrangements for follow-up care and/or hemodialysis.

FLUID BALANCE

Diagnosis/Stabilization Phase		Acute Management Phase		Recovery Phase	
Outcome	Interventions	Outcome	Interventions	Outcome	Interventions
Patient will achieve optimal renal/fluid and electrolyte status as evidenced by: • normovolemic state (adequate circulatory volume) • optimal achievable renal function • normal electrolytes (including calcium and phosphorus) • normal serum glucose • normal hematologic parameters such as Hgb, platelets, and WBCs	Monitor renal parameters including: • UO • BUN • serum creatinine • BUN/serum creatinine ratio • serum electrolytes • acid-base status • urine electrolytes • urine osmolality • specific gravity Monitor fluid status, including I & O (fluid restriction), daily weights, UO trends, VS, CVP, and PCWP. Monitor for signs and symptoms of hypervolemia such as hypertension, tachycardia, pulmonary edema, peripheral edema, distended neck veins, and elevated CVP. Monitor and treat cause of acute renal dysfunction including: • hypoperfusion (prerenal) states • obstructions in the outflow of urine from the body (postrenal states) • nephrotoxic agents and/or severe renal ischemia Direct treatment goals with aim toward maintaining glomerular filtration and urine flow. Monitor patient closely for response of fluid and/or diuretic challenges. Support and monitor patient closely during the three typical phases of acute renal failure: • oliguric phase • diuretic phase • recovery phase	Patient will achieve optimal renal/fluid and electrolyte status.	Continue as in Diagnosis/Stabilization Phase. Monitor, support, and treat during dialysis treatments. Assess patient's response to dialysis therapies. Begin teaching patient and family about renal function, current clinical problems, current treatment, and expected clinical course.	Patient will maintain optimal renal/fluid and electrolyte status.	Continue as in Acute Management Phase. Prepare and instruct patient on necessary ongoing therapies (peritoneal dialysis vs. hemodialysis). Instruct patient in follow-up care indicated. Teach patient/family signs and symptoms of fluid overload and/or electrolyte disturbances. Teach patient/family about fluid retention. Teach patient importance of daily weights.

Acute Renal Failure Interdisciplinary Outcome Pathway (continued)

FLUID BALANCE (continued)

Diagnosis/Stabilization Phase		Acute Management Phase		Recovery Phase	
Outcome	Interventions	Outcome	Interventions	Outcome	Interventions
	Monitor and treat for signs of complications that can occur with acute renal failure: hypertension, cardiac dysfunction, pulmonary edema, dysrhythmias, lethargy, decreased LOC, electrolyte disturbances, acid-base disturbances, abnormal glucose metabolism, anemia, thrombocytopenia, leukopenia, N & V, and subcutaneous edema.				
	Monitor, support, and treat patient with dialysis therapies if indicated.				
	Assess VS, fluid status, CVP, PCWP, and patient response to dialysis therapies.				
	Hemodialysis: Assure that vascular access to hemodialysis remains patent: • palpate the thrill and auscultate buzzing sound over shunt periodically • avoid constrictions above access such as tourniquets or BP cuffs • assure that access is free from infection • monitor perfusion (color, temperature, and sensation) of related extremity				
	Peritoneal dialysis • warm dialysate to body temperature and slowly infuse. • monitor dialysate infusion and drainage closely to evaluate effectiveness of peritoneal dialysis. • weigh patient daily after the drain cycle is complete.				

- monitor for signs and symptoms of fluid overload.
- monitor closely for signs and symptoms of infection. Report cloudiness or color change in drained fluid. Culture drainage daily.

Continuous ultrafiltration:
- monitor and regulate ultrafiltration rate hourly based on patient's response and fluid status
- assess and troubleshoot hemofilter and blood tubing hourly
- monitor closely for signs and symptoms of infection

NUTRITION

Diagnosis/Stabilization Phase		Acute Management Phase		Recovery Phase	
Outcome	Interventions	Outcome	Interventions	Outcome	Interventions
Patient will be adequately nourished as evidenced by: • stable weight not >10% below or >20% above IBW • albumin 3.5–4.0 g/dL • total protein 6–8 g/dL • total lymphocyte count 1,000–3,000	Consult dietitian to direct/coordinate nutritional support. Monitor caloric intake and percentages of fats, carbohydrates, and proteins closely. • protein intake should be somewhat restricted (sufficient yet not excessive; usually 20–30 g/day but will vary from patient to patient) • carbohydrates 100 g/day • assess need for essential and nonessential amino acids Restrict potassium and sodium intake. Restrict fluid intake. Monitor serum protein, albumin, Hct, and urea levels and daily weight to assess effectiveness of nutritional therapy.	Patient will be adequately nourished.	Continue as in Diagnosis/Stabilization Phase. Monitor patient's response to dietary restrictions. Consider activity level when assessing caloric need. Consider calorie count to make certain patient is receiving adequate calories. Teach patient/family rationale for diet restrictions.	Patient will be adequately nourished.	Teach patient/family protein, carbohydrate, and potassium requirements and sodium/fluid restrictions. If patient is diabetic, include carbohydrate restriction as well.

Acute Renal Failure Interdisciplinary Outcome Pathway (continued)

MOBILITY

Diagnosis/Stabilization Phase		Acute Management Phase		Recovery Phase	
Outcome	Interventions	Outcome	Interventions	Outcome	Interventions
Patient will achieve optimal mobility.	Consult PT to assess muscle strength, flexibility, tone, ambulation, and mobility. Begin passive/active-assist ROM exercises. Consult OT to assess functional ability.	Patient will achieve optimal mobility.	PT/OT to help direct and determine activity goals. Progress exercise as tolerated. Dangle, OOB for meals, and walking 50 feet. Monitor patient's response to activity. Decrease if adverse events occur (tachycardia, dyspnea, syncope, ectopy, hypo/hypertension). Provide physical support as needed.	Patient will achieve optimal mobility.	Assist patient/family in developing a home exercise program.

OXYGENATION/VENTILATION

Diagnosis/Stabilization Phase		Acute Management Phase		Recovery Phase	
Outcome	Interventions	Outcome	Interventions	Outcome	Interventions
Patient will have adequate gas exchange as evidenced by: • SaO_2 >90% • SpO_2 >92% • ABGs WNL for patient (CO_2 decreased to compensate for metabolic acidosis) • clear breath sounds • respiratory rate, depth, and rhythm WNL • normal CXR Patient will have adequate tissue perfusion as evidenced by:	Monitor and treat oxygenation status per ABGs and/or SaO_2. Involve RCP. Assess sensorium and LOC q1h. Assess evidence of tissue perfusion (pain, pulses, color, temperature, signs of decreased perfusion such as decreased UO, altered LOC, and ileus). Monitor for signs and symptoms of pulmonary distress from fluid overload. Monitor acid-base status per ABGs. Support patient with O_2 therapy and/or mechanical ventilation as indicated.	Patient will have adequate gas exchange and adequate tissue perfusion.	Monitor and treat oxygenation/ventilation disturbances. Continue to involve RCP in care. Wean oxygen therapy and/or mechanical ventilation as tolerated and monitor response. Observe for complications of acute renal failure that may impair oxygenation/ventilation (i.e., CHF, fatigue, lethargy, somnolence).	Patient will have adequate gas exchange.	Monitor and treat oxygenation/ventilation disturbances. Teach patient/family about pulmonary symptoms of fluid overload and what signs and symptoms to report to the physician.

- normovolemic status
- adequate Hgb
- optimal UO depending on phase of ARF
- alert and oriented
- appropriate LOC

COMFORT

Diagnosis/Stabilization Phase		Acute Management Phase		Recovery Phase	
Outcome	Interventions	Outcome	Interventions	Outcome	Interventions
Patient will be as comfortable and pain free as possible as evidenced by: • no objective indicators of discomfort • no complaints of discomfort	Monitor and treat breathing status closely for signs and symptoms of respiratory distress related to fluid overload. Keep HOB elevated and review breathing techniques such as pursed-lip breathing to minimize respiratory distress. Creatively plan fluid restriction over 24h, including periodic sips of water and ice chips to minimize thirst. Offer gum, hard candy, mouth swab, and frequent oral care. Assess quantity and quality of discomfort. Provide a quiet environment and reassurance in a calm, competent, and caring manner. Observe for complications that may cause discomfort: infection of vascular access for hemodialysis, peritonitis, inadequate draining during peritoneal dialysis, nausea, vomiting. Administer analgesics, antiemetics, sedatives, or anxiolytics as needed and monitor response.	Patient will be as comfortable and pain free as possible.	Continue as in Diagnosis/Stabilization Phase. Provide adequate rest periods, especially if patient is anemic. Teach patient relaxation techniques, including complementary therapies such as touch therapy, humor, or music therapy. Involve family in strategies.	Patient will be as comfortable and pain free as possible.	Teach patient/family breathing techniques, relaxation, and complementary therapy techniques. Have patient/family give return demonstration. Teach patient/family creative ways to maintain fluid restriction and alleviate thirst.

Acute Renal Failure Interdisciplinary Outcome Pathway (*continued*)

SKIN INTEGRITY

Diagnosis/Stabilization Phase		Acute Management Phase		Recovery Phase	
Outcome	Interventions	Outcome	Interventions	Outcome	Interventions
Patient will have intact skin without abrasions or pressure ulcers.	Assess skin integrity and all bony prominences q4h. Use superfatted or lanolin-based soap for bathing and apply emollients for itching. Use preventive pressure-reducing devices if patient is at high risk for pressure ulcer development. Treat pressure ulcers according to hospital protocol.	Patient will have intact skin without abrasions or pressure ulcers.	Continue as in Diagnosis/Stabilization Phase.	Patient will have intact skin without abrasions or pressure ulcers.	Avoid tight-fitting shoes or clothing that may create pressure points susceptible to breakdown. Teach patient/family about skin care management after discharge.

PROTECTION/SAFETY

Diagnosis/Stabilization Phase		Acute Management Phase		Recovery Phase	
Outcome	Interventions	Outcome	Interventions	Outcome	Interventions
Patient will be protected from possible harm.	Assess need for wrist restraints if patient is intubated, has a decreased LOC, is unable to follow commands, or for affected extremity during hemodialysis. Explain need for restraints to patient/family. If restrained, assess response to restraints and check q1–2h for skin integrity and impairment to circulation. Follow hospital protocol for use of restraints. Maintain a patent and infection-free vascular access device for hemodialysis or catheter for peritoneal dialysis. Follow seizure precautions.	Patient will be protected from possible harm.	Continue as in Diagnosis/Stabilization Phase. Provide physical support when dangling or beginning progressive exercise program, and monitor response.	Patient will be protected from possible harm.	Teach patient/family about patient's possible physical limitations.

PSYCHOSOCIAL/SELF-DETERMINATION

Diagnosis/Stabilization Phase		Acute Management Phase		Recovery Phase	
Outcome	Interventions	Outcome	Interventions	Outcome	Interventions
Patient will achieve psychophysiologic stability. Patient will demonstrate a decrease in anxiety as evidenced by: • VS WNL • LOC WNL • subjective reports of decreased anxiety level • objective assessment of decreased anxiety level Patient will begin acceptance process of long-term illness.	Assess physiologic effects of critical care environment on patient. If intubated, develop interventions for effective communication. Assess patient for appropriate level of stress. Arrange for flexible visitation to meet needs of patient and family. Assess personal responses and coping ability of patient/family and take appropriate measures to meet their needs and reduce their anxiety (i.e., explain condition and equipment, provide frequent condition reports, use easy to understand terminology, repeat information as needed, allow family to visit, and answer all questions). Use sedatives and antidepressants as appropriate.	Patient will achieve psychophysiologic stability. Patient will demonstrate a decrease in anxiety. Patient will continue acceptance process of acute renal failure and extended illness.	Continue as in Diagnosis/Stabilization Phase. Initiate discharge planning. Include patient/family in decisions concerning care. Provide information on local support groups, kidney centers, and agencies such as the National Kidney Foundation.	Patient will achieve psychophysiologic stability. Patient will demonstrate a decrease in anxiety. Patient will continue acceptance process of acute renal failure and extended illness.	Continue as in Acute Management Phase. Address concerns about impact on daily life: ADLs, return to work, activities, sexual functioning, driving.

End-Stage Renal Disease/Kidney Transplantation Interdisciplinary Outcome Pathway

COORDINATION OF CARE

Diagnosis/Stabilization Phase		Acute Management Phase		Recovery Phase	
Outcome	Interventions	Outcome	Interventions	Outcome	Interventions
All appropriate team members and disciplines will be involved in the plan of care.	Develop a plan of care with the patient, family, primary physician, nephrologist, kidney transplant coordinator, cardiologist, pulmonologist, hematologist, RN, advanced practice nurse, social services, chaplain, dietitian, and dialysis staff.	All appropriate team members and disciplines will be involved in the plan of care.	Update the plan of care with the patient/family, other team members, PT, OT, recreational therapist, and discharge planner.	All appropriate team members and disciplines will be involved in the plan of care.	Provide instructions for continuing care: • physician's office visit and/or clinic visit • medication regimen • signs and symptoms to report to physician Provide patient/family with phone numbers of resources available.

DIAGNOSTICS

Diagnosis/Stabilization Phase		Acute Management Phase		Recovery Phase	
Outcome	Interventions	Outcome	Interventions	Outcome	Interventions
Patient will understand any tests or procedures that must be completed to assess renal function (hemodynamic assessments, frequent VS, serum labs, calcium and phosphate levels, CBC, platelet count, and renal ultrasound). Patient will understand evaluation and assessment for kidney transplantation potential (echocardiogram, cardiac workup, PFTs, histocompat-	Explain procedures and tests to patient/family. Be sensitive to patient/family's individual needs for information.	Patient will understand meaning of diagnostic tests in relation to continuing care.	Review with patient before discharge results of lab tests and renal function postop. Review with patient/family what to expect in renal function/health. Teach patient/family various treatments when rejection is suspected such as ultrasound, renal scan, renal biopsy, and drug regimen.	Patient will understand meaning of diagnostic tests in relation to continuing care.	Continue as in Acute Management Phase.

ibility studies, human leukocyte antigen test, ABO blood typing, mixed lymphocyte culture, serum blood test to assess for cytoxic antibodies, level of suppressor T cells, clotting factors, ABGs, and x-rays).

FLUID BALANCE

Diagnosis/Stabilization Phase		Acute Management Phase		Recovery Phase	
Outcome	Interventions	Outcome	Interventions	Outcome	Interventions
Patient will achieve and maintain stable fluid and electrolyte status with renal replacement therapy as evidenced by: • fluid balance remains at or near baseline • stable hematologic parameters such as Hgb, WBCs, and platelets • optimal cardiopulmonary function • stable hemodynamic status • stable hemodialysis regimen Patient will be evaluated for kidney transplant.	Monitor and treat signs/symptoms of hypervolemia such as hypertension, tachycardia, pulmonary edema, frothy sputum, peripheral edema, JVD, inspiratory crackles, S3, or increased CVP. Monitor renal parameters including UO (if any), BUN, serum creatinine, BUN/Scr ratio, serum electrolytes, and acid-base status. Assess effect of prescribed antihypertensive agents on BP and HR. Assess patient's understanding and compliance with prescribed medication, fluid, and diet regimen. Determine patient's baseline weight. Weigh daily. Maintain patient's fluid and sodium restriction. Assess dysfunction in other organ systems caused by impaired renal function such as pericarditis, dysrhythmias, lethargy, decreased LOC, electrolyte disturbances (especially hyperkalemia, hyperphosphatemia, hypocalcemia), acid-base disturbances, anemia, platelet dysfunction, anorexia, N & V, bleeding tendencies, and subcutaneous edema.	Patient will achieve and maintain stable fluid and electrolyte status after kidney transplant.	Monitor kidney function closely per UO, creatinine clearance, Scr levels, BUN, and BUN/Scr ratio. Anticipate possible acute tubular necrosis secondary to preservation injury. Prepare patient for possible temporary intermittent hemodialysis treatments when necessary. Maintain adequate fluid balance. Monitor for signs and symptoms of fluid volume deficit (CVP < 4 mmHg, PCWP < 6 mmHg, tachycardia, systolic BP < 110 mmHg) that may occur from an osmotic diuresis post-transplant. Monitor for signs and symptoms of fluid overload. Administer diuretics, renal dose dopamine (1–3 mcg/kg/minute), and/or antihypertensives as indicated postop. If kidney function is delayed post-transplant, monitor and treat abnormal electrolytes such as hyperkalemia, hypermagnesemia, hyperphosphatemia, hypocalcemia, and metabolic acidosis. Administer calcium replacements and phosphate binders when indicated.	Patient will maintain stable fluid and electrolyte status after kidney transplant.	Teach patient/family about post-transplant care including: • daily log of weight, temperature, BP, pertinent laboratory data, and exercise regimen • medications, including cardiac medications, antihypertensives, immunosuppressants, and antirejection medications • signs and symptoms of fluid overload and/or electrolyte disturbances

End-Stage Renal Disease/Kidney Transplantation Interdisciplinary Outcome Pathway (continued)

FLUID BALANCE (continued)

Diagnosis/Stabilization Phase		Acute Management Phase		Recovery Phase	
Outcome	Interventions	Outcome	Interventions	Outcome	Interventions
	Minimize number of blood samples drawn. Monitor, support, and treat patient during dialysis therapy. Assess VS, fluid status, and patient response to dialysis. Monitor and treat signs/symptoms of hypovolemia secondary to dialysis. Assess and maintain vascular access device: • palpate the thrill and auscultate bruit over shunt periodically • avoid constrictions above access such as tourniquets or cuffs • ensure that access is free from infection • monitor perfusion (color, temperature, and sensation) of related extremity Assist with pretransplantation screening including: • extensive cardiopulmonary evaluation • psychosocial assessment (rule out psychosis, severe personality disorder, or history of noncompliance) • histocompatibility studies (ABO and human leukocyte antigen) Administer preop immunosuppressive agents if indicated.		Monitor and assess dysfunction in other organ systems that can occur post-transplant such as dysrhythmias, hypotension, EKG changes, vascular thromboses, hypertension, pulmonary edema, ARDS, diarrhea, GI bleeding, or infection. Administer immunosuppressive agents as ordered and monitor closely for infection, rejection, anemia, thrombocytopenia, or leukopenia. Maintain urinary catheter up to 1 week.		

NUTRITION

	Diagnosis/Stabilization Phase		Acute Management Phase		Recovery Phase
	Outcome	**Interventions**	**Outcome**	**Interventions**	**Outcome**	**Interventions**

Diagnosis/Stabilization Phase — Outcome	Diagnosis/Stabilization Phase — Interventions
Patient will be adequately nourished as evidenced by: • stable weight not >10% below or >20% above IBW • albumin >3.0 g/dL • prealbumin >15 g/dL • total protein 6–8 g/dL • total lymphocyte count 1,000–3,000	Consult dietitian to help determine and direct nutritional support. Monitor caloric intake and percentages of fats, carbohydrates, and proteins closely. Dietary recommendations are: • 1 g protein per kg of IBW • 2–3 g sodium • 40–50 mEq potassium (remind patient/family not to use salt substitutes containing potassium chloride) • 1,200 mg phosphorus per day • calcium supplements if needed when phosphorus controlled • vitamin and iron supplements; folate if anemic Restrict fluid intake to 500–1,000 mL/day (plus sum of UO, if any) and weigh daily. Monitor serum protein, albumin, Hct, urea levels, and daily weight to assess effectiveness of nutritional therapy. Keep serum albumin >3.0 g/dL. Medications to improve gastric motility may be necessary to enhance absorption of nutrients and minimize need for antiemetics. Assess oral mucosa and provide frequent oral hygiene. Monitor bowel function and encourage use of laxatives, stool softeners, or high fiber diet when indicated. Administer H_2 antagonists if ordered.

Acute Management Phase — Outcome	Acute Management Phase — Interventions
Patient will be adequately nourished.	Advance to DAT after kidney transplant. Consult dietitian if: • albumin <3.0 • counseling is needed • eating less than half of food on tray Monitor bowel function as described. Monitor and treat anorexia and dysphagia. Encourage PO fluid intake to thirst (not restricted). Teach patient/family to avoid simple sugars and limit sodium intake. Encourage patient to eat a high protein diet up to 4 weeks post-transplant. Consider calorie count to ascertain patient is receiving adequate nutrition.

Recovery Phase — Outcome	Recovery Phase — Interventions
Patient will be adequately nourished.	Teach patient/family to follow low fat diet and limit simple sugars and sodium intake. Teach patient/family to eat less protein after 4 weeks as prednisone is tapered.

End-Stage Renal Disease/Kidney Transplantation Interdisciplinary Outcome Pathway (continued)

MOBILITY

Diagnosis/Stabilization Phase		Acute Management Phase		Recovery Phase	
Outcome	Interventions	Outcome	Interventions	Outcome	Interventions
Patient will achieve optimal mobility.	Monitor patient's tolerance to activity (may be decreased if anemic). Decrease activity if adverse events occur (tachycardia, dyspnea, ectopy, syncope, hypotension). Progress as patient tolerates. Assess for muscle weakness, gait changes, and the presence of joint pain or deep bone pain. PT to assess for ambulation, mobility, ROM, muscle strength, tone, and flexibility. OT to assess functional ability.	Patient will achieve optimal mobility.	PT or OT to help determine and direct activity goals. Increase activity as tolerated post-transplant. Assess for muscle weakness, joint pain, tingling, or numbness on upper thigh on operative side of transplant.	Patient will achieve optimal mobility.	Instruct patient to avoid lifting or strenuous exercise for 3 months. Continue to progress exercise as tolerated and monitor response. Assist patient/family in developing home exercise program.

OXYGENATION/VENTILATION

Diagnosis/Stabilization Phase		Acute Management Phase		Recovery Phase	
Outcome	Interventions	Outcome	Interventions	Outcome	Interventions
Patient will have adequate gas exchange as evidenced by: • SaO_2 > 90% • SpO_2 > 92% • ABGs WNL • clear breath sounds • respiratory rate, depth, and rhythm WNL • normal CXR • thin, white pulmonary secretions Patient will have adequate tissue perfusion as evidenced by:	Monitor and treat oxygenation status per ABGs and/or SpO_2. Assess sensorium and LOC frequently. Monitor for signs and symptoms of pulmonary distress from fluid overload. Monitor acid-base status per ABGs. Monitor for signs and symptoms of pulmonary infection/pneumonia. Support patient with O_2 therapy and/or mechanical ventilation as indicated. Involve RCP. Monitor for complications of chronic renal failure that may impair oxygenation/ventilation status (CHF, pulmonary edema, fatigue, lethargy, somnolence).	Patient will have adequate gas exchange after kidney transplant.	Continue as in Diagnosis/Stabilization Phase. Anticipate complications related to kidney transplantation that may impair oxygenation/ventilatory status (ARDS, sepsis, pulmonary edema, hypoxemia). Wean oxygen therapy and/or mechanical ventilation as tolerated. Continue to involve RCP. Encourage use of IS and/or deep breathing with inspiratory hold q2h.	Patient will have adequate gas exchange.	Teach patient/family abnormal respiratory symptoms such as SOB, dyspnea on exertion, wheezing, chest pain, and tachypnea, and importance of reporting these to physician. Assess need for RCP follow-up after discharge.

- normovolemic status
- adequate Hgb
- alert and oriented
- appropriate LOC

COMFORT

	Diagnosis/Stabilization Phase		Acute Management Phase		Recovery Phase	
	Outcome	Interventions	Outcome	Interventions	Outcome	Interventions
	Patient will be as comfortable and pain free as possible as evidenced by: • no objective indicators of discomfort • no complaints of discomfort	Monitor and treat breathing status closely for signs and symptoms of respiratory distress related to fluid overload. Keep HOB elevated and review breathing techniques such as pursed-lip breathing. Review coughing techniques to minimize respiratory distress. Creatively plan fluid restriction over 24h, including periodic sips of water, ice chips, or popsicles to minimize thirst. Offer gum, hard candy, mouth swab, and frequent oral care. Assess for signs and symptoms of uremic neuropathy or renal osteodystrophy (numbness or burning in feet, restless leg movements, decreased muscle strength, cramps, paresthesias, and decreased tendon reflexes). Avoid unexpected touching of the feet. Keep heavy bed linens off feet. Instruct patient to inspect feet visually daily for signs of injury. Observe patient for complications of end-stage renal disease that may cause discomfort (dyspnea, joint/bone pain, nausea, lethargy, weakness).	Patient will be as comfortable and pain free as possible.	Teach patient to rate pain on 1–10 scale and administer analgesics as indicated postop. Provide adequate rest periods, especially if patient is anemic. Teach patient relaxation techniques, including complementary therapies such as touch therapy, humor, or music therapy. Involve family in strategies.	Patient will be as comfortable as possible.	Teach patient/family about comfort measures including: • breathing exercises to help control dyspnea • relaxation techniques • complementary therapy techniques to decrease dyspnea

End-Stage Renal Disease/Kidney Transplantation Interdisciplinary Outcome Pathway (continued)

SKIN INTEGRITY

Diagnosis/Stabilization Phase		Acute Management Phase		Recovery Phase	
Outcome	Interventions	Outcome	Interventions	Outcome	Interventions
Patient will have intact skin without abrasions or pressure ulcers.	Assess skin integrity and all bony prominences (including feet) q4h. Use superfatted or lanolin-based soap for bathing and apply emollients for itching. Use preventive pressure-reducing devices if patient is at high risk for developing pressure ulcers. Treat pressure ulcers according to hospital protocol. Avoid tight-fitting shoes or clothing that may create pressure points susceptible to breakdown if applicable.	Patient will have intact skin without evidence of wound dehiscence or pressure ulcers. Patient will have healing surgical wounds.	Evaluate patient's skin integrity. Assess healing of transplant incision. Monitor incision site for signs of infection. Use sterile technique with all dressing changes.	Patient will have intact skin without evidence of wound dehiscence or pressure ulcers. Patient will have healing surgical wounds.	Teach patient/family skin care and incision management for after discharge. Remind patient that sutures/staples may be in for 2–3 weeks due to slower healing rate related to prednisone therapy. Teach patient/family not to lift anything over 10 pounds for 3 months. Teach patient/family signs and symptoms of infection and when to call physician.

PROTECTION/SAFETY

Diagnosis/Stabilization Phase		Acute Management Phase		Recovery Phase	
Outcome	Interventions	Outcome	Interventions	Outcome	Interventions
Patient will be protected from possible harm. Patient will maintain a patent and infection-free vascular access device before kidney transplant.	Assess need for wrist restraints if patient is intubated, has a decreased LOC, is unable to follow commands, or for affected extremity during hemodialysis. Explain need for restraints to patient/family. Check skin integrity and circulation q1–2h. Follow hospital protocol for use of restraints. Provide support when dangling or beginning progressive exercise program. Monitor the color, temperature, and sensation of extremity with vascular access. Assess	Patient will be protected from possible harm.	Provide physical support as needed as patient increases activity post-transplant. Provide assistive devices as necessary. Monitor for signs and symptoms of infection (symptoms may be subtle due to immunosuppression). Instruct patient/family to report any vague discomforts, mental status changes, or constant low grade fevers. Teach patient/family early signs of rejection: fever, pain, tenderness, swelling at graft site, weight gain, decrease in UO,	Patient will be protected from possible harm.	Teach patient/family complications of immunosuppressive agents and interventions to alleviate or minimize such complications. Teach patient signs and symptoms of infection. Encourage patient to avoid crowds for first 3 months. If still needed, teach patient proper use of assistive devices. Have patient give return demonstration.

for signs and symptoms of infection and maintain strict sterile technique when assessing the device. Assess patency by palpating thrill and auscultating for the bruit.
Avoid constriction of affected extremity with BP cuff or tourniquet. Avoid venipuncture in affected extremity.

hypertension, and elevation in serum creatinine.
Monitor stools for occult bleeding.

PSYCHOSOCIAL/SELF-DETERMINATION

Diagnosis/Stabilization Phase		Acute Management Phase		Recovery Phase	
Outcome	Interventions	Outcome	Interventions	Outcome	Interventions
Patient will achieve psychophysiologic stability. Patient will demonstrate a decrease in anxiety as evidenced by: • VS WNL • LOC WNL for the patient • subjective report of decreased anxiety • objective assessment of decreased anxiety	Assess physiologic effects of acute care environment on patient. Assess patient for appropriate level of stress. Assess coping mechanisms for chronic illness. Assess personal responses (affective and/or feelings) of patient/family regarding critical illness and their patterns of thinking/communicating. Assess patient/family for signs of depression, anger, withdrawal, and dependent behaviors. Assist patient/family in decision-making process for transplantation as a treatment alternative. Use calm, competent, reassuring approach with interventions. Observe factors that make patient/family anxious and take measures to reduce their anxiety (initiate family conferences, refer support services, and use consistent caregivers). Allow flexible visitation to meet the needs of patient and family. Use sedatives, antidepressants as appropriate.	Patient will achieve psychophysiologic stability. Patient will demonstrate a decrease in anxiety.	Teach patient/family about continuing care. Provide information about local support groups, kidney centers, and agencies such as the National Kidney Foundation.	Patient will achieve psychophysiologic stability. Patient will demonstrate a decrease in anxiety.	Continue as in Acute Management Phase. Address concerns about possible impact on daily life: ADLs, sexual functioning, recreation, driving, return to work.

CHAPTER 6

Endocrine Pathways

Adrenal Crisis
Interdisciplinary Outcome Pathway

COORDINATION OF CARE

Diagnosis/Stabilization Phase		Acute Management Phase		Recovery Phase	
Outcome	Interventions	Outcome	Interventions	Outcome	Interventions
All appropriate team members and disciplines will be involved in the plan of care.	Develop the plan of care with the patient, family, primary physician, endocrinologist, intensivist, other specialists as needed, RN, advanced practice nurse, RCP, chaplain, and social services.	All appropriate team members and disciplines will be involved in the plan of care.	Update the plan of care with the patient/family, other team members, dietitian, discharge planner, OT, PT, and home health.	Patient/family will understand how to maintain optimal health at home.	Provide guidelines concerning follow-up care to patient/family. Provide patient/family with phone numbers of resources available to answer questions. Consult home health to provide continuity of care.

DIAGNOSTICS

Diagnosis/Stabilization Phase		Acute Management Phase		Recovery Phase	
Outcome	Interventions	Outcome	Interventions	Outcome	Interventions
Patient will understand any tests or procedures that must be completed (VS, hemodynamic monitoring, I & O, CXR, O_2 therapy, pulse oximetry, lab work including plasma ACTH levels, cortisol levels, and aldosterone levels, ACTH stimulation tests to confirm presence of adrenal insufficiency).	Explain all tests and procedures to patient/family. Explain what the patient's role in the diagnostic tests will be (i.e., lie still when hemodynamics obtained, keep digit with pulse oximetry straight and relaxed). Be sensitive to individualized needs of patient/family for information.	Patient will understand the meaning of diagnostic tests or procedures that need to be completed.	Continue as in Diagnosis/Stabilization Phase.	Patient will understand the meaning of diagnostic tests in relation to continued health.	Review with patient/family results of tests before discharge. Discuss abnormal findings and appropriate measures patient/family can take to help correct. Review meaning of individual's stress response and necessity to adjust hydrocortisone for high stress times.

FLUID BALANCE

Diagnosis/Stabilization Phase		Acute Management Phase		Recovery Phase	
Outcome	Interventions	Outcome	Interventions	Outcome	Interventions
Patient will achieve and maintain optimal hemodynamic status as evidenced by: • MAP >70 mmHg • hemodynamic parameters WNL for the patient • UO >0.5 mL/kg/hr • normovolemic status (balanced I & O) • adequate LOC • free of cardiac dysrhythmias • VS WNL for the patient Suspect acute adrenal insufficiency in patients with profound hypotension without identifiable cause.	Assess history for use of corticosteroids (more than 20 mg of hydrocortisone for longer than 7–10 days can suppress hypothalamic-pituitary-adrenal axis). Monitor and treat hemodynamic parameters: • BP • HR • I & O • LOC • evidence of tissue perfusion • PA pressures • CO/CI • CVP • SVR/PVR • SvO₂ • temperature • abnormal heart and lung sounds Monitor lab values: electrolytes; bedside glucose checks q2h until stable, then q4h; CBC with differential (eosinophilia may be present in acute exacerbation of a chronic process); ABGs, SpO₂ as indicated. Assess plasma corticotropin, plasma aldosterone, and thyrotropin level. Administer IV hydrocortisone, IV fluids (usually 0.9% sodium chloride and 5% dextrose to increase glucose and vascular volume) and inotropes as indicated. Monitor and treat dysrhythmias. Assess and monitor fluid balance. Assess weight changes from baseline and weigh daily. Determine hydration needs based on hemodynamics, I & O, cardiopulmonary assessment, VS, and electrolytes.	Patient will maintain optimal hemodynamic status.	Continue as in Diagnosis/Stabilization Phase. Maintain optimal hydration, hemodynamics, and tissue perfusion based on cardiopulmonary assessment and laboratory values. Begin teaching patient/family regarding cause of adrenal crisis, precipitating events, and signs and symptoms of adrenal crisis.	Patient will maintain optimal hemodynamic status.	Continue as in Acute Management Phase. Continue teaching patient/family about: • long-term steroid therapy if indicated. Include instruction on increasing hormonal replacement during stressful times. Emphasize danger of stopping drug therapy abruptly. Remind patients that if they vomit and are unable to take the oral dose of corticosteroids, notify physician immediately or go to the ED for parenteral hydrocortisone. • precipitating signs/symptoms of adrenal crisis so patient can seek medical therapy early. • optimal fluid balance and how to maintain it. Review signs and symptoms of fluid overload and dehydration. Remind patient to weigh daily and report sudden changes to physician.

CO_2

Adrenal Crisis Interdisciplinary Outcome Pathway (continued)

FLUID BALANCE (continued)

Diagnosis/Stabilization Phase		Acute Management Phase		Recovery Phase	
Outcome	Interventions	Outcome	Interventions	Outcome	Interventions
	Monitor and treat complications of adrenal crisis such as profound hypotension, hypovolemic shock, generalized weakness, weight loss, confusion, lethargy, hypokalemia, vomiting, and severe dehydration. Assess tissue perfusion (pain, pulses, color, temperature, signs of decreased perfusion such as decreased UO, altered LOC, and ileus).				

NUTRITION

Diagnosis/Stabilization Phase		Acute Management Phase		Recovery Phase	
Outcome	Interventions	Outcome	Interventions	Outcome	Interventions
Patient will be adequately nourished as evidenced by: • stable weight not >10% below or >20% above IBW • albumin >3.5 g/dL • total protein 6–8 g/dL • total lymphocyte count 1,000–3,000	Assess nutritional status. Assess for vomiting, diarrhea, anorexia, nausea, or weight loss. Monitor albumin, cholesterol, prealbumin, total protein, nitrogen balance, phosphate, magnesium, calcium, and lymphocyte count.	Patient will be adequately nourished.	Consult dietitian to help determine and direct nutritional support. Initiate DAT and monitor for response (clear liquids, regular meals, enteral feedings, or parenteral nutrition). Call dietitian if: • albumin <3.0 • eating less than half of food on tray • diet counseling is needed	Patient will be adequately nourished.	Teach patient/family: • recommended daily allowances • daily caloric intake needed • safe weight-reducing or weight-gaining techniques as indicated Teach patient about dietary supplements (i.e., vitamins, minerals).

MOBILITY

Diagnosis/Stabilization Phase		Acute Management Phase		Recovery Phase	
Outcome	Interventions	Outcome	Interventions	Outcome	Interventions
Patient will achieve optimal mobility.	Assess muscle mobility, flexibility, strength, and tone. Assess functional ability. Begin passive/active-assist ROM exercises.	Patient will achieve optimal mobility.	Assess physical limitations of mobility. Involve PT or OT for specific mobility and/or functional limitations. PT/OT will help determine and direct activity goals. Develop progressive activity program. Provide support as needed. Monitor response to activity and decrease if adverse events occur (tachycardia, dyspnea, ectopy, syncope, hypo/hypertension).	Patient will maintain optimal mobility. Patient will develop home exercise plan.	Assist patient/family in developing home exercise plan. Determine a gradually increasing program of aerobic activity such as walking, swimming, and jogging.

OXYGENATION/VENTILATION

Diagnosis/Stabilization Phase		Acute Management Phase		Recovery Phase	
Outcome	Interventions	Outcome	Interventions	Outcome	Interventions
Patient will have adequate gas exchange and adequate tissue perfusion as evidenced by: • SaO_2 >90% • SpO_2 >92% • ABGs WNL • clear lung sounds • respiratory rate, depth, and rhythm WNL • normal CXR • normal Hgb • evidence of tissue perfusion to major organs: UO >0.5 mL/kg/hr, appropriate LOC, skin warm and dry	Monitor respiratory status closely, including respiratory rate, depth, rhythm, lung sounds, ABGs, SpO_2, and CXR. Be prepared for intubation and mechanical ventilation. If on ventilator, monitor settings and hemodynamic variables before, during, and after weaning. Involve RCP. Wean ventilator when appropriate and monitor patient response. Wean FIO_2 to maintain SpO_2 >92%. If not intubated, use supplemental oxygen if indicated. Assess for evidence of tissue perfusion. Monitor lab values: ABGs, Hgb.	Patient will maintain optimal gas exchange and tissue perfusion.	Continue as in Diagnosis/Stabilization Phase. Monitor and treat oxygenation/ventilation disturbances as per ABGs, pulse oximetry, chest assessment, adventitious breath sounds, and CXR. Wean mechanical ventilation/oxygen therapy as indicated. Continue to involve RCP. Assess effects of increased activity on cardiopulmonary function. Observe for complications associated with adrenal insufficiency that may impair oxygenation/ventilation: infection, tuberculosis, hypovolemic shock, or hypotension.	Patient will maintain optimal gas exchange and tissue perfusion.	Continue as in Acute Management Phase. Monitor and treat oxygenation/ventilation disturbances. Instruct patient/family on signs and symptoms of respiratory distress and when to seek medical care.

Adrenal Crisis Interdisciplinary Outcome Pathway (continued)

COMFORT

Diagnosis/Stabilization Phase		Acute Management Phase		Recovery Phase	
Outcome	Interventions	Outcome	Interventions	Outcome	Interventions
Patient will be as comfortable and pain free as possible as evidenced by: • no objective indicators of discomfort • no complaints of discomfort	Assess absence of, or quantity and quality of, pain. Administer sedatives and analgesics as ordered and monitor response. If patient is intubated, establish effective communication technique with which patient can communicate discomfort. Provide reassurance in a calm, caring, and competent manner.	Patient will be as comfortable and pain free as possible.	Continue as in Diagnosis/Stabilization Phase. Instruct patient on relaxation techniques. Have patient give return demonstration. Use complementary therapies such as touch therapy, humor, music, and imagery to promote relaxation. Involve family in strategies.	Patient will be as comfortable and pain free as possible.	Continue as in Acute Management Phase. Teach patient/family complementary methods to promote relaxation once discharged.

SKIN INTEGRITY

Diagnosis/Stabilization Phase		Acute Management Phase		Recovery Phase	
Outcome	Interventions	Outcome	Interventions	Outcome	Interventions
Patient will have intact skin without abrasions or pressure ulcers.	Assess all bony prominences at least q4h and treat if needed. Use preventive pressure-reducing devices if patient is at high risk for developing pressure ulcers. Treat altered skin integrity according to hospital protocol. Assess skin and mucous membranes for dryness. Assess for thirst and/or decreased skin turgor.	Patient will have intact skin without abrasions or pressure ulcers.	Continue as in Diagnosis/Stabilization Phase.	Patient will have intact skin without abrasions or pressure ulcers.	Continue as in Acute Management Phase. Instruct patient/family on skin care management for after discharge.

PROTECTION/SAFETY

Diagnosis/Stabilization Phase		Acute Management Phase		Recovery Phase	
Outcome	Interventions	Outcome	Interventions	Outcome	Interventions
Patient will be protected from possible harm.	Assess need for wrist restraints if patient is intubated, has a decreased LOC, or is unable to follow commands. Explain need for restraints to patient/family. If restraints used, assess response to restraints and check q1–2h for skin integrity and impairment to circulation. Follow hospital protocol for use of restraints. Assess need for assistance with activities and provide physical support as needed. Institute seizure precautions if severe electrolyte imbalances exist.	Patient will be protected from possible harm.	Continue as in Diagnosis/Stabilization Phase.	Patient will be protected from possible harm.	Teach patient/family regarding any physical limitations in activity after discharge. Provide assistive devices as necessary. Consult with PT/OT.

PSYCHOSOCIAL/SELF-DETERMINATION

Diagnosis/Stabilization Phase		Acute Management Phase		Recovery Phase	
Outcome	Interventions	Outcome	Interventions	Outcome	Interventions
Patient will achieve psychophysiologic stability. Patient will demonstrate a decrease in anxiety as evidenced by: • VS WNL for the patient • subjective reports of decreased anxiety level • objective reports of decreased anxiety level	Assess physiologic effects of critical care environment on patient (hemodynamic variables, psychological status, signs of increased sympathetic response). Use calm, caring, competent, and reassuring approach with patient and family. Take measures to reduce sensory overload. If patient is unresponsive, use tactile and verbal stimuli. Arrange for flexible visitation to meet the needs of patient and family. Determine coping ability of patient/family and take measures to help patient cope (allow verbalization of con-	Patient will achieve psychophysiologic stability. Patient will demonstrate a decrease in anxiety.	Continue as in Diagnosis/Stabilization Phase. Initial discharge planning. Teach patient/family about: • home medications: long-term steroid replacement including dose, increase in greater stress periods, and danger in stopping abruptly • signs and symptoms of adrenal crisis • refer to outside services as appropriate	Patient will achieve psychophysiologic stability. Patient will demonstrate a decrease in anxiety.	Continue as in Acute Management Phase. Address concerns about possible effects on aspects of daily life: activities, return to work, sexual functioning.

Adrenal Crisis Interdisciplinary Outcome Pathway *(continued)*

PSYCHOSOCIAL/SELF-DETERMINATION (continued)

Diagnosis/Stabilization Phase		Acute Management Phase		Recovery Phase	
Outcome	Interventions	Outcome	Interventions	Outcome	Interventions
	cerns and fears, provide frequent explanations, encourage family to visit and participate in care, use easy to understand terminology, and utilize support services when indicated). Administer sedatives and anxiolytics as ordered and monitor response. Begin explanation of adrenal insufficiency to patient/family.				

Diabetic Ketoacidosis Interdisciplinary Outcome Pathway

COORDINATION OF CARE

Diagnosis/Stabilization Phase		Acute Management Phase		Recovery Phase	
Outcome	Interventions	Outcome	Interventions	Outcome	Interventions
All appropriate team members and disciplines will be involved in the plan of care.	Develop the plan of care with the patient/family, primary physician(s), endocrinologist, other specialists as needed, RN, advanced practice nurse, RCP, and dietitian.	All appropriate team members and disciplines will be involved in the plan of care.	Update the plan of care with the patient/family and other team members, PT, OT, transplant team, and home health. Initiate planning for anticipated discharge. Consult transplant team if pancreas transplant is an option. Begin teaching patient/family about diabetes diet. Begin teaching patient/family about care at home.	Patient/family will understand how to maintain optimal health at home.	Refer to home health as needed. Provide guidelines concerning follow-up care to patient and family: • diet • medications • exercise program • proper injection of insulin • when to call physician • signs and symptoms of hypo/hyperglycemia and actions to take Provide patient/family with phone number of resources/diabetes education classes/diabetes clinical nurse specialist available to answer questions. Teach patient/family ways to prevent recurrence of diabetic ketoacidosis (DKA). Continue consult with transplant team if pancreas transplant is an option.

DIAGNOSTICS

Diagnosis/Stabilization Phase		Acute Management Phase		Recovery Phase	
Outcome	Interventions	Outcome	Interventions	Outcome	Interventions
Patient/family will understand any tests or procedures that must be completed (hemodynamic monitoring, x-rays, glucose	Explain all procedures and tests to patient/family. Be sensitive to individualized needs of patient/family for information. Repeat information as needed.	Patient/family will understand any tests or procedures that must be completed (lab work, glucose monitoring).	Explain procedures and tests to assess progress and recovery from DKA to patient/family. Assess individualized needs of patient/family for information.	Patient/family will understand meaning of diagnostic tests in relation to continued health (serum glucose monitoring in the home).	Review with patient/family before discharge the results of all tests. Discuss abnormal findings and appropriate measures patient/family can take to return to normal (i.e., hypo/hyperglycemia).

Diabetic Ketoacidosis Interdisciplinary Outcome Pathway (continued)

DIAGNOSTICS (continued)

Diagnosis/Stabilization Phase		Acute Management Phase		Recovery Phase	
Outcome	Interventions	Outcome	Interventions	Outcome	Interventions
	monitoring, lab work, EEG, EKG, ketone levels).		Anticipate need for further diagnostic tests such as EEG, pancreas transplant workup, and any interventions that may result. Begin teaching patient/family about serum glucose monitoring at home. Have patient/family give return demonstration. Arrange for home health care and/or equipment as necessary.		Provide patient/family with guidelines concerning follow-up care: • when to call physician • skin care • foot care • diabetes diet • administration of insulin • medications • home glucose monitoring • physical restrictions • exercise program • signs of hypo/hyperglycemia and actions to take • management of diabetes when ill Continue to teach patient/family technique for home glucose monitoring. Have patient demonstrate procedure several times before discharge. Arrange for home health care if needed. Continue to consult transplant team if appropriate. Teach patient factors that may precipitate further episodes of DKA: stress, trauma, infection, large food intake, low insulin dose. Refer to outpatient diabetes education classes.

FLUID BALANCE

Diagnosis/Stabilization Phase		Acute Management Phase		Recovery Phase	
Outcome	Interventions	Outcome	Interventions	Outcome	Interventions
Patient will achieve optimal hemodynamic status as evidenced by: • MAP >70 mmHg • hemodynamic parameters WNL • adequate LOC • adequate respiratory functioning • neurologic status WNL • UO >0.5 mL/kg/hr • good skin turgor • normal tissue perfusion Patient will achieve a serum glucose level <300 mg/dL. Patient will achieve a normal serum bicarbonate level. Patient will stay well hydrated.	Monitor and treat hemodynamic parameters: • VS • SvO_2 • CVP • JVD • abnormal heart sounds • EKG • PCWP Monitor for signs of dehydration and hypovolemia (loss of skin turgor, dry skin, flushed, hypotension, rapid pulse, thready pulse, sunken eyeballs). Constantly monitor respiratory functioning and anticipate respiratory complications. Be prepared for intubation and mechanical ventilation. Maintain strict I & O. Assess neurologic status q1h and PRN. Administer insulin bolus followed by infusion and monitor response. Administer fast-acting insulin bolus of 0.1 units/kg IV followed by infusion of 0.1 units/kg/hr. Monitor blood glucose levels every 30–60 minutes. Progress to serum glucose and whole blood glucose levels q1–4h and PRN. Assess evidence of tissue perfusion (pain, pulses, color, temperature, signs of decreased perfusion such as decreased UO, altered LOC, and ileus). Anticipate need for vasopressor agents and assess response and titrate accordingly.	Patient will maintain optimal hemodynamic status. Patient will maintain normal serum glucose level. Patient will remain hydrated.	Continue to monitor and treat hemodynamic parameters. Monitor lab values. Monitor for signs and symptoms of dehydration and hypovolemia. Begin teaching patient/family regarding diabetes, symptoms of hypo/hyperglycemia, and blood glucose monitoring. Monitor blood glucose levels q4h and PRN. Be prepared to administer potassium supplements. Be prepared to administer diuretics and/or corticosteroids in the event of cerebral edema. Continue to monitor for complications.	Patient will maintain optimal hemodynamic status. Patient will maintain normal serum glucose level.	Continue diabetes education and tell patient/family when to seek medical attention. Monitor lab values, particularly serum glucose levels. Teach patient/family proper fluid management at home. Teach patient/family how to monitor serum glucose levels at home. Arrange for home health care and equipment as needed. Have patient demonstrate several times before discharge.

Diabetic Ketoacidosis Interdisciplinary Outcome Pathway (continued)

FLUID BALANCE (continued)

Diagnosis/Stabilization Phase		Acute Management Phase		Recovery Phase	
Outcome	Interventions	Outcome	Interventions	Outcome	Interventions
	Initiate IV therapy with an isotonic solution (NS or lactated Ringer's) first, followed with a hypotonic solution (0.45% sodium chloride). This may be followed with D5W or D5 1/2NS once the serum glucose is < 300 mg/dL. Once the serum glucose levels reach 105 mg/dL, change to D10W. Start fluids at 200–1,000 cc/hr as needed.				
	Monitor for possible complications associated with DKA: dysrhythmias, dehydration, renal failure, vascular collapse, decreased LOC, CHF, pulmonary edema, seizures.				
	Monitor lab values: electrolytes, glucose, ABGs, GFR, bicarbonate, UA for ketonuria and glycosuria, CBC, BUN, creatinine.				
	Monitor for signs of fluid overload or deficit and treat accordingly.				
	Anticipate need for potassium replacement therapy.				
	Monitor plasma bicarbonate levels. Given bicarbonate slowly if needed.				
	Assess for other medical conditions: known heart disease, seizures, inability to eliminate CO_2 appropriately, chronic renal disease.				

NUTRITION

Diagnosis/Stabilization Phase		Acute Management Phase		Recovery Phase	
Outcome	Interventions	Outcome	Interventions	Outcome	Interventions
Patient will be adequately nourished as evidenced by: • stable weight not >10% below or >20% above IBW • albumin 3.5–4.0 g/dL • total protein 6–8 g/dL • prealbumin >15 mg/dL • controlled glucose <130 mg/dL Patient will have normal serum electrolyte values.	Assess bowel sounds, abdominal distension, and abdominal pain and tenderness q4h and PRN. NPO until extubated, if applicable. If intubation is delayed >24h, initiate alternative nutritional therapy. Consult dietitian or nutritional support team to coordinate/direct nutritional support. Assess ability to take fluids. If not able, start enteral feedings. If able to take fluids, administer clear to full liquids and assess response. Monitor for polyphagia, N & V, and weight loss. Monitor serum electrolytes. Monitor serum glucose levels q1h until stabilized.	Patient will be adequately nourished.	Advance DAT to diabetes diet. Consult dietitian if: • albumin <3.0 g/dL • eating less than half of food on tray • diet counseling is needed Monitor protein, albumin, and glucose levels. Monitor serum glucose levels q4h and PRN. Calorie count as needed to determine whether intake meets nutritional goals. Begin teaching patient/family about diabetes diet requirements. Involve dietitian. Monitor ketones in serum and urine. Teach patient how to do this at home. Have patient give return demonstration.	Patient will be adequately nourished.	Reinforce teaching patient/family diabetes diet requirements. Teach patient/family how to monitor serum glucose levels in the home. Teach patient about dietary supplements (i.e., vitamins, minerals, antioxidants).

MOBILITY

Diagnosis/Stabilization Phase		Acute Management Phase		Recovery Phase	
Outcome	Interventions	Outcome	Interventions	Outcome	Interventions
Patient will maintain normal muscle strength and tone. Patient will be free of joint contractures.	Assess degree of mobility, functional ability, flexibility, muscle strength, and tone. If comatose, begin passive ROM exercises. If able, begin active-assist ROM exercises.	Patient will achieve optimal mobility. Patient will be free of joint contractures.	If able, continue active-assist ROM exercises and progress activity as tolerated. Monitor response to increased activity. Decrease activity should adverse events occur (tachycardia, dysrhythmias, dyspnea, hypotension). Monitor effects of increased activity on respiratory status. Monitor with pulse oximetry. Apply supplemental oxygen to keep SpO_2 >92%.	Patient will achieve optimal mobility. Patient will be free of joint contractures.	Teach patient/family about recommended exercise program and any activity limitations. Have patient demonstrate exercises.

Diabetic Ketoacidosis Interdisciplinary Outcome Pathway (continued)

MOBILITY (continued)

Diagnosis/Stabilization Phase		Acute Management Phase		Recovery Phase	
Outcome	Interventions	Outcome	Interventions	Outcome	Interventions
			PT/OT consult if indicated to help determine and meet functional activity goals. Monitor effects of exercise on serum glucose level. Provide support as necessary.		

OXYGENATION/VENTILATION

Diagnosis/Stabilization Phase		Acute Management Phase		Recovery Phase	
Outcome	Interventions	Outcome	Interventions	Outcome	Interventions
Patient will have adequate gas exchange as evidenced by: • SaO_2 >90% • SpO_2 >92% • ABGs WNL • clear breath sounds • respiratory rate, depth, and rhythm WNL • CXR WNL • absence of dyspnea, cyanosis, secretions, Kussmaul's respirations • effective cough • LOC WNL	Constantly monitor respiratory status: respiratory muscle strength, ABGs, SpO_2, rate, rhythm, and depth of respiration, lung sounds, coughing ability, CXR, and $PaCO_2$. Be prepared for intubation and mechanical ventilation. Consult RCP as needed. If on ventilator, monitor settings and hemodynamic variables prior to, during, and after weaning. Wean ventilator when appropriate and monitor patient response: • wean FIO_2 to keep SpO_2 >92% • use humidification to keep secretions thin If not intubated, apply supplemental oxygen. Monitor with pulse oximetry. Maintain SpO_2 >92%.	Patient will have adequate gas exchange.	Monitor and treat oxygenation disturbances as per ABGs and/or SpO_2. Monitor and treat ventilation disturbances as per ABGs, chest assessment, adventitious breath sounds, and CXR. Wean oxygen therapy/mechanical ventilation as indicated. Continue to involve RCP. Assess effects of increased activity on respiratory status. Monitor with pulse oximetry. Apply supplemental oxygen to keep SpO_2 >92%. Observe for complications of DKA that may impair oxygenation/ventilation: pneumonia, aspiration, infection. Continue to monitor $PaCO_2$.	Patient will have adequate gas exchange.	Encourage coughing and deep breathing at least q2h. Encourage patient to use breathing exercise especially with activity. Teach patient/family signs and symptoms of infections and when to call the physician.

Assess evidence of tissue perfusion (pain, pulses, temperature, color, signs of decreased perfusion such as altered LOC and decreased UO).
Monitor lab values: ABGs, Hgb.
Assess for Kussmaul's respirations.

COMFORT

Diagnosis/Stabilization Phase		Acute Management Phase		Recovery Phase	
Outcome	Interventions	Outcome	Interventions	Outcome	Interventions
Patient will be as comfortable and pain free as possible as evidenced by: • no objective indicators of discomfort • no complaints of discomfort	Assess absence of, or quantity and quality of, discomfort. Administer sedatives cautiously and monitor effects on respiratory status. If patient is intubated, establish effective communication technique with which patient can communicate discomfort. Assess need for analgesics and administer accordingly. Use a pain scale or visual analogue tool to gauge discomfort. Provide reassurance in a calm, caring, and competent manner. Provide meticulous oral hygiene.	Patient will be as relaxed and comfortable as possible.	Continue as in Diagnosis/Stabilization Phase. Teach patient relaxation techniques. Have patient give return demonstration. Use touch therapy, humor, and/or music therapy and imagery to promote relaxation.	Patient will be as relaxed and comfortable as possible.	Teach patient/family alternative methods to promote relaxation after discharge. Have patient/family give return demonstration. Teach patient/family proper use of analgesics at home, both prescribed and OTC.

SKIN INTEGRITY

Diagnosis/Stabilization Phase		Acute Management Phase		Recovery Phase	
Outcome	Interventions	Outcome	Interventions	Outcome	Interventions
Patient will have intact skin without abrasions or pressure ulcers.	Assess all bony prominences at least q4h and treat if needed. Use preventive pressure-reducing devices if patient is at high risk for developing pressure ulcers.	Patient will have intact skin without abrasions or pressure ulcers.	Continue as in Diagnosis/Stabilization Phase. Begin teaching patient importance of inspecting skin, especially feet, daily.	Patient will have intact skin without abrasions or pressure ulcers.	Teach patient/family proper skin care, particularly of feet. Teach patient/family to inspect all skin daily for any abrasions or nonhealing wounds, especially the feet.

Diabetic Ketoacidosis Interdisciplinary Outcome Pathway (continued)

SKIN INTEGRITY (continued)

Diagnosis/Stabilization Phase		Acute Management Phase		Recovery Phase	
Outcome	Interventions	Outcome	Interventions	Outcome	Interventions
	Treat pressure ulcers according to hospital protocol. Carefully observe all areas of patient's skin for abrasions or nonhealing wounds.				

PROTECTION/SAFETY

Diagnosis/Stabilization Phase		Acute Management Phase		Recovery Phase	
Outcome	Interventions	Outcome	Interventions	Outcome	Interventions
Patient will be protected from possible harm.	Assess need for assistance with activities. Provide physical support as needed. Institute seizure precautions. If intubated, assess need for wrist restraints. If used, explain need for restraints to patient/family. Check area for skin integrity and circulation q2h and PRN. Remove when possible. Follow hospital protocol for restraint use.	Patient will be protected from possible harm.	Maintain seizure precautions. Assess need for support when OOB. Support as needed. Use assistive devices as needed.	Patient will be protected from possible harm.	Teach patient/family about any physical limitations in activity after discharge. Teach patient/family ways to prevent injury. Have patient demonstrate proper use of assistive devices.

PSYCHOSOCIAL/SELF-DETERMINATION

Diagnosis/Stabilization Phase		Acute Management Phase		Recovery Phase	
Outcome	Interventions	Outcome	Interventions	Outcome	Interventions
Patient will achieve psychophysiologic stability. Patient will demonstrate a decrease in anxiety as evidenced by:	Assess physiologic effects of critical care environment on patient (hemodynamic variables, psychological status, signs of increased sympathetic response).	Patient will achieve psychophysiologic stability. Patient will demonstrate a decrease in anxiety.	Continue as in Diagnosis/Stabilization Phase. Initiate discharge planning with instruction to patient/family: activities at home, diabetes diet, proper skin care, foot care, medications, activity, and so on.	Patient will achieve psychophysiologic stability. Patient will demonstrate a decrease in anxiety.	Continue to reinforce positive coping mechanisms for use after discharge. Continue to reinforce previous teaching. Assess knowledge and reinforce as needed. Include family in teaching.

- normal VS
- subjective report of anxiety
- objective signs of anxiety

Patient will demonstrate a decrease in depression as evidenced by:

- subjective report of decreased depression
- objective report of decreased depression

Patient will begin acceptance process of this diabetic complication.

Take measures to reduce sensory overload.

If patient is unresponsive, use verbal and tactile stimuli.

Develop effective interventions to communicate with intubated patient.

Use a calm, caring, competent, and reassuring approach with patient and family.

Arrange for flexible visitation to meet patient and family needs.

Determine coping ability of patient/family and take measures to help patient cope (allow verbalization of concerns and fears, provide frequent explanations, allow family to visit, use easy to understand terminology, support services, etc.).

Begin teaching patient/family about DKA.

Patient/family will continue acceptance process of DKA.

Administer antidepressants/sedatives cautiously if used.

Help patient identify positive coping mechanisms.

Patient/family will continue with acceptance of DKA.

Refer to diabetes education classes, support groups, diabetes clinical nurse specialist, diabetes educator, and so on.

Allow patient/family to verbalize concerns and fears about DKA and living with diabetes.

Address concerns patient may have about impact on daily life.

Transsphenoidal Hypophysectomy Interdisciplinary Outcome Pathway

COORDINATION OF CARE

Diagnosis/Stabilization Phase		Acute Management Phase		Recovery Phase	
Outcome	Interventions	Outcome	Interventions	Outcome	Interventions
All appropriate disciplines and team members will be consulted and involved in the patient's care as needed.	Consult the following disciplines as needed: internist/family practice, cardiologist, endocrinologist, RN, advanced practice nurse, RCP, PT, OT, pastoral care, social services, and dietitian.	All appropriate disciplines and team members will be consulted and involved in the patient's care as needed.	Involve patient and family in the plan of care as well as other disciplines involved in patient's care. Initiate planning for anticipated discharge. Initiate teaching patient/family about home care and follow-up care.	Patient and family will understand how to achieve and maintain optimal health at home.	Provide guidelines to the patient and family upon discharge, including the following: • follow-up medical care, appointments • prescribed medication instructions, including potential side effects • dietary instructions • activity instructions • symptoms to expect and what symptoms should be reported to the physician Patient should be instructed to wear a medical alert bracelet or necklace indicating his or her history as well as any medications that are being taken.

DIAGNOSTICS

Diagnosis/Stabilization Phase		Acute Management Phase		Recovery Phase	
Outcome	Interventions	Outcome	Interventions	Outcome	Interventions
Patient and family will understand any diagnostic tests and/or procedures that need to be completed, including, but not limited to, VS, hemodynamic monitoring, radiographic studies, and lab tests (including hormonal studies).	Explain all procedures and tests to patient and family. Provide individualized education as needed to patient and family. Be sensitive to individualized needs of patient and family for information. Begin preop teaching with explanation of function of pituitary gland, along with what is causing patient's symptoms; also include the following:	Patient and family will understand any tests or procedures to be performed.	Explain all tests and procedures prior to performance; answer any questions that may be asked. Provide individualized assessment of patient and family needs for information pertaining to disease process and diagnostic tests. Anticipate other diagnostic tests that may be needed to accurately diagnose disease	Patient and family will understand significance of results from diagnostic tests performed and their relationship to patient's current and future health status.	Review results of diagnostic tests with patient and family prior to patient's discharge. Educate patient and family regarding appropriate measures to be taken so as to allow patient to return to maximal physical and mental wellness. Provide patient and family with guidelines and/or instructions regarding follow-up care.

- explain that he or she will have nasal packing following surgery
- practice mouth-breathing preop
- caution patient against nose blowing, sneezing, or coughing postop, as these activities may disrupt the muscle graft and cause CSF leak
- perform baseline neurologic assessment

process as well as any resultant treatments and interventions.

Obtain baseline patient weight.

Obtain baseline chemistry and hematologic studies.

Explain the advantages of transsphenoidal hypophysectomy over craniotomy:

- it allows the tumor to be removed, frequently leaving the gland intact so that pituitary function is preserved
- there is no observable incision line
- mortality and morbidity are decreased
- there is no need to cut patient's hair

FLUID BALANCE

Diagnosis/Stabilization Phase		Acute Management Phase		Recovery Phase	
Outcome	Interventions	Outcome	Interventions	Outcome	Interventions
Patient will achieve optimal hemodynamic status as evidenced by: • MAP >70 mmHg • hemodynamic parameters WNL • adequate LOC • adequate respiratory function • neurologic status WNL	Monitor and treat hemodynamic parameters: • BP • I & O • LOC • evidence of tissue perfusion • dysrhythmias Assess amount and character of drainage on nasal packing.	Patient will maintain optimal hemodynamic status.	Continue as in Diagnosis/Stabilization Phase, including assess VS and neurologic functioning q2–4h. Notify neurosurgeon of elevated temperature, altered respiratory patterns, and/or widened pulse pressure. Replace hormones and steroids as ordered by physician. Observe for symptoms of diabetes insipidus (40% may develop transient DI, 10% may develop permanent DI); teach patient symptoms and significance of same: • excessive thirst • excessive urinary output • signs of dehydration, including dry skin and mucous membranes Maintain strict I & O records.	Patient will maintain optimal hemodynamic status.	Report excessive bleeding on packing; observe for any evidence of CSF drainage. Tell patient to report excessive swallowing while packing in place. If diabetes insipidus is encountered, report to physician and: • monitor I & O • monitor serial urine and serum osmolarities • monitor serum and urine sodium levels • observe patient for symptoms of electrolyte disturbances Teach patient and family to report any changes to physician. If diabetes insipidus is encountered postop, advise patient that this may be temporary or permanent and that replace

Transsphenoidal Hypophysectomy Interdisciplinary Outcome Pathway (*continued*)

FLUID BALANCE (continued)

Diagnosis/Stabilization Phase		Acute Management Phase		Recovery Phase	
Outcome	Interventions	Outcome	Interventions	Outcome	Interventions
			Notify physician if UO > 200 cc/hr. Monitor serum and urine osmolarities. Weigh patient daily. Administer exogenous ADH (Pitressin) as ordered. Monitor for hypernatremia. Monitor urine specific gravity q4h and PRN. Ensure adequate fluid intake. If CSF leak is suspected, elevate HOB and notify physician. Inform patient that nasal packing and "moustache" dressing may be in place 2–3 days.		ment hormone therapy may be required. If Pitressin is ordered postop, advise patient to report symptoms of water intoxication (drowsiness, headaches, listlessness). Other effects of Pitressin: • blanching of skin • constriction of smooth muscle resulting in uterine and/or abdominal cramping • nausea • mild elevation of BP • any patient with a history of angina should be warned of the side effects, since this medication may cause constriction of the coronary arteries.

NUTRITION

Diagnosis/Stabilization Phase		Acute Management Phase		Recovery Phase	
Outcome	Interventions	Outcome	Interventions	Outcome	Interventions
Patient will achieve and maintain adequate nutrition to meet body requirements as evidenced by: • stable body weight not > 10% below or > 20% above IBW	Assess patient's nutritional status upon admission, including: • body weight and appropriateness for height and structure • patient's "normal" daily dietary intake • assess bowel sounds and presence of abdominal distension and/or pain • monitor serum albumin and protein	Patient will achieve and maintain adequate nutrition to meet body requirements.	Advance diet as ordered, beginning with ice chips to adequately assess swallowing ability. Remind patient that oral mucosa may be quite tender for several days, but that nutrition needs to be maintained. Maintain strict I & O records, monitoring for diabetes insipidus (or water intoxication if patient is on Pitressin replacement therapy).	Patient will achieve and maintain adequate nutrition to meet body requirements.	Monitor patient's response to diet and dietary intake. Instruct patient and family on diet that is to be followed post discharge. Warn patient that if steroid therapy is required, weight gain may be expected and actions to take to avoid.

- albumin 3.5–4.0 g/dL
- total protein 6–8 g/dL
- total lymphocyte count 1,000–3,000

Consult dietitian to help determine and direct nutritional support.

Consider calorie count to determine if patient is meeting nutritional needs.

MOBILITY

Diagnosis/Stabilization Phase		Acute Management Phase		Recovery Phase	
Outcome	Interventions	Outcome	Interventions	Outcome	Interventions
Patient will achieve optimal mobility. Patient will maintain normal musculoskeletal functioning during period of bed rest.	Assess degree of mobility upon admission, including muscle strength and ROM. Assess potential need for rotational therapy bed. Begin/teach passive/active-assist ROM exercises. Instruct patient that he or she will be expected to turn at least q2h and PRN.	Patient will achieve optimal mobility. Patient will maintain normal musculoskeletal functioning during period of bed rest.	Perform passive/active assist ROM exercises. Monitor patient's compliance with exercise instructions. Assist patient with position changes. Consult PT/OT for specific mobility/functional limitations.	Patient will achieve optimal mobility.	Continue as in Acute Management Phase. Provide assistive devices if needed.

OXYGENATION/VENTILATION

Diagnosis/Stabilization Phase		Acute Management Phase		Recovery Phase	
Outcome	Interventions	Outcome	Interventions	Outcome	Interventions
Patient will have adequate oxygenation and gas exchange, as evidenced by: • SaO_2 >90%, SpO_2 >92%; • ABGs WNL for patient • clear breath sounds • respiratory rate, depth, and rhythm WNL • normal CXR	Monitor functioning of the respiratory system, including: • SpO_2 • breath sounds • serial ABGs • rate, rhythm, and depth of respirations • serial CXRs • evidence of tissue perfusion. Careful monitoring of patient's airway is essential, since nasal packing and trumpets will be in place, as well as the possibility of postop nasotracheal edema. Administer O_2 as needed to keep SpO_2 >92%.	Patient will have adequate gas exchange.	Monitor and treat oxygenation status as per ABGs or SpO_2. Report adventitious breath sounds. Monitor serial CXR reports; inability of the patient to cough postop may lead to atelectasis and/or pneumonia. Administer O_2, as needed; utilize humidification to keep secretions thin. Maintain ongoing assessment of patency of patient's airway, especially while nasal packing and trumpets are in place; assess patency after removal of same.	Patient will have adequate gas exchange.	Educate patient regarding the importance of: • deep breathing • not bending over, sneezing, or coughing until the physician clears him or her to do so • reporting any signs or symptoms of shortness of breath or dyspnea Have patient demonstrate deep breathing techniques.

Transsphenoidal Hypophysectomy Interdisciplinary Outcome Pathway (continued)

OXYGENATION/VENTILATION (continued)

Diagnosis/Stabilization Phase		Acute Management Phase		Recovery Phase	
Outcome	Interventions	Outcome	Interventions	Outcome	Interventions
• absence of dyspnea, cyanosis, and abnormal respiratory secretions • effective deep breathing skills (*no coughing immediately postop*) • VS WNL for patient	Elevate HOB. Maintain adequate humidification. Monitor for signs and symptoms of altered gas exchange: • dyspnea • restlessness • confusion • headache • cyanosis • SpO_2 <90%		Teach appropriate deep breathing techniques and have patient give return demonstration. Assess tissue perfusion (pulse, pain, color, temperature, signs of decreased perfusion and or altered LOC and decreased UO). Involve RCP as needed.		

COMFORT

Diagnosis/Stabilization Phase		Acute Management Phase		Recovery Phase	
Outcome	Interventions	Outcome	Interventions	Outcome	Interventions
Patient will be as comfortable as possible following surgery as evidenced by: • minimal or no complaints of discomfort • no objective indicators of pain or discomfort • VS WNL for patient	Assess quantity and quality of pain; administer pain medications as indicated. Use a pain scale. Assess effects of pain medication on respiratory function and neurologic function, as well as pain control. Administer pain medication cautiously, considering potential alteration in neurological assessment and effects on respiratory status. Provide reassurance in a calm, caring, and competent manner. Allow family to remain with patient if they promote rest.	Patient will be as relaxed and comfortable as possible.	Continue as in Diagnosis/Stabilization Phase. Provide uninterrupted rest periods in a quiet environment. Instruct patient on relaxation techniques; involve family in strategies; have patient give return demonstration.	Patient will be as relaxed and comfortable as possible.	Administer analgesics as ordered by physician; patient may experience discomfort related to headache, incisional pain, and/or nasal packing. Provide quiet, restful environment. Frequent oral hygiene at least q2–4h. Offer ice chips. Teach patient to avoid those activities that involve bending over and/or straining. Advise patient that physician may advise him or her not to brush front teeth for a period of time until gingival mucosa has healed. Teach patient/family alternative methods to promote relaxation after discharge; have patient give return demonstration.

SKIN INTEGRITY

Diagnosis/Stabilization Phase		Acute Management Phase		Recovery Phase	
Outcome	Interventions	Outcome	Interventions	Outcome	Interventions
Patient will have intact skin without evidence of pressure areas, pressure sores, and/or abrasions.	Perform initial assessment of patient's skin, noting any areas of redness or breakdown. Assess all bony prominences. Utilize preventive measures to decrease risk of skin breakdown in those patients determined to be at high risk. If areas of skin breakdown do exist, document same and treat according to hospital protocol.	Patient will have intact skin without evidence of pressure areas, pressure sores, and/or abrasions.	Pay particular attention to occiput, in consideration of patient's positioning during surgery; if pressure area/breakdown discovered, treat according to hospital protocol. Observe skin areas beneath nose while nasal packing and/or trumpets are in place as well as after their removal. Inspect skin q4h and PRN.	Patient will have intact skin without evidence of pressure areas, pressure sores, and/or abrasions.	Teach patient and family about proper skin care after discharge.

PROTECTION/SAFETY

Diagnosis/Stabilization Phase		Acute Management Phase		Recovery Phase	
Outcome	Interventions	Outcome	Interventions	Outcome	Interventions
Patient will be protected from injury and/or harm.	Assess need for assistance. Provide physical support as needed. Allow family to remain with patient if they have calming influence and can promote rest and safety. Use sedation as indicated.	Patient will be protected from injury and/or harm.	Assess need for assistance; provide physical support as needed. Consult other disciplines (PT, OT) as necessary. Monitor I & O; observe patient for symptoms of excessive UO with possible resultant postural and/or orthostatic hypotension. Maintain HOB at 30 degrees postop to decrease swelling and pressure on the sella turcica.	Patient will be protected from injury and/or harm.	Educate patient and family regarding any physical limitations in activity after discharge.

Transsphenoidal Hypophysectomy Interdisciplinary Outcome Pathway *(continued)*

PSYCHOSOCIAL/SELF-DETERMINATION

Diagnosis/Stabilization Phase		Acute Management Phase		Recovery Phase	
Outcome	Interventions	Outcome	Interventions	Outcome	Interventions
Patient will achieve psychophysiologic stability. Patient will demonstrate a low level of anxiety and/or fear as evidenced by: • VS WNL for patient • reported decrease in anxiety from patient or family • comfortable/rested appearance with lack of restlessness • minimal complaints of discomfort and/or pain	Assess effects of critical care environment on patient: • physiological effects (VS, hemodynamic variables) • psychological effects (restlessness, decreased comfort) Provide emotional support as needed. Minimize environmental sensory stimuli. Answer all questions honestly and openly; explain all treatments and diagnostic tests. Give calm, competent, and reassuring approach with all interventions.	Patient will achieve psychophysiologic ability. Patient will demonstrate a low level of anxiety and/or fear.	Provide adequate periods of rest. Allow patient to verbalize fears and/or anxieties. Attempt to involve family in patient's care whenever possible. Maintain ongoing assessment of patient's coping skills and their effectiveness. Involve pastoral care if indicated. Strive to create atmosphere conducive to development of trust and honesty.	Patient will achieve psychophysiologic stability. Patient will demonstrate a low level of anxiety and/or fear.	Continue ongoing assessment of patient/family coping skills and their effectiveness. Keep patient updated on his or her progress as well as anticipated future effects, if any, of illness. Warn patient that reproductive and sexual difficulties, including sterility and decreased libido, are possible after the surgery; supplemental hormone replacement may be necessary, but does not always relieve these symptoms. Address concerns patient may have on impact on daily life.

CHAPTER 7

Miscellaneous Pathways

Acute Pain Management
Interdisciplinary Outcome Pathway

COORDINATION OF CARE

Diagnosis/Stabilization Phase		Acute Management Phase		Recovery Phase	
Outcome	Interventions	Outcome	Interventions	Outcome	Interventions
All appropriate team members and disciplines will be involved in the plan of care.	Develop the plan of care with the patient/family, surgeons, primary physician, consulting physicians, anesthesiologist, RN, advanced practice nurse, clinical pharmacist, RCP, dietitian, PT, and OT.	All appropriate team members and disciplines will be involved in implementation of the plan of care.	Implement and update the plan of care with all appropriate team members. Initiate consultations, if indicated (i.e., social services and chaplain). Assess social support systems. Initiate discharge planning assessment. Initiate home health consult, as needed.	Patient/family will understand discharge plan. Patient will understand how to control/eliminate pain.	Implement and update the plan of care with all appropriate team members. Provide guidelines concerning care at home. Provide phone numbers of resources available to answer questions. Patient/family will verbalize follow-up discharge and pain control plan: • specific pain medications to be taken • frequency of medication administration • precautions to follow when taking pain medications • drug interactions • activity limitations due to pain medications • diet restrictions

DIAGNOSTICS

Diagnosis/Stabilization Phase		Acute Management Phase		Recovery Phase	
Outcome	Interventions	Outcome	Interventions	Outcome	Interventions
Patient/family will understand the purpose of all diagnostic procedures (x-rays, lab work, VS, PFT, etc.).	Explain appropriate procedures to be performed to determine source of pain and extent of disease/illness/injury. Be sensitive to patient/family's individualized needs for information. Establish effective communication techniques with intubated patient.	Patient/family will understand the purpose of all tests and procedures (i.e., lab work, VS, x-rays, analgesia administration, etc.).	Administer analgesics, as needed, to facilitate diagnostic procedures. Teach patient about individualized pain control methods: oral, IV, PCA, intraspinal.	Patient/family will understand the purpose of all post-discharge diagnostic procedures. Patient will understand actions to take should pain recur.	Consider further diagnostic procedures if change in pain pattern or development of new pain. Provide appropriate patient education. Review appropriate diagnostic results with patient/family prior to discharge. Provide guidelines concerning follow-up care.

Provide patient/family with copies of significant diagnostic results to be used in continuing home care.

FLUID BALANCE

Diagnosis/Stabilization Phase		Acute Management Phase		Recovery Phase	
Outcome	Interventions	Outcome	Interventions	Outcome	Interventions
Patient will achieve optimal hemodynamic status as evidenced by: • HR 60–100 bpm • SBP > 90 mmHg • Hgb > 8 • MAP > 70 mmHg • free of dysrhythmias	Assess for cardiovascular signs and symptoms due to acute pain: • tachycardia • hypertension • increased PVR • water and sodium retention • pertinent lab values such as electrolytes and CBC Assess for and treat sources of acute pain: • myocardial infarction • thoracic/abdominal aneurysm • blunt/penetrating trauma • surgery Determine hydration needs based on hemodynamics, I & O, VS, SaO_2, CXR, breath sounds, and electrolytes. Assess weight daily	Patient will maintain optimal hemodynamic status.	Monitor to distinguish between original source of pain and secondary source of pain. Monitor VS when reassessing pain and before and after medication administration. Monitor for changes in drug absorption due to altered cardiovascular function: • CO • venous capacity • fluid shifts Maintain optimal hydration based on continued assessment. Monitor for complications secondary to acute pain: atelectasis, pneumonia, DVT, ileus.	Patient will maintain optimal hemodynamic status.	Monitor patients with renal or liver disease for altered drug metabolism and excretion. Maintain ongoing evaluation of cardiac and renal functioning. Teach patient/family how to maintain optimal fluid balance at home.

NUTRITION

Diagnosis/Stabilization Phase		Acute Management Phase		Recovery Phase	
Outcome	Interventions	Outcome	Interventions	Outcome	Interventions
Patient will be adequately nourished as evidenced by: • stable weight • weight not > 10% below or > 20% above IBW • albumin > 3.5 g/dL	Assess nutritional status. Assess for bowel sounds, abdominal distension, abdominal pain and tenderness q4h and PRN. Assess for and treat GI sources of acute pain: • ulcers • diverticulitis • pancreatitis	Patient will be adequately nourished. Patient will be free from nausea.	Identify and eliminate foods irritating to the GI tract, if applicable. Administer antiemetics and H_2 blockers, if indicated. Maintain naso/orogastric tube, if indicated. Consult dietitian if: • unanticipated weight loss • diet counseling needed	Patient will maintain adequate nutritional status. Patient will remain free from nausea.	Teach patient/family appropriate diet modifications and assess understanding. Monitor for inappropriate use of antacids. Maintain ongoing evaluation of GI function.

Acute Pain Management Interdisciplinary Outcome Pathway (continued)

NUTRITION (continued)

Diagnosis/Stabilization Phase		Acute Management Phase		Recovery Phase	
Outcome	Interventions	Outcome	Interventions	Outcome	Interventions
• total protein 6–8 g/dL • total lymphocyte count 1,000–3,000	• cholecystitis • hiatal hernia • blunt/penetrating trauma • surgery • dental procedures • bowel obstruction Initiate DAT and monitor response. Assess for GI signs and symptoms due to pain: increased gastric secretions, decreased gastric motility, smooth muscle sphincter spasm, hyperglycemia, N & V, and decreased gastric pH.		• eating less than half of food on tray • albumin < 3 g/dL Monitor albumin, prealbumin, and total protein. Monitor response to diet. Adjust nutritional plan for patients with difficulty swallowing to include: • elixir forms of analgesics • liquid/soft diet • use of topical anesthetics		

MOBILITY

Diagnosis/Stabilization Phase		Acute Management Phase		Recovery Phase	
Outcome	Interventions	Outcome	Interventions	Outcome	Interventions
Patient will maintain normal ROM and muscle strength.	Assess physical limitations due to pain. PT to assess ambulation, mobility, muscle flexibility, strength, and tone. OT to assess functional ability. PT/OT to help determine and direct activity goals. Institute progressive activity program (i.e., ROM exercises, bed transfers, increased ambulation as tolerated). Assess for and treat neuro/musculoskeletal sources of pain:	Patient will achieve optimal mobility.	Monitor surgical patient for compartmental syndrome. Teach energy conservation and proper body mechanics during functional activities. Monitor response to increased activity: decrease if increased pain or adverse effects occur (i.e., tachycardia, dyspnea, ectopy, hypotension, and increased discomfort). Use assistive devices (pillows, splints, ambulation devices, etc.).	Patient will maintain optimal mobility.	Continue to evaluate pain level, using a pain scale, as patient returns to ADLs. Modify activity level based on presence of increased pain. Assist patient in developing realistic goals for home exercise program.

- fractures
- strains
- sprains
- muscle spasms
- spinal/head injuries
- joint disease
- surgery

Perform motor, sensory, and reflex exam of extremities q4h and PRN.

Have patient give return demonstration of correct use of assistive devices.
Schedule periods of rest between activities.

OXYGENATION/VENTILATION

Diagnosis/Stabilization Phase		Acute Management Phase		Recovery Phase	
Outcome	Interventions	Outcome	Interventions	Outcome	Interventions
Patient will have adequate gas exchange as evidenced by: • normal CXR • respiratory rate, depth, rhythm WNL • clear breath sounds • SaO$_2$ >90% • SpO$_2$ >92% • ABGs WNL	Assess respiratory functions q2h and PRN: • breath sounds • respiratory muscle strength and movement • splinting or guarding • respiratory rate, depth, and quality • cough ability • SpO$_2$ • ABGs Assess q2–4h for and treat pulmonary sources of acute pain: • pneumo/hemothorax • rib fractures • blunt/penetrating trauma • surgery • pleuritis Assess q2–4h for pulmonary signs and symptoms of pain: • decreased TV • decreased functional capacity • hyperventilation • use of accessory muscles • decreased peak flow • hypoventilation Monitor pulse oximetry. Apply supplemental O$_2$ to keep SpO$_2$ >92%.	Patient will have adequate gas exchange.	Continue as in Diagnosis/Stabilization Phase, decreasing assessments to q4–8h. Provide pulmonary hygiene and IS. Have patient give return demonstration of IS. Assess color, quantity, and quality (thick/thin) of sputum. Administer high flow, humidified oxygen per nasal cannula or mask.	Patient will maintain adequate gas exchange.	Maintain ongoing evaluation of pulmonary status. Have patient demonstrate breathing exercises. Teach patient/family signs and symptoms of respiratory infection and when to report symptoms to physician.

Acute Pain Management Interdisciplinary Outcome Pathway (continued)

COMFORT

Diagnosis/Stabilization Phase		Acute Management Phase		Recovery Phase	
Outcome	Interventions	Outcome	Interventions	Outcome	Interventions
Patient will be as comfortable as possible, in an effort to minimize the incidence and severity of acute pain.	Obtain a thorough pain history: • previous or ongoing pain episodes • previous pain control methods • patient's attitude toward pain medication • any history of substance abuse Assess pain level through patient self-report. Include: • description • location • intensity/severity using a visual analogue scale • aggravating/relieving factors Assess pain level through direct observation for: • splinting or guarding • distorted posture • decreased mobility/restricted movement of limbs • anxiety Develop a proactive pain control plan based on: • stage of illness/disease process • concurrent medical conditions • psychological/cultural characteristics • ethical considerations • gender concerns Administer analgesics as ordered and monitor response. Establish effective communication techniques with intubated patient. Educate patient/family how to communicate unrelieved pain effectively.	Patient's pain will be controlled. Patient will be as comfortable as possible.	Reassess pain level frequently: • routinely at scheduled intervals (at least q2–4h) • with each new report of pain • following pain medication administration Individualize route, dosage, and schedule for analgesics: • mild to moderate pain: NSAIDs • moderate to severe pain: opioid analgesics (IV, IM, transdermal, intraspinal) Establish optimal analgesic dosing by titration. Utilize modalities, electrical stimulation, touch therapy, acupressure or acupuncture for pain control as indicated. Offer PCA, if medically and psychologically indicated. Administer a loading dose prior to the start of a continuous infusion. Teach patient the appropriate use of PCA. Administer analgesics around the clock while continuous pain present. Consider complementary therapies such as guided imagery, music, humor, touch therapy, or hypnosis to enhance comfort. Provide uninterrupted periods of rest. Recognize and treat side effects of analgesics: • sedation • constipation • N & V • pruritus • respiratory depression	Patient will be as pain free as possible.	Monitor patient for the development of tolerance and/or dependence to analgesics. Instruct the patient in nonpharmacological pain control intervention: • relaxation • distraction • imagery • music therapy • biofeedback Have patient give return demonstration of nonpharmacological interventions. Use physical therapeutic interventions: • application of heat/cold • massage • TENS Refer to Chronic Pain Management Outcome Pathway.

SKIN INTEGRITY

Diagnosis/Stabilization Phase		Acute Management Phase		Recovery Phase	
Outcome	Interventions	Outcome	Interventions	Outcome	Interventions
Patient will have intact skin without abrasions or pressure ulcers.	Obtain and document a complete baseline skin assessment. Assess q2h for and treat integumentary sources of pain: • burns • surgical incisions • soft tissue trauma • shingles Assess all bony prominences q4h. Treat pressure ulcers according to hospital protocol.	Patient will have intact skin without abrasions or pressure ulcers. Patient will have healing surgical wounds and be free of infection.	Continue as in Diagnosis/Stabilization Phase, except decrease assessments to q4h. Document size, location, and description of surgical wounds. Maintain sterile technique with all dressing changes. Monitor all incisions for signs and symptoms of infection. Use pressure-reducing devices as appropriate. Facilitate the highest degree of mobility possible.	Patient will have intact skin without abrasions or pressure ulcers. Patient will have healing surgical wounds and be free of infection.	Teach patient/family proper care of surgical wounds. Teach patient/family proper techniques for dressing changes, if applicable. Evaluate patient for the presence of new pain sources: • wound dehiscence • infection • DVT thrombosis

PROTECTION/SAFETY

Diagnosis/Stabilization Phase		Acute Management Phase		Recovery Phase	
Outcome	Interventions	Outcome	Interventions	Outcome	Interventions
Patient will be protected from possible harm.	Administer naloxone 0.4–2 mg in the event of respiratory depression. Follow hospital protocol for the use of restraints. Assess need for wrist restraints. If used, monitor circulation q1–2h. Explain need for restraints to patient/family. Assess patient for contraindications of opioid administration: • altered sensorium • compromising lung disease • near-term pregnancy • inability to monitor side effects Allow family to remain with patient, if they have a calming influence and can promote rest and safety.	Patient will be protected from possible harm.	In patients receiving intraspinal analgesia: • maintain strict sterile technique • use tubing without injection ports • keep HOB elevated during the first hour of treatment Remove restraints as soon as patient is able to follow commands. Provide appropriate physical support to prevent falls while patient is receiving analgesics. Teach proper body mechanics with functional activities to maintain joint integrity and prevent joint strain or injury. Continue to allow family to remain with patient.	Patient will be protected from possible harm.	Review physical limitations associated with analgesic administration with patient/family prior to discharge. Consult PT/OT for home follow-up, if limitations are present.

Acute Pain Management Interdisciplinary Outcome Pathway (continued)

PSYCHOSOCIAL/SELF-DETERMINATION

Diagnosis/Stabilization Phase		Acute Management Phase		Recovery Phase	
Outcome	Interventions	Outcome	Interventions	Outcome	Interventions
Patient/family will demonstrate effective coping skills. Patient will achieve psychophysiologic stability.	Assess patient/family for current level of anxiety and fear. Assess cultural factors associated with pain such as ethical considerations and gender concerns. Reassure patient/family that most pain can be relieved safely and effectively. Assess patient for psychosocial signs and symptoms of pain: <ul><li>loss of hope</li><li>loss of control</li><li>impaired QOL</li><li>helplessness</li><li>anxiety</li><li>depression</li><li>disruption of sleep</li><li>inability to concentrate</li></ul> Take measures to reduce sensory overload. Allow flexible visitation to meet needs of patient/family. Assess effect of critical care environment on patient and how it affects pain perception.	Patient/family will demonstrate effective coping skills. Patient will achieve psychophysiologic stability.	Continue as in Diagnosis/Stabilization Phase. Consider medication to promote sleep and/or decrease anxiety. Use interventions to assist with coping, such as allowing patient to verbalize fears/concerns and be available to answer all questions. Involve patient in decision making concerning health care.	Patient/family will demonstrate effective coping skills. Patient will achieve psychophysiologic stability.	Educate patient/family that pain (or increase in pain) may not mean progression of illness/injury. Assess effect of pain on patient's work, recreation, and role in family/society. Assess patient for changes in ADLs and sexual functioning. Assist patient/family with identification and implementation of role changes. Provide information on coping mechanisms for use after discharge.

Burns
Interdisciplinary Outcome Pathway

COORDINATION OF CARE

Diagnosis/Stabilization Phase		Acute Management Phase		Recovery Phase	
Outcome	Interventions	Outcome	Interventions	Outcome	Interventions
All appropriate team members and disciplines will be involved in the plan of care.	Develop a plan of care with the patient/family, primary physician(s), surgeon, plastic surgeon, infectious disease specialist, pulmonologist, RN, advanced practice nurse, other specialists as needed, RCP, and PT. Take patient's history immediately upon admission. You may need to get this from the family or significant others. Conduct an immediate assessment of all injuries.	All appropriate team members and disciplines will be involved in the plan of care.	Update the plan of care with patient/family, other team members, PT, dietitian, discharge planner, case manager, social worker, recreational therapist, OT, chaplain, and SP if needed. Initiate planning for anticipated discharge and call home medical health and home medical equipment company as needed. Begin teaching patient/family about care at home. Involve patient/family in care.	Patient/family will understand how to maintain optimal health at home.	Provide guidelines concerning care at home: • diet • medications • activity • exercise program • follow-up visits Provide patient/family with phone number of resources/support group available to answer questions.

DIAGNOSTICS

Diagnosis/Stabilization Phase		Acute Management Phase		Recovery Phase	
Outcome	Interventions	Outcome	Interventions	Outcome	Interventions
Patient will understand any tests or procedures that must be completed (hemodynamic monitoring, CXR, carboxyhemoglobin level, lab tests, type and cross-match, UA, wound management, bronchoscopy, and ABGs).	Explain all procedures and tests to patient/family. Be sensitive to individualized needs of patient/family for information. Be prepared to repeat information Answer all questions in easy to understand terminology.	Patient will understand any tests or procedures that must be completed to recover from burns (hydrotherapy, debridement, skin grafting).	Continue as in Diagnosis/Stabilization Phase.	Patient will understand meaning of diagnostic tests and procedures in relation to continued health (wound care, diet, skin grafting, follow-up visits).	Review with patient/family before discharge the results of lab work, CXR, and skin grafting. Discuss any abnormal findings and appropriate measures patient can take to help return to normal. Provide patient with guidelines concerning follow-up care. Provide instruction on care at home and have patient give return demonstration if appropriate: • when to call the physician • wound care, both burns and donor sites

Burns Interdisciplinary Outcome Pathway (continued)

DIAGNOSTICS (continued)

Diagnosis/Stabilization Phase		Acute Management Phase		Recovery Phase	
Outcome	Interventions	Outcome	Interventions	Outcome	Interventions
					• sterile technique • activity limitations • exercise program • use of assistive devices • wearing of pressure garment(s) • dietary needs • medications Provide patient with phone number of resources available to assist if necessary.

FLUID BALANCE

Diagnosis/Stabilization Phase		Acute Management Phase		Recovery Phase	
Outcome	Interventions	Outcome	Interventions	Outcome	Interventions
Patient will achieve optimal hemodynamic status as evidenced by: • MAP >70 mmHg • hemodynamic parameters WNL • UO >0.5 mL/kg/hr • absence of dysrhythmias • adequate LOC • clear lung sounds • adequate I & O • normothermic state Patient will achieve normal fluid balance. Patient will achieve good tissue perfusion.	Assess degree, extent, and severity of burns using the American Burn Association's standards. Monitor and treat hemodynamic parameters: • dysrhythmias • SvO_2 • BP • evidence of tissue perfusion (pain, pulses, color, temperature, signs of decreased perfusion such as decreased UO and altered LOC) • JVD • CVP • CO/CI • SV/SI • PCWP • PA pressures Monitor lab values: electrolytes, CBC, clotting factors, carboxyhemoglobin, ABGs, Hbg, and Hct.	Patient will maintain optimal hemodynamic status. Patient will maintain normal fluid balance. Patient will maintain good tissue perfusion.	Monitor and treat hemodynamic parameters. Assess neurovascular status q2–4h and PRN. Measure circumference of burned areas to determine if edema is present. Elevate burned extremities. Assess fluid status for overload or deficit and treat accordingly. Continue to estimate fluid loss. Stay prepared for mechanical ventilation should respiratory status deteriorate. Anticipate and be prepared for electrolyte replacement therapy. Continue to assess for complications associated with burns: • cardiovascular collapse • septicemia	Patient will maintain optimal hemodynamic status. Patient will maintain normal fluid balance. Patient will maintain good tissue perfusion.	Continue as in Acute Management Phase. IVs may be discontinued when patient is taking adequate fluids and oral analgesics. Teach patient/family proper fluid management at home: • signs and symptoms of fluid overload/deficit • measures to take should overload/deficit occur • weigh daily

- infection
- subacute bacterial endocarditis

Continue to monitor lab values: potassium, sodium, Hct, bicarbonate.
Weigh daily.
Colloids are usually given after 24h.

Monitor respiratory status and be prepared for mechanical ventilation. Assess lung sounds q1–2h.

Establish IV access with large-bore catheter or central line.

Assess fluid deficit and treat accordingly. Administer electrolyte solutions (usually lactated Ringer's) the first 24h after injury.

Monitor for signs of fluid overload: dyspnea, crackles, peripheral edema, tachycardia.

Type and crossmatch.

Carefully monitor I & O with a urinary catheter.

When estimating fluid loss, consider loss through evaporation, blistering, or wound drainage.

Anticipate and be prepared for electrolyte replacement therapy.

Anticipate need for vasopressor agents; assess response and titrate accordingly.

Assess neurovascular status q1h and PRN.

Monitor and treat potentially life-threatening dysrhythmias.

Obtain weight immediately upon admission. Weigh daily.

Obtain 12 lead EKG.

Monitor temperature and take measures to return to normal: hypo/hyperthermia unit, warm blankets, antipyretics.

Monitor for signs of complications that can occur with burns:
- inhalation injuries
- ARDS
- respiratory failure
- renal failure
- liver failure
- infection
- sepsis
- hypovolemia

Burns Interdisciplinary Outcome Pathway (continued)

FLUID BALANCE (continued)

Diagnosis/Stabilization Phase		Acute Management Phase		Recovery Phase	
Outcome	Interventions	Outcome	Interventions	Outcome	Interventions
	• DIC • clotting abnormalities • anemia • atelectasis • bronchospasm • acute airway obstruction • encephalopathy • decreased tissue perfusion • pulmonary edema • ulcers Monitor for hypokalemia and hemolysis of red blood cells. Monitor for metabolic acidosis.				

NUTRITION

Diagnosis/Stabilization Phase		Acute Management Phase		Recovery Phase	
Outcome	Interventions	Outcome	Interventions	Outcome	Interventions
Patient will be adequately nourished as evidenced by: • stable weight • weight not >10% below or >20% above IBW • albumin >3.5 g/dL • total protein 6–8 g/dL • prealbumin at least 15 g/dL • total lymphocyte count 1,000–3,000 • positive nitrogen balance	NPO if intubated or until able to take fluids. Consult dietitian or nutritional support team to determine and direct nutritional support if: • albumin <3.0 • eating less than half of food on tray If intubated >24h, initiate enteral feedings. Enteral is preferred to parenteral. Provide high calorie diet. Calculate calorie and protein requirements based on body weight and body surface burned. Enteral feedings are recommended if >20% BSA is burned. Monitor response to diet.	Patient will be adequately nourished.	Continue as in Diagnosis/Stabilization Phase. Continue enteral diet; progress DAT until patient is able to eat enough calories to meet metabolic needs. Maintain a high calorie, high protein diet. Wait to transition off enteral feedings until patient is taking three-quarters of needs orally. Consider calorie count when patient is eating to determine if intake meets nutritional goals. If not, consider nocturnal enteral feedings to supplement caloric intake.	Patient will be adequately nourished and able to consume at least three-quarters of caloric need.	Monitor response to diet. Instruct patient/family on dietary needs after discharge. Continue high calorie, high protein diet. When completely healed, return to normal calorie intake.

Assess bowel sounds, abdominal distension, and abdominal discomfort and tenderness q4h and PRN.
Check gastric pH q4h.
Check gastric residual q4h.

MOBILITY

Diagnosis/Stabilization Phase		Acute Management Phase		Recovery Phase	
Outcome	Interventions	Outcome	Interventions	Outcome	Interventions
Patient will achieve optimal mobility. Patient will be free of joint contractures. Patient will maintain joint function and mobility.	Consult PT/OT to help assess ambulation, mobility, ROM, muscle strength, flexibility, and tone. PT/OT to help determine and direct activity goals. Turn at least q2h if hemodynamically stable and monitor response. If not stable, consider alternative bed therapy. Institute alternative bed therapy if indicated (i.e., kinetic therapy, Stryker frame). Begin passive/active-assist ROM exercises. Consult OT for splints when necessary to maintain joint integrity and prevent deformities. Change splints according to schedule devised by OT.	Patient will achieve optimal mobility. Patient will be free of joint contractures. Patient will maintain joint function and mobility.	Increase activity as tolerated. Monitor response to increased activity and decrease if adverse events occur (tachycardia, syncope, dysrhythmias, dyspnea, hypotension, ectopy). Provide physical assistance or assistive devices as necessary. Monitor oxygen content with any increase in activity with pulse oximetry. Apply supplemental oxygen to keep SaO_2 >90%. Begin teaching patient/family progressive activity and how to assist patient with program goals. Medicate with analgesics before exercise if needed.	Patient will achieve optimal mobility. Patient will maintain joint function and mobility. Patient will be free of joint contractures.	Continue to progress activity as tolerated and monitor response. Decrease activity if adverse events occur. Continue teaching patient/family about home exercise program. Include energy conservation techniques to enhance function and strength. Continue ROM at least BID. Teach patient ways to decrease scarring such as wearing a pressure garment for up to one year after the injury. This also helps to maintain mobility and muscle function. OT or PT will fit the appropriate pressure garment. Teach patient proper use of assistive devices. Have patient give return demonstration.

OXYGENATION/VENTILATION

Diagnosis/Stabilization Phase		Acute Management Phase		Recovery Phase	
Outcome	Interventions	Outcome	Interventions	Outcome	Interventions
Patient will have adequate gas exchange as evidenced by: • O_2 saturation >90%	Monitor ventilator settings and hemodynamic variables before, during, and after weaning. Avoid prolonged administration of 100% FIO_2.	Patient will have adequate gas exchange.	Monitor and treat oxygenation disturbances. Monitor and treat ventilation disturbances as per chest assessment, ABGs, adventitious breath sounds, and CXR.	Patient will have adequate gas exchange.	Continue as in Acute Management Phase. Obtain CXR before discharge especially if inhalation injury has occurred. Provide instructions to patient on coughing and deep breathing

Burns Interdisciplinary Outcome Pathway (continued)

OXYGENATION/VENTILATION (continued)

Diagnosis/Stabilization Phase	Acute Management Phase	Recovery Phase
• ABGs WNL • clear breath sounds • CXR WNL • respiratory rate, rhythm, and depth WNL • absence of dyspnea, cyanosis, and secretion Note: Oxygen saturation must be measured in a blood gas laboratory and not per pulse oximetry because pulse oximetry does not measure carboxyhemoglobin. Monitor respiratory status constantly, particularly if inhalation injury has occurred—lung sounds, respiratory muscle strength, respiratory rate and depth, coughing ability, ABGs, and CXR. Involve RCP. Anticipate need for hyperventilation and hyperoxygenation, particularly before suctioning. Apply supplemental humidified oxygen if not intubated. Maintain SpO_2 > 92%. Assess evidence of tissue perfusion (pain, pulses, color, temperature, signs of decreased perfusion such as decreased UO and altered LOC). Monitor lab values: Hgb, ABGs, carboxyhemoglobin (should be less than 10%). Assess for other injuries that may impair respiratory function (i.e., smoke inhalation). RCP may be involved with assessment and treatment of respiratory condition secondary to smoke inhalation.	Wean from oxygen therapy/mechanical ventilation as indicated. Involve RCP. Administer warm humidified oxygen. Anticipate and prepare for bronchoscopy in the event of pulmonary/inhalation burns. Assist PT or RCP with postural drainage, percussion and vibration, and deep breathing and coughing. Observe for complications of burns that may impair oxygenation and ventilation: • pneumonia • infection • thrombus formation • embolus • ARDS • sepsis • hypovolemia • V/Q mismatch • atelectasis • bronchopneumonia • respiratory failure Instruct patient on proper coughing and deep breathing and IS techniques. Have patient give return demonstration. PT or RCP will assist with facilitating segmental breathing techniques to maximize inspiratory effort. Teach how to coordinate breathing with activity to conserve energy.	and IS at home. Have patient give return demonstration. Observe effects of increased activity on respiratory status. Continue to assess for complications of burns that may impair oxygenation/ventilation.

COMFORT

Diagnosis/Stabilization Phase		Acute Management Phase		Recovery Phase	
Outcome	Interventions	Outcome	Interventions	Outcome	Interventions
Patient will be as comfortable and pain free as possible as evidenced by: • no objective indicators of discomfort • no complaints of discomfort	Assess quantity and quality of pain. Use a pain scale such as visual analogue scale. Administer IV narcotic analgesics as needed and monitor response. A titrated morphine drip may be used. Lidocaine may be used as a continuous infusion. Establish effective communication technique with intubated patient in an effort to assess need for analgesia. Provide quiet environment to potentiate analgesia. Provide reassurance in a calm, caring, competent manner. Allow flexible visitation if family calms patient.	Patient will be as relaxed and pain free as possible.	Continue as in Diagnosis/Stabilization Phase. Administer narcotic analgesics before any painful procedure, such as wound debridement or dressing changes. Administer analgesics (IV or oral morphine, oral dilaudid) as needed and monitor response. Administer antianxiety agents as needed and monitor response. Use splints when indicated to provide comfort and maintain joint integrity. Teach patient relaxation techniques. Have patient give return demonstration. Electrical modalities such as TENS may be used. Use touch therapy, humor, and/or music therapy and imagery to promote relaxation. Involve family in strategies. Observe for complications of burns that may cause discomfort (embolus, thrombus formation, infection).	Patient will be as relaxed and pain free as possible.	Progress to oral analgesics and non-narcotic analgesics when possible. Monitor response. Continue alternative methods to promote relaxation as described earlier. Teach patient/family alternative methods to promote relaxation at home. Have patient/family give return demonstration. Assess for pruritus. Medications may be needed. Lanolin-based skin lotions may be applied q2h.

SKIN INTEGRITY

Diagnosis/Stabilization Phase		Acute Management Phase		Recovery Phase	
Outcome	Interventions	Outcome	Interventions	Outcome	Interventions
Patient will have intact skin without abrasions or pressure ulcers. Burns will remain free of infection.	Maintain strict aseptic technique. Assess all bony prominences at least q4h and treat if needed. Use preventive pressure-reducing devices/kinetic therapy if patient is at high risk for developing pressure ulcers. Involve PT early in wound management process.	Patient will have intact skin without abrasions or pressure ulcers. Burns will remain free of infection. Patient will have healing wounds.	Continue as in Diagnosis/Stabilization Phase. PT will be involved in day-to-day wound management. Begin teaching patient/family about assessment of burn areas/grafted areas, treatment, skin care, and how to evaluate effectiveness of treatment.	Patient will have intact skin without abrasions or pressure ulcers. Burns will be free of infection. Skin grafts will be free of infection.	Continue teaching patient/family care of burn/skin graft wounds at home: • aseptic technique • dressing changes usually once a day • pressure bandages • assessment of healing progress

Burns Interdisciplinary Outcome Pathway (continued)

SKIN INTEGRITY (continued)

Diagnosis/Stabilization Phase		Acute Management Phase		Recovery Phase	
Outcome	Interventions	Outcome	Interventions	Outcome	Interventions
	Treat pressure ulcers according to hospital protocol. If chemical burn, wash affected area with large amounts of water. Contact poison control center for further directions.		Teach patient ways to decrease scarring such as wearing a pressure garment for up to one year after the injury. Monitor for signs and symptoms of infection. Monitor WBCs if silver sulfadiazine is used. Provide cleansing or hydrotherapy as indicated. Assist with debridement. Prepare for skin grafting.	Scarring will be kept to a minimum. Patient will have healing wounds.	• potential complications (rejection, infection) • staples may still be in place • care of donor site(s) • splints • exercises • massage. Teach patient/family signs and symptoms of infection and when to call the physician. Teach patient/family importance of wearing pressure garment(s) to reduce scarring.

PROTECTION/SAFETY

Diagnosis/Stabilization Phase		Acute Management Phase		Recovery Phase	
Outcome	Interventions	Outcome	Interventions	Outcome	Interventions
Patient will be protected from possible harm. Patient will be protected from infection.	Assess need for restraints if patient is intubated, has a decreased LOC, or is agitated and restless. Explain need for restraints to patient/family. Assess response to restraints, if used, and check q1h for skin integrity and impairment to circulation. Follow hospital protocol for the use of restraints. Remove restraints as soon as patient is able to follow instructions. Provide sedatives as needed and monitor response, especially to the respiratory system. Use sterile technique with all dressing changes. Assess all burn areas for signs of infection.	Patient will be protected from possible harm. Patient will be protected from infection.	If need still exists for restraints, check q1–2h for skin integrity and impairment to circulation. Provide support when activity increases. Monitor response to activity. Teach correct movement and appropriate functional skills to prevent joint stress, strain, or injury. Continue to use sterile technique with dressing changes. Continue to assess all burn areas for signs of infection.	Patient will be protected from possible harm. Patient will be protected from infection.	Provide support with activity increases and monitor response. Teach patient/family about: • physical limitations in activity after discharge • importance of maintaining sterile technique with dressing changes • signs and symptoms of infection • when to call the physician

PSYCHSOCIAL/SELF-DETERMINATION

Diagnosis/Stabilization Phase		Acute Management Phase		Recovery Phase	
Outcome	Interventions	Outcome	Interventions	Outcome	Interventions
Patient will achieve psychophysiologic stability. Patient will demonstrate a decrease in anxiety as evidenced by: • VS WNL • subjective reports of decreased anxiety • objective signs of decreased anxiety Patient will begin acceptance process of burns.	Assess physiologic effects of critical care environment on patient (hemodynamic variables, psychological status, signs of increased sympathetic response). Provide sedatives as needed and monitor response. Take measures to reduce sensory overload. Develop effective interventions to communicate with intubated patient. Use tactile and verbal stimuli if unresponsive. Use calm, caring, competent, and reassuring approach with patient and family. Arrange for flexible visitation to meet patient and family needs. Determine coping ability of patient/family and take appropriate measures to begin acceptance of long-term therapy for burns and long-term results (provide frequent condition reports, provide frequent explanations, encourage patient/family to ask questions, encourage patient/family to verbalize feelings and concerns).	Patient will achieve psychophysiologic stability. Patient will demonstrate a decrease in anxiety. Patient will accept burns and long-term effects. Patient will preserve self-concept.	Continue as in Diagnosis/Stabilization Phase. Determine social support systems for patient. Help patient identify positive coping mechanisms. Consult psychologists and social worker as needed. Encourage patient/family to participate actively in care. Allow patient some control.	Patient will achieve psychophysiologic stability. Patient will demonstrate a decrease in anxiety. Patient will accept burns and long-term effects. Patient will maintain positive self-image.	OT to teach progressive increase in ADLs and IADLs to increase independence and enhance self-esteem. Provide instruction for positive coping mechanisms after discharge. Address concerns about possible effects on sexual function, activities, recreation, return to work. Refer to outside services or agencies as appropriate (chaplain, social services, support group, home health, medical equipment supplier). Continue to assess social support systems. Arrange visit from burn survivor, if feasible.

Chronic Pain Management
Interdisciplinary Outcome Pathway

COORDINATION OF CARE

Diagnosis/Stabilization Phase		Acute Management Phase		Recovery Phase	
Outcome	Interventions	Outcome	Interventions	Outcome	Interventions
All appropriate team members and disciplines will be involved in the plan of care.	Develop the plan of care with the patient/family, primary physician, consulting physicians, anesthesiologist or pain management specialist(s), RN, advanced practice nurse, clinical pharmacist, psychologist, RCP, dietitian, PT, and OT. Educate patient/family concerning pain relief options available such as modalities, analgesics, electrical stimulation, touch therapy, acupressure or acupuncture. Promote active participation of patient in therapy choices.	All appropriate team members and disciplines will be involved in the plan of care.	Implement and update the plan of care with all appropriate team members. Initiate consultations, if indicated, particularly social services and chaplain. Initiate discharge planning assessment. Assess social support systems.	Patient/family will understand the discharge plan. Patient will achieve maximum functional capacity and maintain wellness and health.	Implement and update the plan of care with all appropriate team members. Provide guidelines concerning care at home. Refer to pain clinic, if feasible. Provide phone numbers of resources available to answer questions. Patient/family will verbalize follow-up pain control plan: • analgesics • frequency • precautions • activity limitations • diet restrictions

DIAGNOSTICS

Diagnosis/Stabilization Phase		Acute Management Phase		Recovery Phase	
Outcome	Interventions	Outcome	Interventions	Outcome	Interventions
Patient/family will understand the purpose of all diagnostic procedures such as lab work, x-rays, CT scan, and MRI.	Explain appropriate procedures to be performed to determine sources of pain and extent of disease/illness/injury. Treat procedural-related pain prophylactically. Prepare patient and assist with conscious sedation. Assist in obtaining consents. Minimize delays in procedures to prevent increased anxiety and peaking of analgesia. Be sensitive to patient/family's individualized needs for information.	Patient/family will understand the purpose of test and procedures (VS, lab work, analgesic administration).	Schedule procedures with periods of rest. For repeated procedures, maximize pain management of first procedure to reduce anxiety for further testing.	Patient/family will understand the purpose of all tests and procedures that may occur during hospitalization and after discharge.	Prepare for follow-up procedures to monitor disease progression and the diagnosis of further episodes of pain. Provide appropriate patient/family education. Review appropriate diagnostic results with patient/family prior to discharge. Provide patient/family with copies of significant diagnostic results to be used in continuing home care. Provide guidelines concerning follow-up care.

FLUID BALANCE

Diagnosis/Stabilization Phase		Acute Management Phase		Recovery Phase	
Outcome	Interventions	Outcome	Interventions	Outcome	Interventions
Patient will achieve optimal hemodynamic status as evidenced by: • HR 60–100 bpm • SBP >90 mmHg • Hgb >8 • MAP >70 mmHg • free of dysrhythmias.	Assess cardiac function: • heart sounds • rhythm • central/peripheral pulses • presence or absence of edema • skin color and temperature. Assess for cardiovascular signs and symptoms due to acute pain: • tachycardia • hypertension • increased PVR • water and sodium retention • pertinent lab values such as electrolytes and CBC Assess for and treat cardiothoracic sources of chronic pain: • angina • cancer • PVD Determine hydration needs based on hemodynamics, I & O, VS, SaO$_2$, CXR, breath sounds, and electrolytes. Assess for and treat other sources of chronic pain: • HA • GI sources • musculoskeletal • burns • cancer • arthritis	Patient will maintain optimal hemodynamic status.	Monitor to distinguish between original source of chronic pain and new sources of acute pain. Monitor VS when: • reassessing pain • before and after medication administration Monitor for changes in drug absorption due to altered cardiovascular function: • CO • venous capacity • fluid shifts Maintain optimal hydration based on continued assessment. Monitor for complications secondary to chronic pain: atelectasis, depression, and addiction.	Patient will maintain optimal hemodynamic status.	Monitor patients with renal and liver disease for altered drug metabolism and excretion. Maintain ongoing evaluation of cardiac and renal functioning. Teach patient/family how to maintain optimal fluid balance at home.

Chronic Pain Management Interdisciplinary Outcome Pathway (continued)

NUTRITION

Diagnosis/Stabilization Phase		Acute Management Phase		Recovery Phase	
Outcome	Interventions	Outcome	Interventions	Outcome	Interventions
Patient will be adequately nourished as evidenced by: • stable weight • weight not >10% below or >20% above IBW • albumin >3.5 g/dL • total protein 6–8 g/dL • total lymphocyte count 1,000–3,000	Assess nutritional status. Assess for bowel sounds, abdominal distension, abdominal pain and tenderness q4h and PRN. Assess for and treat GI sources of chronic pain: • ulcers • diverticulitis • pancreatitis • Crohn's disease • ulcerative colitis • cancer Initiate DAT and monitor response. Assess for GI signs and symptoms due to pain: • increased gastric secretions • decreased gastric motility • smooth muscle sphincter spasm • hyperglycemia • N & V • gastric pH	Patient will be adequately nourished. Patient will be free from nausea or abdominal pain.	Estimate caloric and protein needs. Identify and eliminate foods irritating to the GI tract. Administer antiemetics and H_2 blockers, if indicated. Monitor response to diet. Monitor albumin, prealbumin, and total protein. Weigh daily. Consult dietitian if: • weight reducing or enhancing indicated • diet counseling needed for specific diet • albumin <3.0 g/dL	Patient will maintain adequate nutritional status.	Monitor weight to reevaluate nutritional status and weight stability every week. Monitor for inappropriate use of antacids. Teach patient/family about diet modifications: • bland/soft diet • caloric supplement, if indicated • fluid restriction, if indicated • heart healthy diet (low fat, low cholesterol) • vitamin/mineral supplements Assess understanding of diet modifications. Reinforce as necessary.

MOBILITY

Diagnosis/Stabilization Phase		Acute Management Phase		Recovery Phase	
Outcome	Interventions	Outcome	Interventions	Outcome	Interventions
Patient will maintain normal ROM and muscle strength.	Assess physical limitations due to pain. PT to assess ambulation, mobility, muscle flexibility, strength, and tone. OT to assess functional ability. PT/OT to help determine and direct activity goals.	Patient will achieve optimal mobility.	Teach energy conservation and proper body mechanics during functional activities. Monitor response to increased activity: decrease if increased pain or adverse effects occur (i.e., tachycardia, dyspnea, ectopy, hypotension).	Patient will maintain optimal mobility.	Continue to evaluate pain level as patient returns to ADLs. Modify activity level based on presence of increased pain. Instruct patient/family in the use of long-term orthopedic devices.

Assist patient in developing realistic goals for home exercise program.
Refer to pain management clinic, if appropriate.

Use assistive devices (pillows, splints, ambulation devices).
Have patient give return demonstration of current use of assistive devices.
Schedule periods of rest between activities.

Institute progressive activity program (i.e., ROM exercises, bed transfers, and increased ambulation).
Assess for and treat neuro/musculoskeletal sources of chronic pain:
• degenerative joint disease
• osteo/rheumatoid arthritis
• phantom limb pain
• PVD
• low back pain
• headache
Perform motor, sensory, and reflex exam of extremities q4h and PRN.

OXYGENATION/VENTILATION

Diagnosis/Stabilization Phase		Acute Management Phase		Recovery Phase	
Outcome	Interventions	Outcome	Interventions	Outcome	Interventions
Patient will have adequate gas exchange as evidenced by: • normal CXR • respiratory rate, depth, rhythm WNL • clear breath sounds • SaO$_2$ >90% • SpO$_2$ >92% • ABGs WNL	Assess respiratory functions: • breath sounds • respiratory muscle strength and movement • splinting or guarding • respiratory rate, depth, and quality • cough ability • SpO$_2$ • ABGs Assess for and treat pulmonary sources of chronic pain: • lung cancer • arthritis • muscle spasms Assess CXR. Monitor pulse oximetry. Apply supplemental O$_2$ to maintain SpO$_2$ >92%. Assess for pulmonary signs and symptoms of pain q2–4h: • decreased TV • decreased functional capacity • hyperventilation • use of accessory muscles • decreased peak flow • hypoventilation	Patient will maintain adequate gas exchange.	Continue as in Diagnosis/Stabilization Phase, decreasing assessment to q4–8h. Provide pulmonary hygiene and IS. Have patient give return demonstration of IS. Assess color, quantity, and quality (thick/thin) of sputum. Administer high flow, humidified oxygen per nasal cannula or mask.	Patient will have adequate gas exchange.	Maintain ongoing evaluation of pulmonary status. Have patient demonstrate breathing exercises. Teach patient to report signs and symptoms of infection to physician.

Chronic Pain Management Interdisciplinary Outcome Pathway (continued)

COMFORT

Diagnosis/Stabilization Phase		Acute Management Phase		Recovery Phase	
Outcome	Interventions	Outcome	Interventions	Outcome	Interventions
Patient will be as comfortable as possible, in an effort to minimize the incidence and severity of chronic pain.	Obtain a thorough pain history: • previous or ongoing pain episodes • previous pain control methods • patient's attitude toward pain medication Assess pain level through patient self-report. Include: • description • location • intensity/severity using a visual analogue scale • aggravating/relieving factors Assess pain level through direct observation for increased HR and BP, grimacing, posturing, and guarding. Develop an individualized pain management plan based on: • stage of illness/disease process • concurrent medical conditions • psychological/cultural characteristics • ethical considerations • gender concerns Administer analgesics as ordered and monitor response. Educate patient/family how to communicate unrelieved pain effectively.	Patient's pain will be controlled. Patient will be as comfortable as possible.	Reassess pain level frequently: • routinely at scheduled intervals (at least q2–4h) • with each new report of pain • following pain medication administration Individualize route, dosage, and schedule for analgesics: • mild to moderate pain: NSAIDs • moderate to severe pain: opioid analgesics (IV, IM, transdermal, intraspinal) Establish optimal analgesic dosing by titration. Utilize modalities, electrical stimulation, touch therapy, acupressure or accupuncture for pain control as indicated. Administer medications by the least painful route. Consider other medications: • corticosteroids • anticonvulsants • anxiolytics • antidepressants Prepare patient for possible invasive interventions: • excision of tumor • neurolytic blocks • radiation therapy Monitor effectiveness of pain management plan. Consider complementary therapies (see Acute Pain Management Outcome Pathway).	Patient will be as pain free as possible.	Provide copy of pain control plan and instruct patient/family how to continue pain management properly following discharge. Including: • pain assessment • type and amount of medication to be given • when medication is to be given Instruct patient/family in the use of complex medication therapy, such as parenteral or epidural home infusions. Combine other psychological interventions in conjunction with music therapy: • tapping/nodding (distraction) • focusing on an object or image (imagery) • touch therapy Instruct patient/family in the steps of touch/massage therapy: • use warm lotion • use smooth, long strokes • massage 3–10 minutes Instruct patient in simple relaxation exercises: • slow, rhythmic breathing • jaw relaxation • total body relaxation Instruct patient in the steps of imagery: • remembering pleasant past experience • daydreaming Refer to pain management clinic, if feasible.

SKIN INTEGRITY

Diagnosis/Stabilization Phase		Acute Management Phase		Recovery Phase	
Outcome	Interventions	Outcome	Interventions	Outcome	Interventions
Patient will have intact skin without abrasions or pressure ulcers.	Obtain and document a complete baseline skin assessment. Assess for and treat integumentary sources of chronic pain: • burns • shingles Assess all bony prominences q4h. Treat pressure ulcers according to hospital protocol.	Patient will have intact skin without abrasions or pressure ulcers. Patient will have healing surgical wounds and be free of infection.	Document size, location, and description of skin breakdown and surgical wounds. Maintain sterile technique with all dressing changes, if applicable. Monitor all incisions/wounds for signs and symptoms of infection. Use pressure-reducing devices as appropriate. Facilitate the highest degree of mobility possible.	Patient will have intact skin without abrasions or pressure ulcers. Patient will have healing surgical wounds and be free of infection.	Teach patient/family proper care of incisions and wounds. Teach patient/family proper techniques for dressing changes, if applicable. Teach patient/family to report any new sources of pain to physician.

PROTECTION/SAFETY

Diagnosis/Stabilization Phase		Acute Management Phase		Recovery Phase	
Outcome	Interventions	Outcome	Interventions	Outcome	Interventions
Patient will be protected from possible harm.	Monitor patient for oversedation/respiratory depression. Administer naloxone in the event of respiratory depression. Assess need for wrist restraints. If used, monitor circulation q1–2h. Follow hospital protocol for restraint use. Explain the need for restraints to patient/family. Allow family to remain with patient, if they have a calming influence and can promote rest and safety.	Patient will be protected from possible harm.	Provide appropriate physical support to prevent falls while patient is receiving analgesics. Continue to allow family to remain with patient. Remove restraints as soon as patient is able to follow commands. Teach proper body mechanics with functional activities to maintain joint integrity and prevent joint strain with injury.	Patient will be protected from possible harm.	Instruct patient/family in the limitations associated with pain medication: • assistance with ambulation • driving limitations • side effects/adverse reactions Instruct patient/family in the use of complex therapies such as continuous infusion pumps and indwelling CVADs.

Chronic Pain Management Interdisciplinary Outcome Pathway (*continued*)

PSYCHOSOCIAL/SELF-DETERMINATION

Diagnosis/Stabilization Phase		Acute Management Phase		Recovery Phase	
Outcome	Interventions	Outcome	Interventions	Outcome	Interventions
Patient/family will utilize coping skills effectively to keep anxiety at a tolerable level. Patient will achieve psychophysiologic stability. Patient will begin acceptance process of chronic pain.	Assess patient/family for current level of anxiety and fear. Reassure patient/family that most pain can be relieved or controlled safely and effectively. Allow flexible visitation to meet needs of patient/family. Assess mood changes due to pain. Assess patient for psychosocial signs and symptoms of pain: • loss of hope • loss of control • impaired QOL • helplessness • anxiety • depression • disruption of sleep • inability to concentrate Assess patient/family concerns about the use of controlled substances. Assess patient's typical coping response to stress or pain. Assess effect of critical care environment on patient and how it affects pain perception.	Patient/family will demonstrate effective coping skills. Patient will achieve psychophysiologic stability. Patient will continue acceptance process of chronic pain.	Continue as in Diagnosis/Stabilization Phase. Consider medication to promote sleep and/or decrease anxiety. Take measures to reduce sensory overload, such as providing uninterrupted periods of sleep. Use interventions to assist with coping, such as allowing patient to verbalize fears/concerns and be available to answer all questions. Reinforce and reward positive coping strategies by patient/family. Assess ineffective or maladaptive behaviors. Involve patient in decision making concerning health care.	Patient/family will demonstrate effective coping skills. Patient will achieve psychophysiologic stability. Patient will continue acceptance process of chronic pain.	Evaluate recurrence or progression of illness. Assess patient for changes in ADLs and sexual functioning. Assist patient/family with identification and implementation of role changes. Reinforce use of positive coping mechanisms. OT to teach energy conservation techniques and progression of ADLs and IADLs to increase independence and self-esteem.

Disseminated Intravascular Coagulation Interdisciplinary Outcome Pathway

COORDINATION OF CARE

Diagnosis/Stabilization Phase		Acute Management Phase		Recovery Phase	
Outcome	Interventions	Outcome	Interventions	Outcome	Interventions
All appropriate team members and disciplines will be involved in the plan of care.	Develop the plan of care with the patient/family, primary physician(s), hematologist, RN, advanced practice nurse, and other specialists as needed.	All appropriate team members and disciplines will be involved in the plan of care.	Update the plan of care with the patient/family, other team members including PT, RCP, dietitian, and discharge planner. Initiate planning for anticipated discharge and call home health agency if needed. Begin teaching patient/family about care at home.	Patient will understand how to maintain optimal health at home.	Provide guidelines concerning care at home: • medications • diet • physical restrictions • follow-up visits Provide patient/family with phone number of resources available to answer questions. Teach patient/family about need for follow-up visits for necessary lab tests.

DIAGNOSTICS

Diagnosis/Stabilization Phase		Acute Management Phase		Recovery Phase	
Outcome	Interventions	Outcome	Interventions	Outcome	Interventions
Patient/family will understand any tests or procedures that need to be completed: • clotting studies such as PT, PTT, ACT, thrombin time, fibrinogen, platelets, FSP, D-dimer, CBC, plasminogen, protamine • exchange transfusion • administration of fluids and blood products • plasmapheresis	Explain all procedures and tests to patient/family. Be sensitive to individualized needs of patient/family for information. Establish effective communication technique with intubated patient.	Patient will understand any tests or procedures that need to be completed (lab work, clotting studies, plasmapheresis).	Explain procedures and tests needed to assess recovery. Anticipate need for further diagnostic tests or treatments. Provide information on patient's role concerning diagnostic procedures. Be sensitive to individualized needs of patient/family for information.	Patient will understand meaning of diagnostic tests in relation to continued health.	Review with patient/family before discharge the results of all tests. Discuss any abnormal values and appropriate measures patient can take at home to help return to normal (i.e., clotting studies). Provide written instructions on care at home: • when to call the physician • medications • diet • activity restrictions • bleeding precautions • signs and symptoms of spontaneous bleeding (i.e., gums bleeding easily, swollen painful joints, blood in urine or stool, dark or tarry stools)

Disseminated Intravascular Coagulation Interdisciplinary Outcome Pathway (continued)

FLUID BALANCE

Diagnosis/Stabilization Phase		Acute Management Phase		Recovery Phase	
Outcome	Interventions	Outcome	Interventions	Outcome	Interventions
Patient will achieve optimal hemodynamic status as evidenced by: • MAP >70 mmHg • hemodynamic parameters WNL • UO >0.5 mL/kg/hr • free of cardiac dysrhythmias • adequate LOC Patient will maintain a normal cardiac output. Patient will be free of bleeding.	Monitor and treat cardiac parameters: • dysrhythmias • SvO$_2$ • BP • I & O • PA pressure • PCWP • SV • CO/CI • SVR/PVR Assess for common causes of DIC: • sepsis • shock • trauma • malignancies • vascular disorders • obstetric disorders • immunologic disorders • burns • transplant rejection Institute bleeding precautions. Monitor lab values: PT, PTT, platelets, fibrinogen, FSP (D-dimer, FDP), clotting factor analysis. Monitor for signs of fluid overload or deficit and treat accordingly. Anticipate need for vasopressor agents and assess response. Assess LOC q1-2h. Assess evidence of tissue perfusion (i.e., pain, pulses, color, temperature, signs of decreased perfusion such as decreased UO and altered LOC).	Patient will maintain optimal hemodynamic status. Patient will maintain normal CO. Patient will remain free of bleeding.	Continue to monitor and treat cardiac parameters. Continue to monitor for bleeding. Monitor lab values: PT, PTT, platelets, fibrinogen, FSP, clotting studies. Continue to assess for complications of DIC. Assess response to vasopressors and treat accordingly. Assess response to any anticoagulants given. Begin teaching patient/family about DIC, current treatment, and expected outcome. Weigh daily. Maintain bleeding precautions.	Patient will maintain optimal hemodynamic status. Patient will maintain normal CO. Patient will remain free of bleeding.	Continue as in Acute Management Phase. Teach patient/family about anticoagulants: • name of medication • dosage • potential side effects • dietary considerations • importance of clotting studies and follow-up visits • bleeding precautions

Administer anticoagulants and/or antifibrinolytic agents as ordered and monitor response. Keep antidotes on unit.

Anticipate need for transfusions of blood products (whole blood, red blood cells, FFP, cryoprecipitate, platelets). Assess response.

Monitor for complications of blood transfusion therapy:
- hyperkalemia
- hypocalcemia
- hypothermia
- metabolic acidosis
- infection
- coagulopathies
- ARDS
- hypervolemia
- febrile transfusion

Assess for signs and symptoms of occult and/or overt bleeding:
- petechiae
- ecchymosis
- purpura
- hematoma
- gingival bleeding
- oozing from puncture sites
- cyanosis of lips, nose, ears, fingers, and toes
- epistaxis
- hematemesis
- melena
- increased abdominal girth
- HA
- decreased LOC
- tachycardia
- orthopnea
- hypotension
- hypoxemia
- hematuria

Assess for complications of DIC: vascular occlusion, hemorrhage, and shock.

Insert urinary catheter and monitor for hematuria.

Be prepared to institute alternative therapies such as exchange transfusion and plasmapheresis.

Disseminated Intravascular Coagulation Interdisciplinary Outcome Pathway (continued)

NUTRITION

Diagnosis/Stabilization Phase		Acute Management Phase		Recovery Phase	
Outcome	Interventions	Outcome	Interventions	Outcome	Interventions
Patient will be adequately nourished as evidenced by: • stable weight not > 10% above or > 20% below IBW • albumin 3.5–4.0 g/dL • total protein 6–8 g/dL • total lymphocyte count 1,000–3,000	NPO until extubated, if applicable. If extubation is delayed greater than 24h, institute alternative nutritional therapy. Clear/full liquids as tolerated once able to take fluids. Assess response. If unable to take fluids, keep NPO and initiate enteral or IV feeding. Monitor protein and albumin levels. Assess bowel sounds, abdominal distension, tenderness, or pain q4h and PRN. Assess nutritional status. Assess abdominal girth q2h. Assess for diarrhea that could indicate involvement of the GI system.	Patient will be adequately nourished.	Advance DAT and monitor response. Weigh daily. Consult dietitian to help determine and direct nutritional support. Assess bowel sounds, abdominal distension, tenderness, or pain q4h and PRN. Assess abdominal girth q4h. Monitor protein and albumin levels. Consider calorie count to determine if patient is meeting nutritional goals. Monitor stools for bleeding.	Patient will be adequately nourished.	Teach patient/family about heart healthy diet: • total fat < 30% of daily intake • total saturated fat < 10% of daily intake • total cholesterol daily intake < 300 mg • calorie restriction if needed • sodium restriction if needed Teach patient/family any dietary considerations related to anticoagulant therapy. Involve dietitian as necessary on outpatient basis.

MOBILITY

Diagnosis/Stabilization Phase		Acute Management Phase		Recovery Phase	
Outcome	Interventions	Outcome	Interventions	Outcome	Interventions
Patient will maintain normal muscle strength and tone.	Begin passive/active-assist ROM exercises. Turn at least q2h if hemodynamically stable. Monitor response to activity. If not stable, consider alternative bed therapy. Assess muscle mobility, flexibility, strength, tone, and functional ability.	Patient will achieve optimal mobility.	Progress exercise as tolerated: dangle, OOB for meals, up to chair TID to QID while in critical care environment. Monitor response to increased activity. Decrease activity if adverse events occur: tachycardia, dysrhythmias, dyspnea, ectopy, syncope, hypotension. Monitor oxygen content with increased activity. Use supplemental oxygen to maintain SpO$_2$ > 92%.	Patient will achieve optimal mobility.	Continue to progress exercise as tolerated and monitor response. Teach patient/family about home exercise program. Continue with PT and/or OT as needed. Arrange for home health visits with PT and/or OT as needed.

Provide support as necessary. Assess muscle strength and tone. Consult PT and/or OT for specific mobility/functional limitations.

OXYGENATION/VENTILATION

Diagnosis/Stabilization Phase		Acute Management Phase		Recovery Phase	
Outcome	Interventions	Outcome	Interventions	Outcome	Interventions
Patient will have adequate gas exchange as evidenced by: • SaO$_2$ >90% • ABGs WNL • SpO$_2$ >92% • clear breath sounds • respiratory rate, depth, and rhythm WNL • CXR WNL • absence of dyspnea, cyanosis, and secretions • Hgb and Hct WNL	Apply supplemental oxygen and monitor SpO$_2$ with pulse oximetry. Keep SpO$_2$ >92%. Assess respiratory functioning, including lung sounds, respiratory rate and depth, and CXR. Involve RCP. Encourage coughing and deep breathing while on bed rest. Assess evidence of tissue perfusion (i.e., pain, pulses, color, temperature, signs of decreased perfusion such as decreased UO or altered LOC). Monitor lab values: Hgb, ABGs. Be prepared for intubation and mechanical ventilation. Assist with placement and maintenance of artificial airways as needed. Monitor for signs and symptoms of respiratory distress: • weak ineffective cough • dyspnea • use of accessory muscles • adventitious breath sounds • alterations in LOC • PCO$_2$ >50 mmHg • SaO$_2$ <90% • SpO$_2$ <92% Maintain adequate humidification. Assist with monitoring or adjusting of ventilator settings to obtain appropriate level of assistance and mechanical ventilation. Monitor tracheal secretions for bleeding.	Patient will have adequate gas exchange.	Assess respiratory function and intervene as needed. Continue to involve RCP. Assess need for continued supplemental oxygen with use of pulse oximetry. Keep SpO$_2$ >92%. Observe for complications of DIC that may impair oxygenation/ventilation (pulmonary embolus, pulmonary edema, decreased CO). Assess readiness to wean from mechanical ventilation. Measure respiratory mechanics: minute ventilation, NIF, TV, respiratory rate. Assess for improvement in breath sounds, thin white secretions, and adequate cough reflex. Monitor ventilatory status and hemodynamic variables prior to, during, and after weaning from mechanical ventilation. Assist with extubation. Monitor and treat oxygenation/ventilation disturbances.	Patient will have adequate gas exchange.	Continue as in Acute Management Phase. Teach patient/family about home medications and treatments. Teach patient/family signs and symptoms of respiratory infection and when to report symptoms. Instruct on methods for smoking cessation if applicable.

Disseminated Intravascular Coagulation Interdisciplinary Outcome Pathway (continued)

COMFORT

Diagnosis/Stabilization Phase		Acute Management Phase		Recovery Phase	
Outcome	Interventions	Outcome	Interventions	Outcome	Interventions
Patient will be as comfortable and pain free as possible as evidenced by: • no objective indicators of discomfort • no complaints of discomfort	Assess quantity and quality of discomfort using a pain analogue scale. Administer analgesics as needed and monitor response. Provide a quiet environment to potentiate analgesia. Provide supplemental oxygen. Provide reassurance in a calm, caring, and competent manner. Administer sedatives as needed and assess response. If patient is intubated, establish effective communication technique with which patient can communicate discomfort and need for analgesia. Maintain meticulous oral hygiene. Observe for bleeding from gums.	Patient will be as relaxed and pain free as possible.	Continue as in Diagnosis/Stabilization Phase. Observe for complications of DIC that may cause discomfort (pulmonary embolus, pulmonary edema, bleeding, dyspnea). Provide uninterrupted periods of rest. Teach patient/family use of other methods to promote relaxation (i.e., imagery, deep breathing, music therapy). Have patient/family give return demonstration. Use sedatives as indicated and assess response.	Patient will be as relaxed and pain free as possible.	Progress analgesics to oral medications as needed and assess response. Continue alternative methods to promote relaxation as described earlier. Teach these methods to patient/family. Have patient demonstrate relaxation techniques. Teach patient proper use of analgesics, both prescribed and OTC.

SKIN INTEGRITY

Diagnosis/Stabilization Phase		Acute Management Phase		Recovery Phase	
Outcome	Interventions	Outcome	Interventions	Outcome	Interventions
Patient will have intact skin without abrasions or pressure ulcers.	Assess all bony prominences at least q4h and treat as needed according to hospital protocol. Assess skin integrity surrounding all invasive sites. Institute bleeding precautions. Take measures to control bleeding. Use preventive pressure-reducing devices if patient is at high risk for developing pressure ulcers.	Patient will have intact skin without abrasions or pressure ulcers.	Continue as in Diagnosis/Stabilization Phase.	Patient will have intact skin without abrasions or pressure ulcers.	Teach patient/family proper skin care for after discharge.

PROTECTION/SAFETY

Diagnosis/Stabilization Phase		Acute Management Phase		Recovery Phase	
Outcome	Interventions	Outcome	Interventions	Outcome	Interventions
Patient will be protected from possible harm.	Assess need for wrist restraints if patient is intubated, has a decreased LOC, is restless or agitated, or is unable to follow commands. Explain need for restraints to patient/family. If restrained, assess response to restraints. Check for skin integrity and impairment to circulation q1–2h. Follow hospital protocol for use of restraints. Remove restraints as soon as patient is able to follow instructions. Institute bleeding precautions. Provide sedatives as needed and monitor response. Assess patient for altered mental status. Confusion is common in patients with DIC.	Patient will be protected from possible harm.	Provide physical support with all activities as needed. Monitor response. If need still exists for restraints, check q1–2h for skin integrity and impairment to circulation. Continue bleeding precautions. PT consult as indicated.	Patient will be protected from possible harm.	Provide physical support with ambulation and climbing stairs. Teach patient/family activity limitations and bleeding precautions.

PSYCHOSOCIAL/SELF-DETERMINATION

Diagnosis/Stabilization Phase		Acute Management Phase		Recovery Phase	
Outcome	Interventions	Outcome	Interventions	Outcome	Interventions
Patient will achieve psychophysiologic stability. Patient will demonstrate a decrease in anxiety as evidenced by: • VS WNL • subjective response of decreased anxiety • objective report of decreased anxiety	Assess physiologic effect of critical care environment on patient (hemodynamic variables, psychological status, signs of increased sympathetic tone). Take measures to reduce sensory overload. Provide uninterrupted periods of rest. Use calm, caring, competent, and reassuring approach with patient/family. Allow flexible visitation to meet the needs of patient/family.	Patient will achieve psychophysiologic stability. Patient will demonstrate a decrease in anxiety.	Continue as in Diagnosis/Stabilization Phase. Teach patient/family other ways to promote relaxation (i.e., guided imagery, music, humor, deep breathing exercises). Have patient give return demonstration. Continue to assess coping ability of patient/family and take measures as indicated (family conferences, support services, verbalization of concerns and fears). Help patient identify positive coping mechanisms.	Patient will achieve psychophysiologic stability. Patient will demonstrate a decrease in anxiety.	Provide instruction on coping methods. Reinforce positive coping mechanisms. Refer to outside services or agencies as appropriate. Continue to utilize alternative methods to assist with relaxation. Address concerns of patient about effects DIC may have on home life (activities, work, sexual functioning, ADLs).

Disseminated Intravascular Coagulation Interdisciplinary Outcome Pathway (*continued*)

PSYCHOSOCIAL/SELF-DETERMINATION (continued)

Diagnosis/Stabilization Phase		Acute Management Phase		Recovery Phase	
Outcome	Interventions	Outcome	Interventions	Outcome	Interventions
	Determine coping ability of patient/family and take appropriate measures to meet their needs (i.e., explain condition, equipment, and medications; provide frequent condition reports; use easy to understand terminology; repeat information as needed; answer questions). Provide sedatives as needed and monitor response.		Provide adequate rest periods. Continue to include family in all aspects of care. Maintain a quiet environment. Allow patient/family to ventilate/communicate feelings of anxiety and fear.		

HIV
Interdisciplinary Outcome Pathway

COORDINATION OF CARE

Diagnosis/Stabilization Phase		Acute Management Phase		Recovery Phase	
Outcome	Interventions	Outcome	Interventions	Outcome	Interventions
All appropriate disciplines will be involved in the plan of care.	Develop a plan of care with patient/family, infectious disease and primary physician, RN, advanced practice nurse, and other specialists as needed including RCP, chaplain, social worker. Discuss any concerns regarding attitudes, stigmas, and discrimination. Refer patient to appropriate support groups.	All appropriate team members and disciplines will be involved in plan of care.	Update the plan of care as patient's status and T4 cell counts fluctuate and opportunistic infections occur. Teach patient how to decrease incidence of infection: no live flowers, no fresh fruits, and stay away from infection, crowds. Give information on when to notify doctor or nurse regarding restrictions, medications, side effects, and symptoms to report. Prepare patient/family for discharge to home, extended care, and/or rehabilitation.	Patient/family will understand how to maintain optimal health.	Provide educational materials on HIV infection. Teach patients about their disease. Provide instructions for follow-up. Provide information on support groups.

DIAGNOSTICS

Diagnosis/Stabilization Phase		Acute Management Phase		Recovery Phase	
Outcome	Interventions	Outcome	Interventions	Outcome	Interventions
Patient/family will understand the indications for tests or procedures that need to be completed: • VS • I & O • hemodynamic monitoring • lab tests • x-rays/CT scan • LP • EKG • EEG • endoscopy procedures	Assess patient/family's ability to understand procedures. Explain all procedures and tests specific to HIV infection: • Elisa • Western Blot • viral culture • CBC • polymerase chain reaction • liver function tests • absolute T4 lymphocyte • bronchoscopy • sputum C & S Perform physical exam including pelvic and rectal exam. Be sensitive to patient/family's individualized need for information.	Patient/family will understand any tests or procedures performed.	Assess need for information. Teach patient about the immune system and the effects of HIV and opportunistic infection. Anticipate need for further diagnostic tests. Explain to patient/family. Establish effective communication with patient if intubated.	Patient will discuss the meaning of positive results of diagnostic tests performed: • + HIV test • opportunistic infections • decreased T4 count Patient will follow up on results and consult with MD/RN regarding questions or concerns.	Discuss abnormal findings before discharge. Identify resources and measures family can take to return or regain previous ADLs. Prepare family for patient's possible feelings of depression, suicide, and hopelessness.

HIV Interdisciplinary Outcome Pathway (continued)

FLUID BALANCE

Diagnosis/Stabilization Phase		Acute Management Phase		Recovery Phase	
Outcome	Interventions	Outcome	Interventions	Outcome	Interventions
Patient will achieve optimal hemodynamic status as evidenced by: • MAP > 70 mmHg • hemodynamic parameters WNL • alert and oriented • adequate respiratory function • UO > 0.5 mL/kg/hr • normothermic • absence of thirst	Monitor and treat hemodynamic parameters: • HR • UO • BP • GCS/LOC • weight loss > 10% body weight Monitor and treat fluid/electrolyte imbalances. Monitor temperature and watch for signs of shivering. Administer antipyretics. Monitor CBC with differential including absolute T cell count. Maintain I & O. Provide oral care. Administer antiviral agents. Monitor for side effects. Monitor levels. Monitor lab values for indications of: • hepatitis • pancreatitis • anemia • neutropenia • thrombocytopenia • hyperglycemia	Patient will be free of infectious diarrhea. Patient will remain afebrile and free of night sweats. Patient will maintain optimal hemodynamic status.	Same as Diagnosis/Stabilization Phase. Maintain meticulous I & O records; replace fluid loss through IV fluids and oral supplementation. Provide special skin protecting rectal care at least BID. Administer antimotility drugs PRN. Monitor for occult blood. Perform surveillance cultures and repeat with every temperature spike. Provide incontinent care. Weigh daily. Administer antibiotics as ordered. Follow universal (standard) precautions when handling any contaminated items.	Patient will remain adequately hydrated. Patient will recognize signs and symptoms of impending dehydration. Patient will follow up with physician or nurse practitioner. Patient will maintain optimal hemodynamic status.	Provide information to patient and significant others on dehydration. Consider need for consultation with home health nurse for teaching and follow-up.

NUTRITION

Diagnosis/Stabilization Phase		Acute Management Phase		Recovery Phase	
Outcome	Interventions	Outcome	Interventions	Outcome	Interventions
Patient will be adequately nourished as evidenced by: • stable weight not > 10% below or > 20% above IBW	Assess bowel sounds, abdominal distension, pain, or tenderness. Assess nutritional status. Consult dietitian or nutritional support team to determine and direct nutritional support.	Patient will not have anorexia or dysphasia. Patient will have no oral lesions. Patient will be adequately nourished.	Same as Diagnosis/Stabilization Phase. Administer antiemetics PRN. Weigh daily. Provide oral care with soft toothbrush and bactericidal agent TID.	Patient will maintain adequate nutrition and appropriate weight. Patient will consult doctor or nurse for: • dysphasia	Social services to evaluate family dynamics and resources. Provide information on high protein, high lipid, low microbial diet. Consider need for home health teaching and follow-up.

Diagnosis/Stabilization Phase		Acute Management Phase		Recovery Phase	
Outcome	Interventions	Outcome	Interventions	Outcome	Interventions
• albumin > 3.5 g/dL • prealbumin > 15 • total protein 6–8 g/dL	Administer prophylactic oral antifungal. Culture oral lesions. Encourage use of oral nonabsorbable anesthetics: viscous lidocaine, benzocaine, or benadryl. Administer saliva substitute. Use gloves when encountering oral secretions. Monitor albumin, prealbumin, and total protein values. Perform calorie count to ensure patient's intake is meeting nutritional goals.	• weight loss >10% • anorexia • fever • N & V	Assess temperature. Prepare food aesthetically. Encourage family and friends to bring in food and eat with patient. Administer yogurt or acidophilus milk to maintain normal flora. Maintain low microbial diet. Monitor response to nutrition given (i.e., residual, weight gain/loss). Monitor albumin, prealbumin, and total protein values.		Teach patient to eat properly prepared food. No fresh fruits or inadequately cooked or mass-prepared foods. Use caution with spices, pepper, and nuts.

MOBILITY

Diagnosis/Stabilization Phase		Acute Management Phase		Recovery Phase	
Outcome	Interventions	Outcome	Interventions	Outcome	Interventions
Patient will achieve optimal mobility.	Assess neurologic status q2–4h: • orientation • motor activity • strength • memory Consult PT to assess ambulation, mobility, muscle flexibility, strength, and tone. OT to assess functional ability. Promote rest.	Patient will achieve optimal mobility. Patient will be less fatigued as evidenced by increasing daily activity.	Assist patient with passive/active-assist ROM. PT/OT to help determine functional activity goals. Provide diversional activities when patient is able to participate. Coordinate efforts to assist with advanced directives and medical power of attorney. Monitor response to increased activity. Modify if adverse events occur. Teach energy conservation techniques. Perform daily activities in small increments throughout the day. Provide adequate uninterrupted sleep.	Patient will deny fatigue. Patient will maintain optimal mobility.	Identify need for consultation with social worker if patient develops AIDS dementia. Teach general infection prevention measures. Teach patient and significant others about important neurologic symptoms such as profound fatigue, confusion, and decreased LOC requiring medical attention. Encourage interdisciplinary conferences on a regular basis. Assist family in development of home exercise program.

HIV Interdisciplinary Outcome Pathway (continued)

OXYGENATION/VENTILATION

Diagnosis/Stabilization Phase		Acute Management Phase		Recovery Phase	
Outcome	Interventions	Outcome	Interventions	Outcome	Interventions

Patient will have adequate gas exchange as evidenced by:
• SpO_2 > 90%
• ABGs WNL
• clear breath sounds
• rate and depth of breathing WNL
• CXR: no acute changes
• absence of dyspnea
• effective cough
	Respiratory assessment q2–4h.
	Supplemental oxygen for hypoxemia and increased effort.
	Obtain culture and sensitivity of sputum for mycology, virus, and acid-fast bacilli.
	Monitor and treat ABGs.
	Assess temperature.
	Administer expectorant.
	Maintain respiratory isolation if:
	  • community-acquired pneumonia
	  • tuberculosis
	  • Pneumocystis carinii
	Elevate HOB for dyspnea.
	Maintain adequate humidification.
		Patient will have adequate gas exchange.	Same as Diagnosis/Stabilization Phase.
			Respiratory assessment q4h.
			Monitor oxygenation and ABGs, SpO_2, and effort.
			Monitor for patent airway.
			Administer prophylactic antibiotics or those noted to cause susceptibility.
			Note sputum characteristics.
			Assess readiness to wean oxygen and ventilator as tolerated. (SpO_2 > 90, stable VS, normal effort).
			Consult respiratory therapy for pulmonary toilet and airway maintenance.
			Encourage coughing and deep breathing q2h.
			Maintain respiratory isolation as needed.
			Monitor patient for signs and symptoms of altered gas exchange:
			  • dyspnea
			  • restlessness
			  • decreased LOC
			  • confusion
			  • HA
			  • acidosis
				Patient will maintain adequate gas exchange.	Assess respiratory status and intervene as indicated.
					Encourage cough and deep breathing q2h.
					Continue to assess for complications that may impair oxygenation/ventilation.
					Assess patient/family understanding of home care needs.
					No live flowers or standing water in room.
					Support prophylactic antibiotics against PCP, TB, CMV.
					Consider need for home health nurse for teaching and follow up with medical regimen.
					Teach patient effective cough techniques.
					Teach patient signs and symptoms of respiratory infection and when to call doctor or nurse.

COMFORT

Diagnosis/Stabilization Phase		Acute Management Phase		Recovery Phase	
Outcome	Interventions	Outcome	Interventions	Outcome	Interventions
Patient will be as pain free and comfortable as possible as evidenced by: • optimal hemodynamic status • no complaints of discomfort	Teach patient to acknowledge situations that cause pain. Assess quality and quantity of pain as identified by patient. Administer analgesics as ordered. Plan interventions to provide rest and diversion. Provide a calm and quiet environment to enhance comfort. Establish methods for communication of discomfort if patient intubated. Observe for complications of HIV that can cause discomfort: • shingles or herpes zoster • esophagitis related to candida • Kaposi's sarcoma • enterocolitis • pancreatitis	Patient will be as comfortable and pain free as possible.	Teach patient relaxation techniques and other activities to enhance comfort: • music • touch therapy • guided imagery • water therapy • range of motion Monitor side effects of analgesics (i.e., constipation, respiratory distress).	Patient will be as comfortable and pain free as possible.	Patient/family will demonstrate techniques used for relaxation and comfort. Patient/family will understand the indications and side effects of analgesics.

SKIN INTEGRITY

Diagnosis/Stabilization Phase		Acute Management Phase		Recovery Phase	
Outcome	Interventions	Outcome	Interventions	Outcome	Interventions
Patient will have intact skin without lesions. Patient will have absence of: • reddened areas • skin discomfort at pressure areas • Kaposi's sarcoma • rashes • pruritis • immobility	Assess total body cutaneous areas daily. Culture all existing lesions. Treat pressure ulcers per institution policy. Wound and dressing care as with neutropenia every 24–48h PRN. Sketch location and size of lesion in daily assessment. Use air mattress or other protective mattress for skin. Maintain cool environment. Follow universal precautions when handling any contaminated materials.	Patient will have intact skin. Patient will deny itching/pruritis.	Same as Diagnosis/Stabilization Phase. Apply anti-itch ointment. Administer antihistamines. Use condom catheters or fecal incontinence bags as indicated.	Patient will maintain intact skin.	Teach patient/family proper skin care. Begin plans for transfer to extended care, physical rehabilitation, or home.

HIV Interdisciplinary Outcome Pathway (continued)

PROTECTION/SAFETY (continued)

Diagnosis/Stabilization Phase		Acute Management Phase		Recovery Phase	
Outcome	Interventions	Outcome	Interventions	Outcome	Interventions
Patient will be protected from harm.	Seizure precautions for HIV encephalopathy. Assess need for restraints. Monitor for restraints q1h for skin integrity/circulation. Introduce self at each interaction. Assess neurologic function and document changes. Administer antivirals and monitor for for side effects. Allow family/friends to remain at bedside if they have a calming effect.	Patient will be protected from harm. Patient will identify personal risk factors for infection.	Monitor for confusion/anxiety. Remove restraints when patient able to follow instructions. Assess need for assistance with activities. Provide support as necessary. Culture workup for any of the following: • chills for any reason • fever >99.6°F • hypotensive event • change in mental status • sputum production	Patient will be protected from harm. Family will recognize limitations and seek consultation for resources.	Teach patient/family about any physical limitations in activity. Teach patient/family the side effects of medications and signs of toxicities. Outline resources available when patient unable to care for self or meet needs. Consult social services. Significant other/family will consult with appropriate MD or NP for concerns regarding altered thought processes and drug toxicities.

PSYCHOSOCIAL/SELF-DETERMINATION

Diagnosis/Stabilization Phase		Acute Management Phase		Recovery Phase	
Outcome	Interventions	Outcome	Interventions	Outcome	Interventions
Patient will achieve psychophysiologic stability. Patient will demonstrate decrease in anxiety as evidenced by: • no change in baseline VS • no subjective complaints of anxiety	Assess effects of stress and anxiety. Administer sedatives PRN. Take measures to decrease fear by informing patient of tests performed, results, and routines. Allow flexible visitation to meet psychosocial needs of patient/family.	Patient will maintain psychophysiologic stability.	Provide truthful information and feedback to patient. Note number of visitors and relationship between family/patient. Provide adequate rest. Arrange for flexible visits with family.	Patient will have realistic expectations of self, disease, and therapies. Patient will achieve independence and maintain ADLS. Patient/family will seek assistance with drug addiction and/or self-destructive behaviors.	Involve social support for crisis counseling, legal and financial assistance, and family dynamics. Refer to support for HIV. Refer patient to mental health provider if necessary as indicated by depressive or self-destructive behaviors. Provide information regarding sexual functioning. Address concerns patient may have about impact on daily life.

Obstetric Crises
Interdisciplinary Outcome Pathway

COORDINATION OF CARE

	Diagnosis/Stabilization Phase	Acute Management Phase		Recovery Phase	
Outcome	Interventions	Outcome	Interventions	Outcome	Interventions
All appropriate disciplines and team members will be involved in the plan of care.	Develop a plan of care with patient/family, primary physician(s), obstetrician, neonatologist, pediatrician, other specialists as needed, RN, advanced practice nurse, RCP, dietitian, and chaplain.	All appropriate team members and disciplines will be involved in the plan of care.	Update the plan of care with the patient/family, team members, PT, OT, discharge planner, support groups, social worker, and lactation specialist if indicated. Initiate consults as needed. Initiate planning for anticipated discharge. Begin teaching patient/family about care at home.	Patient will understand how to maintain optimal health at home.	Provide guidelines concerning care at home for mother and/or baby: • diet • medications • baby care • activity • follow-up visits Provide patient/family with phone numbers of resources available to answer questions for mother regarding self-care and/or infant care. Provide information concerning breastfeeding and any potential complications/concerns of lactation.

DIAGNOSTICS

	Diagnosis/Stabilization Phase	Acute Management Phase		Recovery Phase	
Outcome	Interventions	Outcome	Interventions	Outcome	Interventions
Patient will understand any tests or procedures that need to be completed (hemodynamic monitoring, x-rays, care of baby if applicable, clotting studies, chemistries, ultrasounds, CBC, liver enzymes, ABGs, proteinuria, urine specific gravity, fetal monitoring).	Explain all procedures and tests to patient/family. Explain procedures and tests needed to care for baby, if applicable. Be sensitive to individualized needs of patient/family for information. Establish effective communication technique with intubated patient.	Patient will understand any tests or procedures that must be completed to recover from obstetric crisis (hemodynamic monitoring, lab work, radiologic procedures, tests baby may need).	Anticipate need for further diagnostic tests or procedures and prepare patient for these. Anticipate diagnostics tests or procedures baby may need and explain to patient/family. Explain care of baby to patient/family (neonatal intensive care, well baby care, other tests or care as needed).	Patient will understand meaning of diagnostic tests and procedures in relation to continued health for self and baby.	Review with patient before discharge the results of lab tests, procedures, and so forth, as they relate to patient/baby. Discuss any abnormal findings and appropriate measures patient can take to help return to normal. Discuss long-term care needs if appropriate. Refer to home health agency as needed. Teach patient/family about care after discharge: • diet (both mother and baby) • medications

Obstetric Crises Interdisciplinary Outcome Pathway (continued)

DIAGNOSTICS (continued)

Diagnosis/Stabilization Phase		Acute Management Phase		Recovery Phase	
Outcome	Interventions	Outcome	Interventions	Outcome	Interventions
					• activity • exercise program • care of baby • when to call the physician • follow-up visits • immunization schedule • safety measures for baby

FLUID BALANCE

Diagnosis/Stabilization Phase		Acute Management Phase		Recovery Phase	
Outcome	Interventions	Outcome	Interventions	Outcome	Interventions
Patient will achieve optimal hemodynamic status as evidenced by: • MAP > 70 mmHg • hemodynamic parameters WNL • UO > 0.5 mL/kg/hr • absence of dysrhythmias • adequate LOC • clear lung sounds • adequate I & O • good tissue perfusion	Monitor and treat cardiac parameters: dysrhythmias, BP, SvO$_2$, JVD, CO, PCWP. Monitor lab values: Hgb, Hct, electrolytes, BUN, creatinine, ABGs, platelets, liver enzymes, renal function, urine specific gravity, proteinuria, PT, PTT, glucose, and uric acid. Monitor respiratory status and be prepared for mechanical ventilation. Assess lung sounds q1–2h. Maintain strict I & O. Assess fluid overload or deficit and treat accordingly. For fluid deficit, crystalloids are usually given at 80–125 mL/hr. However, the rate may vary from patient to patient. Anticipate need for vasopressor agents and assess response and titrate accordingly.	Patient will maintain optimal hemodynamic status.	Monitor and treat hemodynamic parameters. Assess neurologic status q2–4h and PRN. Stay prepared for mechanical ventilation should respiratory status deteriorate. Continue seizure precautions for severe preeclampsia. Continue magnesium sulfate if ordered. Weigh daily. Continue to assess lab values. Continue to assess for complications associated with obstetric crisis. Monitor for postpartum hemorrhage. Assess uterus and lochia q2h and PRN. Be prepared for a large diuresis after delivery. Assess for petechiae, oozing from puncture sites, hematuria, and ecchymoses.	Patient will maintain optimal hemodynamic status.	Continue to assess and treat hemodynamic parameters. Continue seizure precautions and administration of magnesium sulfate if ordered. Assess neurologic status q4–8h and PRN. Assess follow-up care postdischarge and teach patient signs and symptoms for which to seek medical attention: • bleeding • acute dyspnea • dizziness • seizures • other neurologic changes • daily weight Continue to monitor blood pressure for several weeks after delivery.

Assess for hypertension, edema, proteinuria, and seizures.

Institute seizure precautions for severe preeclampsia. Magnesium sulfate may be administered prophylactically. Observe for respiratory depression if magnesium is given. The antidote is calcium gluconate. Also, if receiving magnesium sulfate, assess deep tendon reflexes q1h and PRN and assess UO q1h.

Assess neurologic status q1h and PRN.

Monitor for signs of complications that can occur with obstetric crises:

- DIC
- amniotic fluid embolus
- ARDS
- renal failure
- hypovolemia
- sepsis
- pulmonary edema
- HELLP syndrome

Assess evidence of tissue perfusion (pain, pulses, temperature, color, signs of decreased perfusion such as decreased UO and altered LOC).

Observe for signs of bleeding and administer blood products as needed. Monitor response.

Assess uterus and lochia every 15 minutes during the immediate postpartum periods.

Assess for edema in all areas of the body.

Check protein levels in the urine q4h.

Place patient on her left side to promote venous return to the heart.

Obstetric Crises Interdisciplinary Outcome Pathway (continued)

NUTRITION

	Diagnosis/Stabilization Phase		Acute Management Phase		Recovery Phase	
Outcome	Interventions	Outcome	Interventions	Outcome	Interventions	
Patient will be adequately nourished as evidenced by: • adequate weight for pregnancy or postpartum • albumin > 3.5–4 g/dL • total protein 6–8 g/dL • total lymphocyte count 1,000–3,000	NPO if intubated or until able to take fluids. If extubation is delayed > 24h, initiate alternative nutritional therapy. Consult dietitian to help determine and direct nutritional support. Initiate enteral or intravenous feedings as necessary. Monitor response. If able to swallow, provide clear liquids and monitor response. Provide supplements as needed. Assess bowel sounds q4h and PRN. Monitor serum glucose levels q4h. Treat levels < 80 mg/dL.	Patient will be adequately nourished.	Progress DAT and monitor response. Consult dietitian if albumin < 3.0 g or if eating less than half of food on tray. Assess bowel sounds q4h and PRN. Provide supplements as needed. Maintain IV and enteral feedings as needed. Maintain high caloric diet. Consider calorie count to ascertain nutritional needs are met. Monitor protein, albumin, and glucose levels.	Patient will be adequately nourished.	Teach patient/family about dietary needs for mother and/or baby after discharge. Stress need for well-balanced diet with increased calorie intake particularly if breastfeeding. Stress need for a healthy diet: • total fat intake < 30% of all calories • total saturated fat intake < 10% of all calories • total cholesterol intake < 300 mg/day • sodium restriction • weight loss if applicable • vitamin and mineral supplements	

MOBILITY

	Diagnosis/Stabilization Phase		Acute Management Phase		Recovery Phase	
Outcome	Interventions	Outcome	Interventions	Outcome	Interventions	
Patient will maintain muscle strength and tone.	Bed rest if preeclamptic or hemodynamically unstable. Begin passive/active-assist ROM exercises.	Patient will achieve optimal mobility.	Increase activity as tolerated. Monitor response to increased activity and decrease if adverse effects occur (tachycardia, dyspnea, syncope, dysrhythmias, hypotension). Monitor effects of increased activity on respiratory status. Monitor with pulse oximetry. Apply supplemental oxygen to keep SpO$_2$ > 92%. Provide physical support as needed. Continue passive/active-assist ROM exercises. Obtain PT/OT consult if indicated to address mobility/functional limitations.	Patient will achieve optimal mobility.	Continue to monitor response to activity. Teach patient/family about home exercise program or activity restrictions.	

OXYGENATION/VENTILATION

Diagnosis/Stabilization Phase		Acute Management Phase		Recovery Phase	
Outcome	Interventions	Outcome	Interventions	Outcome	Interventions
Patient will have adequate gas exchange as evidenced by: • SaO_2 >90% • SpO_2 >92% • ABGs WNL • clear breath sounds • CXR WNL • respiratory rate, depth, and rhythm WNL • absence of dyspnea, cyanosis, and secretions	Monitor ventilator settings (if used) and hemodynamic variables before, during, and after weaning. Avoid prolonged administration of 100% FIO_2. PEEP will be needed for the patient in severe respiratory failure. Involve RCP in plan of care. Monitor respiratory status: • lung sounds • respiratory muscle strength • respiratory rate and depth • coughing ability • ABGs • CXR • SpO_2 Anticipate need for hyperventilation and hyperoxygenation, particularly before suctioning. If not intubated, apply supplemental oxygen. Monitor with pulse oximetry and keep SpO_2 >92%. Assess evidence of tissue perfusion (pain, pulses, temperature, color, signs of decreased perfusion such as decreased UO and altered LOC). Monitor lab values: ABGs, Hgb, magnesium levels if magnesium sulfate is infusing. Assess for dyspnea and cyanosis.	Patient will have adequate gas exchange.	Monitor and treat oxygenation status as per ABGs and/or SpO_2. Monitor and treat ventilation disturbances as per chest assessment, ABGs, adventitious breath sounds, and CXR. Continue to involve RCP. Wean oxygen therapy/mechanical ventilation as indicated. Apply supplemental oxygen to keep SpO_2 >92%. Encourage coughing and deep breathing and/or IS q2h. Observe for complications of obstetric crises that may impair oxygenation/ventilation: • pneumonia • infection • sepsis • DIC • embolus • pulmonary edema • ARDS • thrombus formation • atelectasis • hypovolemia • amniotic fluid embolus Monitor effects of increased activity on respiratory status with pulse oximetry. Apply supplemental oxygen to keep SpO_2 >92%.	Patient will have adequate gas exchange.	Continue to assess complications of obstetric crisis that may impair oxygenation/ventilation. Instruct patient to call physician for any sudden shortness of breath or upper respiratory infection. Teach patient to continue cough and deep breathing and IS at home.

Obstetric Crises Interdisciplinary Outcome Pathway (continued)

COMFORT

Diagnosis/Stabilization Phase		Acute Management Phase		Recovery Phase	
Outcome	Interventions	Outcome	Interventions	Outcome	Interventions
Patient will be as comfortable and pain free as possible as evidenced by: • no objective indicators of discomfort • no complaints of discomfort	Assess quantity and quality of pain with a pain scale or visual analogue tool. Administer IV narcotic analgesics as needed and monitor response. Also monitor fetal HR. Consider fetal response to narcotic analgesics. Provide uninterrupted periods of rest in a quiet environment to potentiate analgesia. If patient is intubated, develop effective interventions with which patient can communicate discomfort. Use sedatives as indicated and monitor response. Observe for complications of obstetric crisis that may cause discomfort: thrombus, embolus, infection, episiotomy. Provide reassurance in a calm, caring, and competent manner. Assess for HA and right upper quadrant or epigastric discomfort.	Patient will be as relaxed and pain free as possible.	Continue as in Diagnosis/Stabilization Phase. Teach patient relaxation techniques. Have patient give return demonstration. Use touch therapy humor, music therapy, and imagery to promote relaxation. Involve family in strategies. Use sedatives as indicated and monitor response. Continue to observe for complications of obstetric crisis that may cause discomfort.	Patient will be as relaxed and pain free as possible.	Progress to oral analgesics and non-narcotic analgesics when possible. Monitor response. Continue alternative methods to promote relaxation as described. Teach patient/family alternative methods to promote relaxation at home. Have patient/family give return demonstration.

SKIN INTEGRITY

Diagnosis/Stabilization Phase		Acute Management Phase		Recovery Phase	
Outcome	Interventions	Outcome	Interventions	Outcome	Interventions
Patient will have intact skin without abrasions or pressure ulcers.	Assess all bony prominences at least q4h and treat if needed. Use preventive pressure-reducing devices if patient is at high risk for developing pressure ulcers. Treat pressure ulcers according to hospital protocol.	Patient will have intact skin without abrasions or pressure ulcers. Patient will have healing wounds/incisions (i.e., Caesarean section).	Continue as in Diagnosis/Stabilization Phase. Monitor wounds/incisions for signs and symptoms of infection. Use sterile technique with all dressing changes.	Patient will have intact skin without abrasions or pressure ulcers. Patient will have healing wounds/incisions.	Teach patient/family proper skin care for both mother and baby after discharge. Teach patient/family proper care of incisions.

PROTECTION/SAFETY

Diagnosis/Stabilization Phase		Acute Management Phase		Recovery Phase	
Outcome	Interventions	Outcome	Interventions	Outcome	Interventions
Patient will be protected from possible harm.	Assess need for restraints if patient is intubated, has a decreased LOC, or is agitated and restless. Explain need for restraints to patient/family. Assess response to restraints, if used, and check q1–2h for skin integrity and impairment to circulation. Follow hospital protocol for use of restraints. Remove restraints as soon as patient is able to follow instructions. Institute seizure precautions and administer magnesium sulfate if ordered. If patient has seizures, other medications may be given with magnesium sulfate. If patient has had seizures, plan for diagnostic tests to determine cause (i.e., CT scan, LP, lab work). Assess for the following symptoms: HA, trauma, infection, other system illnesses, fever, drug use, lack of sleep, lack of food, nausea. Provide sedatives as needed and monitor response, especially to respiratory system. Take measures to lessen the chance of seizures: • quiet environment • no bright lighting in room • use indirect lighting • allow adequate periods of rest	Patient will be protected from possible harm.	If need still exists for restraints, check q1–2h for skin integrity and impairment to circulation. Provide physical support when activity increases. Monitor response to activity. Continue seizure precautions. Continue to decrease stimulation from lights and noise.	Patient will be protected from possible harm.	Provide physical support with increased activity and monitor response. Instruct patient/family about any physical limitations in activity after discharge. Arrange for help at home as needed. Consult home health agencies.

Obstetric Crises Interdisciplinary Outcome Pathway (continued)

PSYCHOSOCIAL/SELF-DETERMINATION

Diagnosis/Stabilization Phase		Acute Management Phase		Recovery Phase	
Outcome	Interventions	Outcome	Interventions	Outcome	Interventions
Patient will achieve psychophysiologic stability. Patient will demonstrate a decrease in anxiety as evidenced by: • VS WNL • subjective reports of decreased anxiety • objectives signs of decreased anxiety Patient will begin acceptance process of obstetric crisis.	Assess physiologic effects of critical care environment on patient: hemodynamic variables, psychological status, signs of increased sympathetic response. Assess psychological effects of obstetric crisis on patient (miscarriage, stillbirth, unable to see baby). Arrange for flexible visitation to meet patient/family needs, especially husband or significant other. Provide sedatives as indicated. Take measures to reduce sensory overload. If patient is intubated, develop effective interventions to communicate with her. If unresponsive, use tactile and verbal stimuli. Use calm, caring, competent, and reassuring approach with patient/family. Assess social support systems. Determine coping ability of patient/family and take appropriate measures (encourage verbalization of fears and concerns, encourage questions, provide information frequently in easy to understand terminology, allow family to visit). If feasible, allow patient to see baby. If not appropriate, provide frequent condition updates. Take pictures of the baby to show to the mother.	Patient will achieve psychophysiologic stability. Patient will demonstrate a decrease in anxiety. Patient will continue acceptance process of obstetric crisis.	Continue as in Diagnosis/Stabilization Phase. Continue to assess coping ability of patient/family and take measures as indicated (counseling, psychiatric consult, verbalization of fears/concerns, social worker, family conferences). Initiate discharge planning. Utilize patient's social support systems. Help patient identify positive coping mechanisms. Take a picture of the newborn if appropriate.	Patient will achieve psychophysiologic stability. Patient will demonstrate a decrease in anxiety. Patient will continue acceptance process of obstetric crisis.	Provide instruction on coping mechanisms after discharge. Reinforce use of positive coping mechanisms. Refer to outside services or agencies as appropriate (chaplain, home health, social services). Utilize patient's social support systems. If appropriate, continue to allow patient to see baby or provide frequent condition updates. Address concerns patient may have about impact of obstetric crisis on ADLs, activities, work, sexual function, and baby care.

Sepsis/Systemic Inflammatory Response Syndrome Interdisciplinary Outcome Pathway

COORDINATION OF CARE

Diagnosis/Stabilization Phase		Acute Management Phase		Recovery Phase	
Outcome	Interventions	Outcome	Interventions	Outcome	Interventions
All appropriate team members and disciplines will be involved in the plan of care.	Develop plan of care with patient, family, primary physician, pulmonologist, infectious disease physician, RN, advanced practice nurse, RCP, social services, chaplain, and outcome manager.	All appropriate team members and disciplines will be involved in the plan of care.	Update plan of care with patient/family, other staff members, PT, OT, dietitian, physical rehabilitation staff (if indicated), home health, medical equipment company (if home supplies necessary—i.e., home oxygen, nebulizer), and discharge planner. Assess social support systems. Initiate planning for anticipated discharge and arrange any equipment that may be needed at home. Assess ability to manage care at home. Begin home care teaching with patient/family.	Patient will understand how to maintain optimal health at home.	Instruct patient/family on any follow-up visits and/or rehabilitation. Provide guidelines concerning care at home such as: • oxygen therapy • medications (indication, dose, and potential side effects) • when to call physician (fever, increased SOB, chest pain, malaise, fatigue) Coordinate home care with continuing care agency. Provide patient/family with phone number of resources available to answer questions and provide support. Remind patient/family that it takes at least a few months to recuperate from significant infectious response and bodily defenses are typically still low. The patient may be very susceptible to further infections for a few months and have a low amount of energy.

Sepsis/Systemic Inflammatory Response Syndrome Interdisciplinary Outcome Pathway (continued)

DIAGNOSTICS

Diagnosis/Stabilization Phase		Acute Management Phase		Recovery Phase	
Outcome	Interventions	Outcome	Interventions	Outcome	Interventions
Patient will understand any tests or procedures that must be completed (VS, hemodynamics, I & O, CXR, intubation, mechanical ventilation, suctioning, lab work, ABGs, SpO$_2$, collection of sputum, blood, and/or urine culture, EKG, cardiac monitoring).	Explain all procedures and tests to patient/family. Be sensitive to individual needs of patient/family for information. Establish effective communication technique with patient if intubated.	Patient will understand any tests or procedures that must be completed (removal of ETT, mechanical ventilation, ABGs, pulse oximetry, removal of urinary catheter, lab work, CXR).	Explain procedures and tests needed to assess organ function/dysfunction as related to sepsis (i.e., pulmonary function: respiratory mechanics, ABGs, SpO$_2$, CXR; cardiovascular: hemodynamics, cardiac enzymes, echocardiogram [if indicated]; renal: BUN, creatinine, urine electrolytes, urine osmolarity; liver: enzymes, bilirubin).	Patient will understand any tests or procedures that must be completed (lab tests, CXR, follow-up ABGs).	Review with patient/family prior to discharge the results of significant tests, especially if any organ dysfunction remains (i.e., pulmonary: ABGs, SpO$_2$) and impact on continuing care. Make sure patient has a copy of tests that may be significant to continuing care. Provide patient with guidelines concerning follow-up care.

FLUID BALANCE

Diagnosis/Stabilization Phase		Acute Management Phase		Recovery Phase	
Outcome	Interventions	Outcome	Interventions	Outcome	Interventions
Patient will achieve optimal hemodynamic status as evidenced by: • MAP >70 mmHg • normal hemodynamic parameters • free from dysrhythmias • optimal hydration • UO >0.5 mL/kg/hr • normothermia	Monitor and treat hemodynamic parameters. Evaluate cardiac function closely (myocardial depressant factor released early in septic shock has been shown to play a role in myocardial dysfunction). Cardiac output (CO) is usually elevated in sepsis. However, evaluate CO based on end organ perfusion and oxygen delivery, not on whether it is high, low, or normal. Monitor oxygen delivery/consumption balance by attempting to normalize the SvO$_2$ to 60–75%. Usually the SvO$_2$ in sepsis is also elevated (>80%).	Patient will maintain optimal hemodynamic status.	Continue as in Diagnosis/Stabilization Phase. Monitor for complications that may occur such as hypoxemia, hypoxia, ARDS, dysrhythmias, acute respiratory failure, pneumothorax, liver failure, pancreatitis, gastritis, renal failure, thrombocytopenia, bleeding disorders, thrombotic events, ischemia, multiple organ dysfunction syndrome (MODS), and septic shock. Maintain optimal hydration based on continued assessment. Maintain optimal oxygen delivery by monitoring SvO$_2$.	Patient will maintain optimal hemodynamic status.	Teach patient/family: • optimal fluid balance and how to maintain it • signs and symptoms of fluid overload or hydration • importance of daily weight • importance of reporting changes in weight/fluid status to health care providers • signs and symptoms to report to physician such as fever, malaise, low energy

indicating low oxygen extraction in tissue beds. Normalizing SvO_2 to 60–75% indicates return of normal oxygen extraction and improved end organ perfusion.

Also monitor and treat:
- BP
- PA systolic and diastolic values
- PCWP
- RA
- SVR/PVR
- dysrhythmias

Monitor for fluid volume deficit related to fever and diaphoresis.

Weigh daily.

Determine hydration needs based on hemodynamics, I & O, viscosity of secretions, vital signs, CXR, breath sounds, SpO_2, SvO_2, and electrolytes.

Monitor for infectious process in blood, sputum, or lungs. Culture of sputum and blood should be obtained, if possible, prior to initiation of antimicrobial therapy. Monitor response to antibiotics.

Monitor lab values: SMA-18, ABGs, CBC with differential, PT, PTT, DIC profile (fibrinogen level, fibrin degradation products, and d-dimer), platelet count, antithrombin III levels, Protein C levels, Factor VIII or IX levels, plasminogen levels, and reticulocyte count, and lactic acid level. Inflammatory mediators that can currently be measured and monitored are activated complement proteins (split products), endotoxin, arachidonic acid metabolites, prothrombin, and certain cytokines (including TNF and IL-1 [interleukin 1]).

Sepsis/Systemic Inflammatory Response Syndrome Interdisciplinary Outcome Pathway (continued)

FLUID BALANCE (continued)

Diagnosis/Stabilization Phase		Acute Management Phase		Recovery Phase	
Interventions	Outcome	Interventions	Outcome	Interventions	Outcome

Administer medications as indicated to stop and/or reverse inflammatory process. Many of these medications are still under clinical investigation. The most common medications used to block or reduce the inflammatory mediators are:
1. Monoclonal antibodies
  • Anti-TNF monoclonal antibodies
  • Anti-endotoxin monoclonal antibodies
2. Anti-cytokine therapy
  • IL-1 receptor antagonist
  • Pentoxyfylline (Trental)
3. Antioxidant therapy
  • Allopurinol
  • Mannitol
4. Miscellaneous anti-inflammatory therapy
  • NSAIDs (ibuprofen, indomethacin, Naprosyn)
  • Protease inhibitors
  • Complement inhibitors
  • Arachidonic acid inhibitors
5. Modulators of coagulation
  • Antithrombin III
  • Protein C
  • Heparin
Administer colony-stimulating factors (CSF) such as filgrastim (Neupogen) if patient is neutropenic to enhance neutrophil production.
Administer vasopressors as indicated.					

Administer blood products, clotting factors (fresh frozen plasma, cyroprecipitate = Factor VIII, fibrinogen, and fibronectin), platelets, and/or heparin (to block thrombin formation) if indicated.

Monitor patient for bleeding tendencies such as disseminated intravascular coagulation (DIC). Also monitor medications closely that interfere with coagulation.

NUTRITION

Diagnosis/Stabilization Phase		Acute Management Phase		Recovery Phase	
Outcome	Interventions	Outcome	Interventions	Outcome	Interventions
Patient will be adequately nourished as evidenced by: • stable weight • weight not >10% below or >20% above IBW • albumin >3.5 g/dL • total protein 6–8 g/dL • prealbumin >15 • total lymphocyte count 1,000–3,000 • positive nitrogen balance	Consult dietitian or nutritional support team to determine and direct nutritional support. Monitor albumin, prealbumin, total protein, cholesterol, triglycerides, and lymphocytes. Monitor gastric pH when possible. Changes in gastrointestinal pH can sometimes lead to translocation of gram negative bacteria or endotoxin across the gastrointestinal wall setting off the sepsis cascade. Other conditions thought to be associated with endotoxin gastrointestinal translocation include viral or bacterial infection, mucosal injury, trauma, burns, radiation therapy, nutritional compromise, immunosuppression, or episodes of shock/mesenteric ischemia. Begin nutritional support as soon as possible. Body's ability to respond to hypoxemia and hypercapnea is impaired after	Patient will be adequately nourished. Patient will be free of bowel and elimination problems.	Same as in Diagnosis/Stabilization Phase. Dietitian to continue to estimate caloric need and best route to achieve. Weigh daily. Advance DAT and monitor response. Consider calorie count if patient taking oral diet. Continue enteral nutrition until patient consuming three-quarters of caloric need. May need nocturnal enteral feedings to meet nutritional goals. Treat diarrhea, constipation, or ileus as indicated.	Patient will be adequately nourished and able to consume at least three-quarters of caloric need.	Assess effectiveness of patient/family teaching. Reinforce as needed. Teach patient/family about: • food pyramid • suggested servings per day • daily caloric requirements • weight-reducing or weight-gaining techniques if needed • vitamin and mineral supplements

Sepsis/Systemic Inflammatory Response Syndrome Interdisciplinary Outcome Pathway (continued)

NUTRITION (CONTINUED)

Diagnosis/Stabilization Phase		Acute Management Phase		Recovery Phase	
Outcome	Interventions	Outcome	Interventions	Outcome	Interventions
	5 days without nutrition. Use the GI tract if at all possible to prevent bacterial translocation and potential compromise of hepatic and mesenteric function. If total parenteral nutrition (TPN) is used, monitor serum glucose q2h.				

MOBILITY

Diagnosis/Stabilization Phase		Acute Management Phase		Recovery Phase	
Outcome	Interventions	Outcome	Interventions	Outcome	Interventions
Patient will achieve optimal mobility.	PT consult to assess ambulation, mobility, muscle flexibility, strength, and tone. OT consult to determine functional ability for ADLs and IADLs. PT/OT to help determine and direct activity goals. Begin passive/active-assist ROM exercises. Allow frequent rest periods.	Patient will maintain optimal mobility.	Develop individualized progressive activity program and advance as tolerated. Use oxygen if necessary to enhance exercise capability and monitor SpO$_2$. Consult physiatrist for rehabilitation if appropriate. Monitor response to increased activity. Decrease if adverse events occur (dyspnea, syncope, ectopy, tachycapnea, tachycardia, hypo/hypertension). Teach energy conservation techniques to enhance functioning and strengthening. Provide physical assistance or assistive devices as necessary.	Patient will maintain optimal mobility.	Continue PT/OT in home if indicated. Assist patient in developing realistic goals for home exercise plan. Refer to rehabilitation program if applicable.

OXYGENATION/VENTILATION

Diagnosis/Stabilization Phase		Acute Management Phase		Recovery Phase	
Outcome	Interventions	Outcome	Interventions	Outcome	Interventions
Patient will have a patent airway and optimal ventilation/gas exchange as evidenced by: • normal CXR • respiratory rate, depth, and rhythm WNL for patient • clear breath sounds bilaterally • SaO₂ >90%; SpO₂ >92% • ABGs, VS, mental status, and pulmonary function tests WNL for patient • demonstrated ability to cough and clear secretions • normal Hgb • normal degree of intrapulmonary shunting or WNL for patient • UO >0.5 mL/kg/hr	Monitor breath sounds, respiratory pattern, SpO₂ and/or ABGs. Determine causative organism if possible by blood, urine, and sputum cultures. Analyze sensitivities for appropriate antibiotic coverage. Be prepared for intubation and mechanical ventilation. Monitor and adjust ventilator settings to obtain appropriate level of assistance and minute ventilation. Maintain adequate humidification. Monitor quantity, color, and consistency of secretions. Observe sputum for rusty color or blood streaked due to DIC. Monitor for signs/symptoms of respiratory distress: • weak ineffective cough • dyspnea, SOB • use of accessory muscles • adventitious breath sounds • alterations in LOC • PCO₂ >50 mmHg or above normal limits for patient • SaO₂ <90% or SpO₂ <92% Administer antibiotics, bronchodilators, and drugs to counter inflammatory mediators as indicated. Monitor patient for signs/symptoms of altered gas exchange: • dyspnea • restlessness • confusion • headache • central cyanosis (not peripheral)	Patient will have optimal ventilation and gas exchange.	Continue as in Diagnosis/Stabilization Phase. Monitor culture results closely and reaffirm proper antibiotic coverage. Assess for improvement in gas exchange (decreased intrapulmonary shunting), breath sounds, thin white secretions, and adequate cough reflexes. Assess readiness to wean from mechanical ventilation if intubated. • measure respiratory mechanics: minute ventilation, negative inspiratory force, RR, tidal volume, and vital capacity • assess hemodynamic stability and factors that increase metabolic demand (fever, increased WBCs, hypo/hyperthyroid) • monitor electrolytes including calcium, magnesium, and phosphorous Monitor ventilatory and hemodynamic variables prior to, during, and after weaning from mechanical ventilation. Assist with extubation. Teach patient effective cough techniques such as cascade coughing and huff technique if indicated to facilitate secretion clearance. Change medications to oral route and monitor response. Begin smoking cessation program if indicated. Determine motivation level of quitting (precontemplator, contemplator, or action) in order to provide appropriate support.	Patient will have optimal ventilation and gas exchange.	Teach patient/family home medications, oxygen therapy (if indicated), breathing exercises, relaxation exercises, energy conservation techniques, daily fluid intake requirements, cough techniques, signs and symptoms of respiratory infection, and symptoms to report to health care provider. Assist with getting home oxygen and/or home nebulizer therapy if indicated. Inform patient/family that energy may be low and susceptibility to other infections may last for 2–3 months. Continue smoking cessation counseling if indicated. Refer to rehabilitation program if indicated.

Sepsis/Systemic Inflammatory Response Syndrome Interdisciplinary Outcome Pathway (continued)

OXYGENATION/VENTILATION (continued)

Diagnosis/Stabilization Phase		Acute Management Phase		Recovery Phase	
Outcome	Interventions	Outcome	Interventions	Outcome	Interventions
	• PaO_2 <50 mmHg on room air • PaO_2/PAO_2 ratio <60, PaO_2/FiO_2 <300, or Q_sQ_t >30 • PCO_2 >50 mmHg • SaO_2 <90% or SpO_2 <92% • use of accessory muscles • dysrhythmias • hypo/hypertension Administer optimal PEEP level. Try to get highest PaO_2 without decreasing CO/SV or increasing peak airway pressures above 40 or 45 cm H_2O pressure. Assess for evidence of adequate tissue perfusion in all organ systems (normal BP, SvO_2, LOC, UO, and normal liver enzymes). Monitor and treat complications such as hypoxemia, hypercapnea, acid-base disturbances, headache, restlessness, tachycardia, bronchospasm, hypo/hypertension, pleural effusion, or pneumothorax. Assist patient to change position at least q2h to ventilate different components of lung to minimize intrapulmonary shunting. Consider CLRT if: PaO_2/PAO_2 ratio is <0.25, PaO_2/FIO_2 ratio is <200, or Q_sQ_t >30).		Wean oxygen therapy as gas exchange improves. Evaluate need for oxygen with activity. Begin teaching patient/family on sepsis and effect on major body systems, especially pulmonary system, current condition, treatment, expected clinical course, and future health implications.		

COMFORT

Diagnosis/Stabilization Phase		Acute Management Phase		Recovery Phase	
Outcome	Interventions	Outcome	Interventions	Outcome	Interventions
Patient will be as comfortable and pain free as possible as evidenced by: • no objective indicators of discomfort • no complaints of discomfort	Plan interventions to provide optimal rest periods. Assess amount and degree of discomfort. Use a pain scale (visual analogue scale from 1–10) to help evaluate pain status. Administer analgesics/sedatives when indicated. Use visual analogue scale to monitor response. Provide reassurance in a calm, caring, and competent manner. Keep HOB elevated to enhance breathing comfort. If intubated, establish effective communication methods. If patient has bleeding tendencies, the following are indicated to prevent discomfort: • limit venipunctures; if venipuncture is necessary, hold all sticks for at least 5 minutes to prevent hematomas • take extra care to prevent breaks in skin and mucous membranes • avoid invasive procedures when possible • insert long-term access device (arterial line and/or central venous catheter if multiple blood sampling is anticipated) • maintain good oral hygiene; use extra soft toothbrush or swab • reduce frequency of dressing changes by using clear dressings (Tegaderm) when possible	Patient will be as comfortable as possible.	Continue as in Diagnosis/Stabilization Phase. Teach patient relaxation techniques. Have patient give return demonstration. Use complementary therapies such as guided imagery, music, humor, or touch therapy to enhance patient's comfort. Involve family in strategies. Consider OT consult for splinting, positioning of extremities for joint protection and comfort.	Patient will be as comfortable as possible.	Continue as in Acute Management Phase. Instruct patient/family on alternative methods to promote relaxation after discharge.

Sepsis/Systemic Inflammatory Response Syndrome Interdisciplinary Outcome Pathway (continued)

COMFORT (continued)

Diagnosis/Stabilization Phase		Acute Management Phase		Recovery Phase	
Outcome	Interventions	Outcome	Interventions	Outcome	Interventions
Patient will have intact skin without abrasions or pressure ulcers.	• administer stool softeners to prevent constipation • use electric razor to shave patient • avoid taking rectal temperatures Observe for complications of sepsis that can cause discomfort (respiratory failure, renal failure, liver failure, heart failure, bleeding into body cavities or joints, tissue ischemia).				

SKIN INTEGRITY

Diagnosis/Stabilization Phase		Acute Management Phase		Recovery Phase	
Outcome	Interventions	Outcome	Interventions	Outcome	Interventions
Patient will have intact skin without abrasions or pressure ulcers.	Assess all bony prominences q4h. Use preventative pressure-reducing devices when patients are at high risk for developing pressure ulcers. Treat pressure ulcers (if present) per hospital protocol.	Patient will have intact skin without abrasions or pressure ulcers.	Continue as in Diagnosis/Stabilization Phase.	Patient will have intact skin without abrasions or pressure ulcers.	Instruct patient/family on proper skin care postdischarge.

PROTECTION/SAFETY

Diagnosis/Stabilization Phase		Acute Management Phase		Recovery Phase	
Outcome	Interventions	Outcome	Interventions	Outcome	Interventions
Patient will be protected from possible harm.	Assess need for wrist restraints if patient is intubated. Balance the need to protect patient from dislodgment of ET with additional fear and anxiety that might be caused by restraints. Follow hospital protocol for use of restraints, if indicated. Assess response to restraints and check skin integrity/potential for impairment to circulation q1–2h. Explain need for restraints to family.	Patient will be protected from possible harm.	Assess need for assistance with activities. Provide physical support as needed. OT to teach correct movement and appropriate functional skills to prevent joint stress, strain, or injury. Splinting to prevent joint deformities and maintain joint integrity when indicated. Continue to allow family to stay with patient.	Patient will be protected from possible harm.	Review with patient/family any physical limitations in activity prior to discharge. Consult PT and/or OT for home follow-up if indicated.
	Monitor peak airway pressures closely and attempt to keep <45 cm H_2O pressure to prevent barotrauma.				
	Use sedatives/anxiolytics as indicated.				
	Allow family to remain with patient if they have calming influence and can promote rest and safety.				
	If patient has bleeding tendency, follow precautions listed under "Comfort" section and				
	• use low suction (<100 mmHg) for gastric and endotracheal suction				
	• pad rails to prevent injury				

Sepsis/Systemic Inflammatory Response Syndrome Interdisciplinary Outcome Pathway (continued)

PSYCHOSOCIAL/SELF-DETERMINATION

Diagnosis/Stabilization Phase		Acute Management Phase		Recovery Phase	
Outcome	Interventions	Outcome	Interventions	Outcome	Interventions
Patient will achieve psychophysiologic stability. Patient will demonstrate a decrease in anxiety as evidenced by: • VS WNL • subjective report of decreased anxiety • objective signs of decreased anxiety	Assess physiologic effect of environment on patient/family. Assess patient for appropriate level of stress. Monitor for delirium, anxiety, or depression. Observe patient's patterns of thinking and communicating. Use calm, competent, reassuring approach to all interventions. Take measures to reduce sensory overload such as providing uninterrupted periods of rest. Allow flexible visiting patterns to meet the psychosocial needs of patient/family.	Patient will achieve psychophysiologic stability. Patient will demonstrate a decrease in anxiety.	Same as in Diagnosis/Stabilization Phase. Provide adequate rest periods. OT to teach progressive increase in ADLs and IADLs to increase independence and self-esteem.	Patient will achieve psychophysiologic stability. Patient will demonstrate a decrease in anxiety.	Refer to outside agencies (Better Breathers Club, American Lung Association) or services as appropriate. Address concerns patient may have about impact on daily life.

Trauma
Interdisciplinary Outcome Pathway

COORDINATION OF CARE

	Diagnosis/Stabilization Phase		Acute Management Phase		Recovery Phase	
Outcome	Interventions	Outcome	Interventions	Outcome	Interventions	
All appropriate team members and disciplines will be involved in the plan of care.	Develop the plan of care with the prehospital providers, patient/family, ED physician, surgeons, primary physician(s), consulting physicians, radiologist, RN, advanced practice nurse, pharmacist, dietitian, RCP, and chaplain.	All appropriate team members will be involved in the plan of care.	Implement and update plan of care with all appropriate team members. Include PT, OT, and social services.	Patient/family will understand how to continue rehabilitation process.	Implement and update plan of care with all appropriate team members. Include plastic surgeon, SP, and psychologist as indicated.	
	Assess severity of injuries using an established trauma scale; revise trauma score as needed.		Continue consultations, as indicated.	Patient will achieve maximum level of recovery.	Develop rehabilitation plan and make referrals to appropriate community services for ongoing health care needs, including:	
	Identify mechanisms of injury.		Assess social support systems.	Patient will maintain optimal level of health.	• functional cognition	
	Identify actual and potential injuries.		Initiate discharge planning assessment.		• communication	
	Perform primary and secondary physical assessment.		Begin planning for rehabilitation by identifying type of program needed:		• self-care	
	Obtain AMPLE history from patient/family/prehospital providers:		• spinal cord injury		• mobility	
	• allergies		• brain injury		• hygiene	
	• medications		• orthopedic and soft tissue injury		• vocation	
	• past medical history		• multiple trauma		• family role	
	• last meal/liquid ingested				• coping abilities	
	• events prior to and of the accident				Assist patient/family for reintegration into the home, workplace, and social activities.	
	Stabilize and assist with transfer to Level I trauma center, if appropriate.				Patient/family will verbalize follow-up plan and supportive resources:	
	Prepare patient for surgery, if indicated.				• access to health care	
					• community resources	
					• home modifications	
					• accessible transportation	
					• vocation and leisure opportunities	
					• financial assistance	
					Assist with transfer plans to rehabilitation facility, if indicated.	
					Provide patient/family with phone number of resources available to answer questions.	

Trauma Interdisciplinary Outcome Pathway (continued)

DIAGNOSTICS

Diagnosis/Stabilization Phase		Acute Management Phase		Recovery Phase	
Outcome	Interventions	Outcome	Interventions	Outcome	Interventions
Patient/family will understand the purpose of all diagnostic procedures such as lab work, x-rays, CT scan, MRI, and possible surgery.	Prepare patient for full radiology series based on mechanism of injury: cross table lateral cervical spine (through C7), skull series, KUB/flat plate abdomen and extremity series. Assist with peritoneal lavage. Assist with explanation of all procedures and obtaining consents. Establish effective communication techniques with intubated patient. Keep explanation short and simple in an emergency situation.	Patient/family will understand the purpose of all diagnostic procedures and treatments.	Explain all applicable procedures/tests needed to evaluate recovery of injuries. Anticipate need for further procedures to evaluate injuries and recovery process. Be sensitive to patient/family's individualized needs for information. Be prepared to repeat information frequently.	Patient/family will understand the purpose of all post-discharge diagnostic procedures in relation to continued health.	Review appropriate diagnostic results with patient/family prior to discharge. Provide patient/family with copies of significant diagnostic results to be used in continuing home care. Explain all follow-up procedures as applicable: • pulmonary function studies • tracheostomy closure • wound reconstruction Provide instructions on care at home: • when to call physician • activity limitations • late complications • diet • medication • whom to call with questions

FLUID BALANCE

Diagnosis/Stabilization Phase		Acute Management Phase		Recovery Phase	
Outcome	Interventions	Outcome	Interventions	Outcome	Interventions
Patient will achieve optimal hemodynamic status as evidenced by: • HR 60–100 bpm • MAP > 70 mmHg • Hgb > 8 • normal hemodynamic parameters • UO ≥0.5 mL/kg/hr	Assess for signs of shock: • altered LOC • anxiety, fear, and apprehension • prolonged capillary refill • pallor, mottling, and cyanosis • tachycardia • dysrhythmias • narrowed pulse pressure • tachypnea • quality, rate, and regularity of pulses • JVD	Patient will maintain optimal hemodynamic status.	Obtain complete lab profile: • CBC • electrolytes • chemistry profile • PT, PTT, ACT • blood and urine toxicology • UA Repeat Hgb and Hct, clotting studies, and electrolytes q12h until stable. Type and cross-match for six units of RBCs or whole blood. Type-specific blood may be given until cross match completed.	Patient will maintain optimal hemodynamic status.	Maintain fluid intake: • to thin pulmonary secretions • until all wounds are closed • to maintain normovolemic state • to maintain adequate UO Instruct patient/family on the prevention and signs and symptoms of edema in dependent extremities and orthostatic hypotension.

• free of dysrhythmias
• no bleeding

Treat life-threatening conditions:
• cardiac tamponade
• profuse bleeding
• tension pneumothorax
• aortic dissection
Apply direct pressure to control bleeding and/or elevate extremities.
Measure body fluid loss including blood loss, excess wound drainage, and insensible fluid loss.
Monitor EKG and treat serious dysrhythmias.
Obtain peripheral venous access with two large-bore lines for volume replacement.
If peripheral access unobtainable, assist central venous line insertion or venous cutdown.
Insert urinary catheter.
Use warming measures to prevent hypothermia, such as warmed IV fluids and warm humidified oxygen.
Assess for signs and symptoms of increased ICP:
• decreased LOC
• decreased motor function
• decreased pupillary activity
• abnormal VS
• posturing
• HA
• N & V
Take measures to decrease increased ICP:
• elevate HOB 15–30 degrees
• prevent hyperextension, flexion, or rotation of head
• limit suctioning to 15 seconds
• decrease metabolic activity by barbiturate coma, hypothermia, and/or paralyzing agents.
Assist with bur holes, if indicated.
Prevent and/or treat seizures.

Initiate autotransfusion, if applicable.
Initiate volume replacement based on clinical presentation and hemodynamic profile:
• Phase I/II shock: crystalloids and colloids
• Phase III shock: add blood products
Warm fluids to maintain body temperature.
Assist with insertion of PA catheter and central venous catheter.
Assist with insertion of or insert arterial line for BP monitoring and to obtain blood samples.
VS, PAP, PCWP, CVP, SVR/PVR q15 mins–1h and CO/CI, SV/SI q1–2h until stable; progress to q4h until lines discontinued.
I & O q1h until stable; progress to q8h.
Apply pneumatic leg compression devices to prevent DVT.
Weigh daily.

Trauma Interdisciplinary Outcome Pathway (continued)

NUTRITION

Diagnosis/Stabilization Phase		Acute Management Phase		Recovery Phase	
Outcome	Interventions	Outcome	Interventions	Outcome	Interventions
Patient will be adequately nourished as evidenced by: • stable weight not > 10% below or > 20% above IBW • albumin > 3.5 g • prealbumin > 15 g • total protein 6–8 g • total lymphocyte count 1,000–3,000	Assess nutritional status: • weight • hydration status • signs of vitamin and mineral deficiencies Assess for bowel sounds, abdominal distension, abdominal pain and tenderness q4h and PRN. Assess KUB/flat plate abdominal series for abdominal injuries. Keep patient NPO until injuries are assessed. Maintain naso/orogastric tube to suction, if needed. Consult dietitian to help determine and direct nutritional support.	Patient will be adequately nourished. Patient will remain free of nausea.	Estimate caloric and protein needs. Perform calorie count. Initiate parenteral nutrition and fat emulsion via central circulation (no later than 3–4 days postinjury), if enteral route nonfunctional. Initiate earlier, if patient is intubated > 24h. Monitor glucose q6–8h, while on parenteral nutrition. When GI tract functional, initiate enteral nutrition. • start feedings with low volumes; increase to estimated requirements (based on the type of injury) • use intermittent gastric feedings or continuous duodenal or small bowel feedings When enteral nutrition discontinued, initiate progressive oral feedings; advance DAT (pureed or mechanical soft may be used if indicated). Monitor serum electrolytes, protein, nitrogen balance, and prealbumin, albumin. Weigh daily.	Patient will maintain adequate nutritional status.	Weigh daily. Monitor progress toward preinjury nutritional status and body weight. Teach patient/family about dietary requirements: • increased calorie intake • caloric supplement, if needed • fluid restriction, if indicated • increased vitamin and mineral supplements, if indicated • healthy diet Continue dietary supplements as needed.

MOBILITY

Diagnosis/Stabilization Phase		Acute Management Phase		Recovery Phase	
Outcome	Interventions	Outcome	Interventions	Outcome	Interventions
Patient will maintain normal ROM and muscle strength.	Establish and maintain proper bone alignment. Stabilize fractures, if applicable. Assess physical limitations to mobility.	Patient will achieve optimal mobility. Patient will maintain normal ROM and muscle strength.	Initiate passive/active-assist ROM. PT/OT to help determine and direct activity goals.	Patient will achieve optimal mobility.	Implement long-range PT/OT plan. In spinal cord injury patients: • encourage patient to assist to fullest potential

Consult OT to assess functional ability.
Consult PT to assess muscle mobility, flexibility, strength, and tone, and alteration in sensation.
Institute progressive mobilization.

Monitor response to increased activity and decrease if increased pain or adverse effects occur (i.e., tachycardia, dyspnea, hypotension, ectopy).
Use assistive devices (pillows, splints, ambulation devices) as indicated.
Schedule periods of rest between activities (1:3 rest period/activities).
Assess for and take measures to prevent DVT such as anticompression devices and antithrombolytic stockings.

- initiate bowel and catheterization program
- initiate sitting program

Implement training for use of long-term orthopedic devices.
Teach patient/family about home exercise program.
Refer to inpatient/outpatient program, if appropriate.

OXYGENATION/VENTILATION

Diagnosis/Stabilization Phase		Acute Management Phase		Recovery Phase	
Outcome	Interventions	Outcome	Interventions	Outcome	Interventions
Patient will have adequate gas exchange as evidenced by: • $PaCO_2$ 25–30 mmHg • PaO_2 >90 mmHg (or baseline for patient) • normal CXR • respiratory rate, depth, rhythm WNL • clear breath sounds • SaO_2 >90% • SpO_2 >92% • ABGs WNL	Maintain a patent airway. Intubate and mechanically ventilate, if necessary. Involve RCP. Correct acid-base imbalance, if indicated. Assess respiratory functions: • breath sounds • respiratory muscle strength and movement • respiratory rate, depth, and quality • tracheal deviation • subcutaneous emphysema • cough ability • CXR Monitor patient for signs and symptoms of altered gas exchange: • decreased LOC • dyspnea • restlessness • confusion • HA • central cyanosis Treat life-threatening condition(s):	Patient will have adequate gas exchange.	Monitor CXR. Monitor chest tube drainage and function, if used. Assess for air leaks. Reassess for tension pneumothorax. Monitor oxygenation by continuous pulse oximetry and intermittent ABGs. Apply supplemental O_2 to keep SpO_2 >92%. Continue to involve RCP. Continue to monitor for pulmonary complications (i.e., pneumonia, atelectasis, and fat embolism). Provide pulmonary hygiene, IS, and chest physiotherapy. Assess color, quantity, and quality (thick/thin) of sputum. Assess patient for posttraumatic respiratory distress syndrome. Initiate weaning and monitor patient response: • wean FIO_2 to keep SpO_2 >92%	Patient will maintain adequate gas exchange.	If long-term mechanical ventilation required, assist with patient placement in appropriate facility and/or home respiratory therapy program. Instruct patient/family in tracheostomy care and safety measures to be taken, if applicable. Monitor patient for development of further complications, such as retained secretions and infection. Evaluate patient for long-term effects of posttraumatic respiratory distress syndrome, such as abnormalities in lung volumes and changes in respiratory mechanics.

Trauma Interdisciplinary Outcome Pathway (continued)

OXYGENATION/VENTILATION (continued)

Diagnosis/Stabilization Phase		Acute Management Phase		Recovery Phase	
Outcome	Interventions	Outcome	Interventions	Outcome	Interventions
	• tension pneumothorax • flail chest • open pneumothorax • massive hemothorax • tracheobronchial injury Assist with chest tube insertion, as needed. Administer high flow, humidified oxygen (unless contraindicated).		• after extubation, apply supplemental O$_2$. Maximize oxygen conservation. Provide tracheostomy care, if applicable.		

COMFORT

Diagnosis/Stabilization Phase		Acute Management Phase		Recovery Phase	
Outcome	Interventions	Outcome	Interventions	Outcome	Interventions
Patient will be as comfortable and pain free as possible as evidenced by: • decreased incidence of pain • decreased severity of pain • normal VS	Perform pain assessment by direct patient report and observation. Develop a proactive individualized pain management plan, including: • medication, route, dosing, and frequency • alternative therapies Perform a complete neurologic exam. Educate patient/family to communicate unrelieved pain effectively. Administer analgesics and monitor response using a pain scale or visual analogue tool. Establish effective communication techniques with intubated patients to ensure the ability to communicate discomfort and the need for analgesics. Refer to Acute Pain Management Outcome Pathway as needed.	Patient will be as relaxed and as comfortable as possible.	Reassess pain level frequently at scheduled intervals, such as: • q2h • with any complaint of pain • after administration of analgesia Individualized route, dosage, and schedule for analgesics: • mild to moderate pain: NSAIDs • moderate to severe pain: opioid analgesics (IV, IM, transdermal, intraspinal) Offer PCA, if medically and psychologically indicated. Teach patient the appropriate use of PCA. Administer a loading dose prior to the start of a continuous infusion. Evaluate pain management therapy by patient self-report and/or observation of physical symptoms.	Patient will be as pain free as possible.	Continue to monitor pain level and reassess to rule out new pain sources (i.e., infection, inflammation, or osteoarthritis). Instruct the patient in the use of relaxation exercises, distraction, and imagery and have patient give return demonstration. Pain lasting longer than 6 months following injury should be considered chronic pain. Refer to Chronic Pain Management Outcome Pathway as needed.

Switch medication route using equianalgesia dosing.
Monitor for side effects of analgesia:

- sedation
- mood changes
- respiratory depression
- decreased gastric mobility
- N & V
- drowsiness
- clouding of mentation
- orthostatic hypotension

Assess for complications of pain:

- anxiety
- sleep disturbances/psychosis
- decreased TV and functional capacity
- tachycardia
- hypertension
- increased PVR
- increased gastric secretions
- decreased gastric motility
- smooth muscle sphincter spasm
- water and sodium retention
- hyperglycemia

Provide uninterrupted periods of rest.

SKIN INTEGRITY

Diagnosis/Stabilization Phase		Acute Management Phase		Recovery Phase	
Outcome	Interventions	Outcome	Interventions	Outcome	Interventions
Patient will have intact skin without abrasions or pressure ulcers.	Remove debris, bacteria, foreign bodies, and necrotic tissue. Debride, irrigate, and cover wounds with sterile gauze. Obtain and document a complete baseline skin assessment. Document size, location, and description of wounds.	Patient will have intact skin without abrasions or pressure ulcers. Patient will have healing wounds (surgical and traumatic). Patient will be free of infection.	Reassess skin based on initial assessment. Maintain sterile technique with all dressing changes. Monitor all incisions/wounds for signs and symptoms of infection. Monitor for signs and symptoms of compartment syndrome: increased swelling, absence of pulses, pain. Prepare for fasciotomy, if needed.	Patient will have intact skin without abrasions or pressure ulcers. Patient will have healing wounds (surgical and traumatic). Patient will be free of infection.	Teach patient/family proper care of incisions and wounds. Teach patient/family proper techniques for dressing changes, if applicable. Monitor patient for poor cosmetic/reconstructive results of wound healing and facilitate early intervention; consult plastic surgeon, if indicated. Monitor patient for signs and symptoms of infection in:

Trauma Interdisciplinary Outcome Pathway (continued)

SKIN INTEGRITY (continued)

Diagnosis/Stabilization Phase		Acute Management Phase		Recovery Phase	
Outcome	Interventions	Outcome	Interventions	Outcome	Interventions
			Maintain aseptic conditions around immobilization pins. Prevent/correct abdominal distension to prevent wound dehiscence. OT to assess for need for splints or assistive devices. Use pressure-relieving devices as appropriate. Facilitate the highest degree of mobility possible. Assess all bony prominences at least q4h; treat if indicated according to hospital protocol. Use bagging technique for draining wounds.		• all wounds • old chest tube sites • incisions • old drain sites Prepare patient for reconstructive procedures. Schedule follow-up appointment for suture/cast removal, if applicable.

PROTECTION/SAFETY

Diagnosis/Stabilization Phase		Acute Management Phase		Recovery Phase	
Outcome	Interventions	Outcome	Interventions	Outcome	Interventions
Patient will be protected from possible harm.	Paralyzing agents may be needed in the combative or severely restless patient. Administer naloxone in the event of respiratory depression. Follow hospital protocol for restraint use. Assess the need for soft restraints to prevent dislodgment of tubes/drains; explain need to patient/family. If restraints used, monitor skin integrity and circulation q1–2h. Carefully monitor the use of NSAIDs and aspirin in the trauma patient due to increased bleeding tendencies.	Patient will be protected from possible harm.	Pad side rails and other firm surfaces, if combative or head injury. Monitor patient for signs and symptoms of sensory deprivation: • confusion • disorientation • hallucinations • restlessness • combativeness In patients receiving intraspinal analgesia: • maintain strict sterile technique • use tubing without injection ports	Patient will be protected from possible harm.	Review physical limitations with patient/family prior to discharge. Instruct patient/family on the signs and symptoms of infection: • unusual redness/swelling • increased pain • foul drainage or odor from wound • temperature elevation Instruct patient/family on actions to take if signs and symptoms of infection occur. Assess patient/family for understanding of all instructions. Reinforce as needed.

- keep HOB elevated during the first hour of treatment.

Avoid extreme temperatures to extremities.

Provide appropriate physical support to prevent falls.

PSYCHOSOCIAL/SELF-DETERMINATION

Diagnosis/Stabilization Phase		Acute Management Phase		Recovery Phase	
Outcome	Interventions	Outcome	Interventions	Outcome	Interventions
Patient/family will utilize coping skills effectively to keep anxiety at a tolerable level. Patient will achieve psychophysiologic stability.	Assess patient/family for: • current level of anxiety and fear • support systems (or lack of) • reactions to stress Recognize defensive coping mechanisms such as repression, denial, regression, projection, and anger. Be honest when giving information regarding patient's condition. Immediately identify patient's religion/spiritual needs and have support available. Provide short and concise explanations.	Patient/family will demonstrate effective coping skills. Patient will achieve psychophysiologic stability. Patient will demonstrate a decrease in anxiety. Patient will begin acceptance process of injuries.	Support patient through stages of loss and grieving. Assist patient with adaptation to altered body functions and body image. Reinforce and reward positive coping strategies by patient/family. Assess ineffective or maladaptive behaviors. Allow flexible visitation to meet patient/family's needs. Involve patient/family in all decisions regarding care. Provide adequate rest periods. Identify and eliminate stressors.	Patient/family will maintain effective coping skills. Patient will achieve psychophysiologic stability. Patient will begin acceptance process of injuries.	Assess patient for current stage of perception of injuries and adaptation. Assess for signs and symptoms of posttraumatic stress disorder (PTSD). Educate patient/family on signs of PTSD and the appropriate interventions such as ventilation, relaxation, and imagery. Assist patient/family with identification and implementation of role changes. Assist patient with reconstruction of traumatic event. Address concerns patient may have on impact of trauma on daily life: ADLs, return to work, sexual functioning, recreation. Refer to outside agencies as appropriate.

PATIENT EDUCATION OUTCOME PATHWAYS

CHAPTER 8

Patient Education Outcome Pathways

Asthma

Patient Education Outcome Pathway

Asthma is a very common lung disease affecting millions of people. In asthma, the airways become swollen and sensitive, causing them to narrow and breathing to become difficult. Symptoms of asthma include wheezing, cough (sometimes lasting for up to one week), chest tightness, and shortness of breath.

The exact cause of asthma is not known. The airways are more sensitive and they may react to many substances or things called *triggers*. Triggers vary from person to person. Some common triggers are cold weather, hot weather, air pollution, cigarette smoke, perfumes, exercise, a cold or flu, and allergic reactions to dust, mold, pets, food, or medications.

Although there is no cure for asthma, it can usually be controlled. This requires teamwork between you and your health care providers. Asthma can be controlled. It does not have to control you.

ASTHMA

In the Emergency Room		During Your Hospital Stay		After You Are Discharged	
Goal	Activities	Goal	Activities	Goal	Activities
You will understand the care you receive in the emergency room.	The purposes of treatment in the emergency room are: • relax the airways and relieve the bronchospasm (narrowing or tightness) in the airways • help you relax • improve the oxygen content in your blood • give you fluids to keep you well hydrated • prevent further problems	You will understand the care you receive in the hospital.	The purposes of treatment during the hospital stay are to: • improve the oxygen content in your blood • identify and treat the trigger of the episode • teach you how to manage your asthma • improve your diet and hydration (fluids) • prevent further problems • allow adequate rest • initiate an exercise/pulmonary rehabilitation program • teach you about your medication regimen	You should understand how to control your asthma. You should understand how to prevent future episodes.	Know your triggers of acute episodes and take measures to avoid them. Common triggers include: • cold air • hot weather • humidity • dust • pets • cigarette smoking • air pollution • odors • perfumes • medications • certain foods • exercise • upper respiratory infection Demonstrate proper use of your inhaler(s) with and without a spacer device. Know your medications: name, purpose, dosage, how to take, and potential side effects. Recognize the signs and symptoms of infection and when to call the doctor.

Follow your home exercise program or enroll in an outpatient pulmonary rehabilitation program.

Practice pursed-lip breathing and diaphragmatic breathing. Use pursed-lip breathing when you are short of breath and to prevent shortness of breath, such as when you are climbing stairs.

Practice your relaxation exercises.

Join an asthma support group if one is available in your area.

Monitor your peak flow at least once a day and record. Know your danger zone and what measures to take. This level will vary from person to person. Ask your doctor, nurse, or respiratory therapist. Your own medication plan will be based on your own personal best peak flow number. To find out your personal best peak flow, take peak flow readings:

- every day for two weeks
- mornings and evenings
- before and after taking inhaled bronchodilators

Once you know your personal best peak flow, your doctor will give you a medication care plan based on changes in your peak flow. For example:

- *Green zone* (80–100% of your personal best) signals all clear. No asthma symptoms are present and you may take your medications as usual.

- *Yellow zone* (50–80% of your personal best) signals caution. You may be having an episode of asthma that requires an increase in your medication or your overall

Asthma Patient Education Outcome Pathway (continued)

ASTHMA (continued)

In the Emergency Room		During Your Hospital Stay		After You Are Discharged	
Goal	Activities	Goal	Activities	Goal	Activities
					asthma may not be under control. Call your doctor. Your medication plan may need to be changed.
					• *Red zone* (less than 50% of your personal best) signals a medical alert. You must take your bronchodilator right away and call your doctor immediately if the peak flow number does not return to the yellow or green zone and stay there. Continue to drink lots of fluids unless your doctor tells you otherwise. Recognize the signs of an impending acute episode and seek treatment immediately. Asthma can kill if not treated promptly and accurately. Keep your appointments for follow-up visits. Asthma can be controlled but it requires teamwork by you, your doctor, and your other health care providers.

TESTS

In the Emergency Room		During Your Hospital Stay		After You Are Discharged	
Goal	Activities	Goal	Activities	Goal	Activities
You and your family will understand the tests that will be done in the emergency room.	You will be placed on a cardiac monitor to watch your heart rate and rhythm. Your blood pressure will be checked frequently.	You will understand any tests that may be done during your hospital stay.	After you are admitted, the following tests may be done: • blood work • arterial blood gases • x-rays • pulse oximetry	You and your family should understand any tests that may be done after you leave the hospital.	After you are discharged, you may need to return to either the hospital or your doctor for further testing: • pulmonary function tests • peak flow

An IV will be started in your arm to give you medications to help you breathe easier.

The oxygen content of your blood will be monitored with a device called pulse oximetry. This involves placing a small sensor on your finger, earlobe, or toe.

Oxygen will be started either with a cannula (small tube in your nose) or mask. In some severe cases, you may have to be placed on a respirator (ventilator) to help you breathe until the crisis is over. This will involve placing a large tube through your mouth into your lungs.

Blood will be drawn for several lab tests.

You will be encouraged to drink fluids. If you are unable to do so, they will be given through your IV.

A chest x-ray will be done.

Your peak flow will be measured. This tells the doctors and nurses the severity of the episode. You will be asked to take a deep breath and blow as hard and fast as you can into a small hand-held meter. Peak flow is the volume of air that you can blow out. Each person's asthma is different, and peak flow is based on your height, weight, and sex. This means it is important for you to find out your personal best peak flow.

Your family will be kept informed of your condition and will be allowed to see you as soon as possible.

You may be on a heart monitor for a few days.

If you are on a ventilator (respirator), it will gradually be weaned and removed as your condition improves.

You will have oxygen either by a nasal cannula (small tube) or mask.

The nurses will watch your fluid intake (both by mouth and through the IV) and how much you urinate.

You will still have an IV. You will receive fluids and medications through the IV.

It is important for you to drink fluids. This will help keep your mucus thin and easier to cough up.

You may have pulmonary function tests done as you improve.

Your peak flow (as described earlier) will be measured frequently during your hospital stay.

- allergy testing
- pulse oximetry
- arterial blood gases
- exercise stress test
- bronchial provocation

Before you leave the hospital, the nurse or respiratory therapist will teach you how to use your peak flow meter properly.

Asthma Patient Education Outcome Pathway (continued)

DIET AND FLUIDS

In the Emergency Room		During Your Hospital Stay		After You Are Discharged	
Goal	Activities	Goal	Activities	Goal	Activities
You will have an IV started in the emergency room. You may have only clear liquids in the emergency room.	It is important that you drink many fluids to keep your mucus thin. Thin mucus is easier to cough up. You will be encouraged to drink lots of fluids and an IV will be started. You may have clear liquids in the emergency room. Blood may be drawn to check your nutritional status.	You will start on a healthy diet. You will stay well hydrated.	You will still be encouraged to drink lots of fluids. You will still have an IV. Your diet may progress as tolerated. The nurse will keep track of how much you drink and how much you urinate. You will be weighed daily. A dietitian may see you before you are discharged.	You should continue a healthy diet. You should stay well hydrated.	You should still drink lots of fluids unless your doctor tells you otherwise. You should follow a healthy diet: • keep fat intake less than 30% of your diet • keep saturated fat intake less than 10% of your diet • keep cholesterol intake to less than 300 mg per day • follow a low salt diet. Do not add salt to your food and be sure to read labels. Avoid foods with sodium added (for example, processed meats, canned goods, chips, pickles, etc.). • restrict calories if needed In some people, dairy products (milk, cheese, ice cream) can cause extra mucus production. Report any of the following to your doctor: • any sudden weight gain • swelling • shortness of breath Avoid foods that may trigger attacks. You may need to see an allergy specialist to determine if there are any foods you should avoid.

ACTIVITY

	In the Emergency Room		During Your Hospital Stay		After You Are Discharged	
Goal	Goal	Activities	Goal	Activities	Goal	Activities
You will remain on bed rest in the emergency room.		You will be on bed rest in the emergency room. The head of your bed can be elevated for comfort and to help you breathe. Do not expend any more energy than you have to. It is taking all of your energy to breathe during an acute attack. The nurse or respiratory therapist may coach you through some relaxation exercises. If you know any relaxation exercises, try them. Deep breathing can be very helpful.	You will start on an exercise program. You will maintain/regain muscle strength.	Your activity level will be whatever you can handle without problems. You will start gradually with dangling at the bedside, to sitting in a chair for meals, to walking in the hallway. The head of your bed may be raised for comfort and to help you breathe. The physical therapist or nurse may show you some arm and leg exercises. You may start a pulmonary rehabilitation program while you are still in the hospital. You will be taught the technique of pursed-lip breathing, which can be done any time you are short of breath and to help prevent shortness of breath. The nurse or respiratory therapist will demonstrate for you. You must practice. You may also be taught the technique of diaphragmatic breathing. The diaphragm is a large muscle located just under your rib cage. Its main purpose is to aid in breathing. Many people with lung disease do not use their diaphragm and use their chest muscles instead. This uses up a lot of energy. You must practice using your diaphragm to breathe so that it will become second nature. Your oxygen content will be monitored while you exercise. You may be seen by a physical therapist or occupational therapist.	You should maintain/regain muscle strength. You should continue an exercise program at home.	You may be referred to an outpatient pulmonary rehabilitation program. You should continue your exercise program at home. Aerobic activity is best and includes walking, jogging, bicycling, swimming, tennis, or water aerobics. Any activity that gets you up and moving is all right. You should continue using pursed-lip breathing, diaphragmatic breathing, and relaxation exercises. If you have exercise-induced asthma, use your medications as prescribed before exercising. You will be asked to see your doctor to have the oxygen level in your blood monitored either by arterial blood gases or pulse oximetry. Monitor your body's reaction to exercise or activity. Report any of the following to your doctor: • fast heart rate • irregular heart rate • palpitations • skipped beats • fainting • dizziness • wheezing • weakness • decreased peak flow

Asthma Patient Education Outcome Pathway (continued)

ACTIVITY (continued)

In the Emergency Room		During Your Hospital Stay		After You Are Discharged	
Goal	Activities	Goal	Activities	Goal	Activities
			You will be taught relaxation exercises to help prevent episodes and to help you through an acute episode. You will be asked to practice these exercises. You may be given an inspiratory muscle trainer. If you are, the respiratory therapist will show you how to use it.		

MEDICATIONS

In the Emergency Room		During Your Hospital Stay		After You Are Discharged	
Goal	Activities	Goal	Activities	Goal	Activities
You will receive medications in the emergency room to help relieve the bronchospasm (wheezing) and help you breathe easier.	You may receive the following medications in the emergency room: • bronchodilators (oral, IV, or inhaled) to help widen the airways • steroids (oral, IV, or inhaled) to help decrease swelling or inflammation in the airways • oxygen • antibiotics to fight infection Response to the medications will be monitored by a peak flow and pulse oximeter (to monitor the oxygen content in your blood).	You will receive medications during your hospital stay to help relieve the bronchospasm (wheezing, tightness, or narrowing) and help you breathe easier. You will receive medications to help prevent future episodes.	You may receive the following medications while you are in the hospital: • oxygen • same as listed earlier • vitamins Response to the medications will be monitored by a peak flow and pulse oximeter (to monitor the oxygen content in your blood).	You should know the medications you are taking at home: • name • dosage • proper use • side effects You will demonstrate proper use of an inhaler.	Medications that may be prescribed after discharge from the hospital include: • antibiotics • steroids (either oral or inhaled) • bronchodilators (either oral or inhaled) • oxygen in some cases • medications to help dry secretions • allergy shots • allergy medications You will demonstrate the proper use of an inhaler with and without a spacer device before you leave the hospital. The nurse and respiratory therapist will show you how to use and take care of an inhaler properly.

You will be given a medication care plan to follow based on your peak flow numbers.

The nurse will review with you:

- names of your medications
- purposes of your medications
- how to take
- potential side effects
- when to call the doctor

Ask your doctor, nurse, or pharmacist any questions about your medications.

Cardiac Catheterization

Patient Education Outcome Pathway

A cardiac catheterization (cath) is a dye test in which a catheter (hollow tube) is placed into the arteries and chambers of your heart. The test is done to:

- determine how well the heart is pumping
- determine the condition of the heart valves
- determine if there are any blockages in the coronary arteries

PROCEDURE

Before		During		After	
Goal	Activities	Goal	Activities	Goal	Activities
You will understand what happens before the cardiac cath.	The entry site for the catheter (hollow tube), usually the groin, will be washed with an antibacterial soap. In some cases, the arm may be used. The area may be shaved.	You will understand what happens during the cardiac cath.	You will receive some medication to help you relax. The doctor will numb the entry site with a medication called xylocaine or lidocaine, which is similar to novacaine, the medicine the dentist uses to numb your gums. If you have had a reaction to either novacaine or lidocaine before, tell your doctor or nurse. You can be given medication to prevent a reaction. The doctor will make a small hole into the artery and thread several catheters or wires into your heart. You may be asked to cough, hold your breath, or turn your head to the left or right. Dye will be injected into each of the arteries of your heart to locate blockages. Dye will also be injected into the left ventricle, the main pumping chamber of the heart, which will show how well your heart is pumping. You will feel hot all over for about 30 seconds when this picture is taken. In some cases, catheters are placed into the right side of the heart to measure pressures inside the heart.	You will understand what happens after the cardiac cath.	Once the catheters are removed, pressure will be applied to the entry site for 15–20 minutes to stop any bleeding. In some cases, the sheaths or guiding tubes are left in if you and your doctor decide to proceed with a cardiac intervention such as a balloon angioplasty. A tight bandage will be applied to the entry site for several hours. This will be replaced by an adhesive bandage. The nurse will check your heart rate, blood pressure, and the pulses in your feet frequently for several hours. If your arm was used as the entry site, the nurse will check the pulse in your wrist frequently. You will be encouraged to drink lots of fluids, at least 1 glass every hour for 6–8 hours. You should also drink more fluid at home for at least one week unless your doctor tells you otherwise. Pain medication will be available. You will remain in bed 4–8 hours.

TESTS

	Before		During		After	
	Goal	Activities	Goal	Activities	Goal	Activities
	You and your family will understand the tests that will be done before the cardiac cath.	Blood will be drawn to determine your complete blood cell count, clotting studies, and electrolytes. You may have a chest x-ray. A 12 lead EKG will be done. You will be asked to provide a urine sample.	You and your family will understand any tests that may be done during the cardiac cath.	You may feel some extra heartbeats during the cath. Information about the heart valves may be collected. The procedure lasts about 30 minutes. Your heart rate and blood pressure will be monitored throughout the procedure. Pressures inside your heart will be recorded during the procedure. The pulses in your feet/wrist will be checked frequently.	You and your family will understand any tests that may be done after the cardiac cath.	You may be discharged a few hours after the procedure or the next day unless further treatment is needed. Avoid lifting over 10 pounds for one week. A 12 lead EKG may be repeated. Blood may be drawn to check your complete blood count, clotting, and cardiac enzymes. Your heart rate and rhythm will be monitored closely after the procedure for several hours.

DIET AND FLUIDS

	Before		During		After	
	Goal	Activities	Goal	Activities	Goal	Activities
	You will take nothing by mouth for at least 6 hours before the procedure.	You may take nothing by mouth after midnight the night before your procedure. Your doctor or nurse will let you know if you can take your usual medications with a small sip of water the morning of your cardiac cath. If your cardiac cath is scheduled for later in the day, you may be able to have a clear liquid breakfast. Your doctor or nurse will let you know. An IV will be started in your arm and fluids given.	You will not take anything by mouth during the procedure.	You will still not take any fluids by mouth during the cardiac cath. You may be given some oral medications during the procedure to either place under your tongue or swallow with a small sip of water. IV fluids will be continued.	You will begin taking fluids in order to stay well hydrated and to help flush the dye from your system. You will progress to a heart healthy diet as tolerated.	You should drink at least 8 ounces of fluid per hour for 6–8 hours after the cardiac cath. The IV will be removed once you are taking fluids well. You should drink extra fluids for several days after the procedure. You will be able to eat after the procedure. You should follow a heart healthy diet: • limit your fat intake to less than 30% of calories per day • limit your saturated fat intake to less than 10% of calories per day

Cardiac Catheterization Patient Education Outcome Pathway *(continued)*

DIET AND FLUIDS *(continued)*

Before		During		After	
Goal	Activities	Goal	Activities	Goal	Activities
					• limit your cholesterol intake to less than 300 mg per day • restrict calories if needed • restrict salt if needed

ACTIVITY

Before		During		After	
Goal	Activities	Goal	Activities	Goal	Activities
You should maintain your current activity level.	Maintain your current activity level as directed by your doctor.	You will remain flat during the cardiac cath.	During the procedure you will remain flat on your back on a hard table. If you have any back discomfort, let the nurse know. Pain medication will be available.	You will remain flat for 4–8 hours after the procedure. You will return to your pre-cardiac cath activity level. You may begin an exercise program upon the recommendation of your doctor.	After the cardiac cath, you will remain in bed for 4–8 hours to reduce the chance of bleeding. After 3–4 hours, you may be able to raise the head of the bed 30 degrees. The nurse will let you know. A tight bandage will be applied where the catheter was inserted (usually the groin). You may have a 5 pound sandbag placed over the bandage. Do not get up the first time without help. Call for the nurse. If you must cough or sneeze, place your hand over the bandage and apply pressure. If you feel a sensation of warmth or wetness at the bandage, apply pressure with your hand and call for the nurse. You may be referred to an outpatient cardiac rehabilitation program.

MEDICATIONS

	Before		During		After	
	Goal	Activities	Goal	Activities	Goal	Activities
	You should be able to state your medications to the doctor and the nurse before the cardiac cath.	The nurse and the doctor will ask you about your medications. Be sure to know the name and dosage of all of your medicines. You may want to bring them to the hospital with you. You may be able to take your medications the morning of the cardiac cath with a small sip of water. Ask your doctor or nurse about this. An IV will be started in your arm. A sedative may be given either orally or through the IV to help you relax before the procedure.	You will be kept as comfortable as possible during the cardiac cath.	If needed, a sedative or pain medication may be given through the IV during the procedure. The IV is also maintained in case medications must be given to you quickly.	You will be able to start back on or start new medications before discharge.	The IV will be removed when you start drinking fluids. You will receive teaching about the medications you will take at home: • name • dosage • when to take • special instructions • side effects You may have a prescription for pain medication if needed.

DISCHARGE PLANNING

	Before		During		After	
	Goal	Activities	Goal	Activities	Goal	Activities
	You will begin planning your discharge as soon as you are admitted.	The nurse will ask you about your home life when you are admitted. Let the nurse know if someone will be with you when you are discharged.	Discharge planning will be started as soon as you are admitted.	You may be discharged within a few hours or the next day.	You will understand the results of the procedure. You will understand care needed after discharge.	Make an appointment with your doctor as instructed for follow-up. Maintain a heart healthy diet. Gradually increase your activities. You may be referred to a cardiac rehabilitation program. The doctor will discuss the findings of the cardiac cath with you and make recommendations for future treatment. Ask for a phone number to call if you have questions after discharge. Plan to have someone with you the day you are going home.

Coronary Artery Bypass Grafting

Patient Education Outcome Pathway

Open heart surgery can be extremely frightening for you and your family. In many cases, people do not even realize they have heart disease until they have a heart attack or cardiac catheterization, and then suddenly are faced with needing open heart surgery. It is usually quite a shock, to say the least. Knowing what is going to happen can help you be prepared and participate in your care instead of being a passive bystander. The more you know and can do for yourself, the more quickly your healing process will be.

Coronary artery bypass surgery involves using an artery from your chest or a vein from your leg to actually bypass the coronary artery on your heart that is blocked by plaque and cholesterol. One end of the artery or vein attaches to the aorta and the other end is sewn directly into the coronary artery past the blocked area so that blood may flow freely from the aorta through the coronary artery, thus bypassing the blocked area.

Coronary artery bypass surgery is one of the most common surgeries performed in the United States. Complication rates are between 2 and 5% depending on your age and condition.

PROCEDURE

	Before		During		After	
	Goal	Activities	Goal	Activities	Goal	Activities
You and your family will understand what happens before the procedure.	You and your family will understand what happens before the procedure.	You will be seen by your cardiologist, heart surgeon, and an anesthesiologist before your surgery. A nurse will explain what will happen to you. You may be able to watch a videotape explaining open heart surgery. You will take a shower the night before your surgery and use a special antimicrobial soap. Just before your surgery, a technician will scrub your chest, groin, and legs again using the special soap. Your chest, groin, and legs will also be shaved or clipped. An intravenous (IV) line will be started if you don't already have one. Once in the operating room, an anesthesiologist will begin inserting other lines that help the nurses and physicians monitor your condition constantly. A small catheter	You and your family will understand what happens during the procedure.	The surgeon will begin by making an incision on your chest. The breastbone will be cut so the surgeon can work on your heart. The surgeon will assess your heart and begin taking down the artery from your chest wall. At the same time, a surgical technician will begin taking the vein out of your leg. Once the artery and vein(s) are ready, the team will prepare to attach them to the heart and bypass the blockage(s). The team cannot sew onto the heart while it is pumping and beating. A tube is placed into the right atrium, which drains blood out of the heart and then takes it to a bypass machine that functions as an artificial heart and lung. The blood is oxygenated and then put back into the body by way of another tube, which is placed into the aorta. The blood then goes to the rest of the body normally. Once the blood is	You and your family will understand what happens after the procedure.	You will be taken to an open heart recovery or intensive care unit for the first 6–24 hours after surgery. The nurses will closely monitor your pulse (heart rate), blood pressure, the pressures in your heart, your breathing, your heart and lung sounds, how much urine is produced by your kidneys, and how much fluid/blood is draining from your chest tubes. As you begin to awaken from the anesthesia, the ventilator will be turned down as you do more of your breathing on your own. By the time you are totally awake, usually the breathing tube can be removed. The chest tubes will be removed typically by the next morning after your surgery. You will begin getting up out of bed as soon as possible after surgery.

(about 1.5 inches long) will be placed into an artery in your wrist and be connected to a pressure tubing that attaches to the monitor so your blood pressure can be monitored. A yellow IV line will be put into one of your large veins (usually in the neck). This catheter goes through the right atrium and right ventricle of your heart and sits in the pulmonary artery (a vessel that carries blood from your heart to your lungs). The nurses and physicians can monitor several pressures in and around your heart and how much blood your heart is actually pumping per beat. This information allows the nurses/doctors to know if you need more or less fluid, medications to increase or decrease your blood pressure, and/or medications to help your heart beat stronger. Next the anesthesiologist will give you medicines to help you go to sleep during the surgery. After you are put under anesthesia, a breathing tube will be placed in your throat so your breathing can be controlled while you are under anesthesia.

A catheter will also be placed in your bladder so the amount of urine that your kidneys are producing can be measured.

rerouted through the heart/lung machine, the heart is stopped and the surgical team sews the new artery and veins around the blocked areas. Once they are finished, the heart is restarted and the tubes from the heart/lung bypass are removed. The surgery usually takes 3–5 hours depending on the number of bypasses. The surgeon will usually attach pacemaker wires from the heart muscle to a pacemaker generator box in case the heart has an irregular rhythm after surgery. These wires are removed prior to going home. Chest tubes are also placed in the front of the chest to drain any extra blood or fluid that may drain from the chest in the first 12–24 hours after surgery. The breastbone is wired together to help the bone fuse back together, and the skin is sewn up. Bandages are placed on your incisions and your surgery is completed.

The catheter in your artery and the large yellow tube in your vein will be removed.

You will be transferred to a progressive care unit or telemetry floor where the nurses can continue to monitor your heart rate and rhythm.

As you become more mobile and can walk to the bathroom, the catheter will be removed from your bladder.

The day before you go home, the pacemaker wires will be removed from your chest. You will also be able to take a shower once these pacemaker wires are out.

Coronary Artery Bypass Grafting Patient Education Outcome Pathway (continued)

TESTS

Before		During		After	
Goal	Activities	Goal	Activities	Goal	Activities
You and your family will understand the tests that will be done before your surgery.	Blood will be drawn to measure your complete blood count, clotting studies, electrolytes, and to determine your blood type. You will have a chest x-ray. Blood will be drawn from your artery to measure your oxygen level and carbon dioxide levels, which tells the physician and nurses about the adequacy of your breathing. A 12 lead EKG will be done. You will be asked to provide a urine sample. You will be taught how to use an incentive spirometer, a device that measures how much air you can inhale in one breath. You will be taught to take a deep breath and hold it up to 5 seconds with the device.	You and your family will understand any tests that will be done during your surgery.	Your pulse (heart rate), blood pressure, the pressures in your heart, and your breathing will be monitored constantly by the surgical team. Blood will be drawn throughout your surgery to check your blood count and how well your blood is clotting. Blood will also be drawn to measure your oxygen/carbon dioxide levels to check your breathing status. Any blood that you lose will be collected through a cell saver machine, filtered, and given back to you so that you shouldn't need any additional blood transfused.	You and your family will understand any tests that may be done after surgery.	The nurses will closely monitor your pulse (heart rate), blood pressure, the pressures in your heart, your breathing, your heart and lung sounds, how much urine is produced by your kidneys, and how much fluid/blood is draining from your chest tubes. A device will be placed on your finger/earlobe/toe that will measure the oxygen content of your blood. The next morning after surgery, a chest x-ray and a 12 lead EKG will be performed, and more blood will be drawn to check your blood count, clotting ability, and oxygen/carbon dioxide levels. Once you are moved to the telemetry floor, the nurses will continue to monitor your heart rate and rhythm.

DIET AND FLUIDS

Before		During		After	
Goal	Activities	Goal	Activities	Goal	Activities
You will take nothing by mouth at least 6 hours before surgery.	You may take nothing by mouth after midnight the night before your surgery. Your doctor or nurse will let you know if you can take your usual medications with a small sip of water the morning of the surgery. Most of the time, you will be allowed to take your heart medications.	You will not take anything by mouth during the surgery.	You will take nothing by mouth during the surgery. IV fluids will be continued. A tube will be placed in your stomach to keep your stomach empty and prevent vomiting while you are on the breathing machine (ventilator).	You will begin taking fluids and advance your diet slowly until you are eating a heart healthy diet.	Once your breathing tube and the tube in your stomach are removed, you will be able to take ice chips and sips of water. You will progress slowly to clear liquids, full liquids, and finally to a heart healthy diet. Slow progression is recommended.

mended to decrease stomach and intestinal discomfort. The IV fluids will be removed and the IV will be capped with a saline lock once you are taking fluids well. Few dietary restrictions are enforced in the first four to six weeks as you are healing from open heart surgery. However, as you recover completely, you should follow a heart healthy diet:

- limit your fat intake to less than 30% of your calories for the day
- limit your saturated fat intake to less than 10% of your calories for the day
- limit your cholesterol intake to less than 300 mg per day
- restrict calories if needed
- restrict salt if needed

You will see a dietitian before discharge.

One or two IV lines will be started in your arm and fluids will be given. A sedative will be given before the surgery to help you relax. However, you will still be awake.

ACTIVITY

Before		During		After	
Goal	Activities	Goal	Activities	Goal	Activities
You will conserve your energy until after your surgery.	You will be on bed rest or just up to go to the bathroom before surgery.	You will remain flat on the operating table during the procedure.	During the procedure, you will remain flat on the operating table.	You will gradually increase your activity until you have reached and/or surpassed your presurgery activity level. You will be referred to cardiac rehabilitation.	You will stay on bed rest until your breathing tube is removed (some hospitals will allow you to sit on the side of the bed and dangle your feet). You will begin a progressive exercise program. • first you will get up in the chair three times a day • next you will begin simple stretching exercises and walk around in your room • you will continue to increase how far you walk until you can walk 300 feet, three times a day

Coronary Artery Bypass Grafting Patient Education Outcome Pathway (continued)

ACTIVITY (continued)

Before		During		After	
Goal	Activities	Goal	Activities	Goal	Activities
					• you will walk up and down a flight of stairs prior to being discharged You will be visited by the cardiac rehabilitation staff. You will begin outpatient cardiac rehabilitation three times a week, three to six weeks after you are discharged from the hospital. You will have a low level stress test (treadmill) before you start an outpatient cardiac rehabilitation program. You will not be able to lift or pull anything heavier than 5–10 pounds for four to six weeks. It takes at least this long for the breastbone to set and begin to fuse together. Avoid lifting grocery bags, laundry baskets, young children, or pets. Purchase your milk or juice in half gallon containers (a full gallon weighs close to 10 pounds).

MEDICATIONS

Before		During		After	
Goal	Activities	Goal	Activities	Goal	Activities
You should be able to state the medications you take and why you take them.	The nurses and doctors will ask you what medications you currently take. Be sure to know the name and dosage of all your medications. You may want to bring them to the hospital with you.	You will be kept under anesthesia during the surgery.	Anesthesia will be given through the IV lines and the tube in your lungs during the procedure. The IV is maintained during and after the surgery in case medications must be given quickly.	You will be able to state your medications that you will take after discharge.	Some of your heart medications may be able to be stopped after open heart surgery. Some of the medications that help to keep your blood pressure normal, however, will need to be continued.

You should be able to take your medications the morning of your surgery with a small sip of water. Ask your doctor or nurse about this.

A sedative may be given either orally or through the IV line to help you relax before the surgery.

You will receive teaching about the medications you will take at home including:

- name
- dosage
- side effects
- special instructions

You will have a prescription for pain medication.

DISCHARGE PLANNING

Before		During		After	
Goal	Activities	Goal	Activities	Goal	Activities
We will begin planning for your discharge as soon as you are admitted.	The nurse will ask you about your home life when you are admitted. Let the nurse know if someone will be with you when you are discharged. It is recommended that someone stay with you at least two weeks after discharge.	Discharge planning will continue.	The nurses or social services department may talk to your family to ensure that you will have everything that you need after discharge.	You will understand the results of the surgery. You will understand care needed after discharge.	Make an appointment with your primary doctor, your cardiologist, and your surgeon as instructed for follow-up. Continue your exercise plan with daily stretches and walking. Gradually increase the distance you are walking. Cleanse your incisions with soap and water. Allow the steri-strips to come off your chest incision naturally. Call your surgeon if your incisions become extremely painful, red, have pus coming from them, or if you have a fever. Continue to wear your antithrombotic hose at night for at least two weeks. This helps your circulation while you are not as active as normal. Begin your cardiac rehabilitation program when instructed by your doctors. Ask questions if there is anything you do not understand. Ask for a phone number to call if you have questions after discharge.

Dysrhythmias

Patient Education Outcome Pathway

Dysrhythmias are abnormalities in the heart's rhythm. Normally, your heart beats 60–100 times a minute at a regular pace. It can be normal, however, to have a lower resting heart rate in a healthy individual. This is particularly common in an athlete.

Some of the more common causes of dysrhythmias are heart disease, side effects of medications (such as digoxin, stimulants, and beta-blockers), endocrine disorders (such as thyroid disease), and postoperative chest or heart surgery. It is very common for adults to have an occasional irregular heartbeat.

When the irregular heartbeats become too frequent, totally irregular, too fast or too slow, you will probably start feeling bad and seek treatment. The usual symptoms experienced are palpitations, chest pain, shortness of breath, and dizziness. Some tests are common to all dysrhythmias. Other tests, as well as treatments, are specific to one particular dysrhythmia, or to rhythms too slow or too fast.

TESTS AND PROCEDURES

Before		During		After	
Goal	Activities	Goal	Activities	Goal	Activities
You and your family will understand the tests that will be done before they are performed.	A 12 lead EKG will be done. EKG (or ECG) stands for *electrocardiogram.* An EKG records the electrical activity in your heart. It shows your heart rate and rhythm. It also shows any strain or damage to your heart. Blood will be drawn to determine your complete blood count (to check for anemia or infection), electrolytes (such as potassium), and measurement of cardiac enzymes released into your blood from damaged heart muscle. An echocardiogram may be performed. This test shows the chambers, valves, and movement of your heart. Your chest will need to be exposed, and a quiet, dimmed room is needed. It is an ultrasound of your heart. A Holter monitor may be used. This test records your heart rhythm continuously for 24 hours. The hair on your chest	You and your family will understand how the tests and procedures are performed.	A 12 lead EKG will be done. This test is not painful. Several sticky electrodes will be placed on your chest, arms, and legs. Cable wires are hooked to the electrodes, which are connected to the EKG machine. You will be asked to lie still until a rhythm without artifact (interference) can be detected on the machine. An EKG report will print out, and the electrodes will be removed from your body. Blood will be drawn from your arm for lab work. This procedure might produce discomfort during the needle stick. An echocardiogram will be done in a darkened, quiet room. This test is not painful. A transducer (like a microphone) is passed across your chest. It picks up sound waves and is then translated into a picture of your heart on a large monitor screen. It shows the chambers and valves of	You and your family will understand the interpretation of these tests and what happens after the cardiac procedure.	For the 12 lead EKG, blood tests, echocardiogram, and Holter monitor, you will be told if they are normal or abnormal and the significance of these abnormalities on your dysrhythmia. Your heart may be monitored continuously while you are in the hospital. After the EP study, your heart rate, rhythm, and pulses in your feet will be monitored closely. A 12 lead EKG will be done. You will be returned to a holding area or your room. You will lie flat in bed for 3–4 hours. You may raise the head of your bed 30 degrees after this time. The nurse will let you know when. You will have a tight bandage over your groin or catheter insertion site. If you need to cough or sneeze, apply pressure with your hand over the bandage. If you feel any warmth or wetness in the area, apply pressure and call

your heart and also how your heart is pumping. You will be asked to lie still during the test.

A Holter monitor may be worn. This test is not painful. Electrodes on your chest will be attached to wires from a portable heart monitor. Usually you wear the heart monitor for 24 hours. It will record your heart rhythm continuously. You will be asked to document in a diary your activities and any symptoms experienced, such as palpitations, chest discomfort, or dizziness. A cardiologist will then examine the recording and compare it to your activities and symptoms to see if any of your symptoms can be attributed to dysrhythmias.

An electrophysiology (EP) study may be done. You will be taken to a heart catheterization room. You will lie on a table during the procedure. Your heart rate, rhythm, blood pressure, and pulses in your feet will be monitored throughout the procedure. Your groin will be numbed with lidocaine, a medication similar to novocaine. This will burn or sting until the area is numb. The physician will make a small incision into the artery (usually in your groin) and thread a catheter into your heart. Your heart will be electrically stimulated in order to locate the irritable focus causing the dysrhythmia. Frequently this study is combined with treatment. The cardiologist can destroy the irritable focus by ablation therapy: the electrical path-

may need to be shaved or clipped to obtain good contact with the electodes.

A pacemaker may need to be inserted if your heart rate is too slow. This is a small device inserted below your collarbone that will keep your heart rate normal. In some cases, pacemakers are implanted to treat fast heart rhythms.

An electrophysiology study (EP study) may be performed. This test is done in the cardiac catheterization lab. Its purpose is to locate the irritable electrical focus in your heart that's causing your dysrhythmia. This test is not as common as the other tests because it is not needed for every dysrhythmia. The entry site for the catheter, usually the groin, will be washed with an antibacterial soap. The area may be shaved. One or two IV lines will be started. You will be given a sedative to help you relax.

An implantable defibrillator (cardioverter defibrillator) may need to be inserted for some serious dysrhythmias. A small device is implanted that will deliver shocks to your heart when dangerous rhythms occur. The incision site for insertion of the cardioverter defibrillator (usually below your left collarbone) will be washed with an antibacterial soap. You will be given a sedative to help you relax.

for a nurse. Also call for a nurse if you have any pain. You will need to avoid lifting anything over 10 pounds for one week. Your physician will discuss the findings of the study with you and let you know when you can return to work.

After a cardioverter defibrillator is implanted, your heart rate and rhythm will be monitored closely. Your breathing and blood pressure will also be monitored closely until you awaken fully and are stable. You will be returned to a holding area or your room. You will remain on bed rest until you are fully awake and can tolerate activity. Walking is usually well tolerated within 24 hours. Your arm may be immobilized up to 24 hours. Avoid above the shoulder arm movements for four weeks. Pain medication will be available to you if you need it. You will stay in the hospital for a few days after the device is implanted. The device will be tested before you leave the hospital.

Dysrhythmias Patient Education Outcome Pathway (continued)

TESTS AND PROCEDURE (continued)

Before		During		After	
Goal	Activities	Goal	Activities	Goal	Activities
			way of the irritable focus is destroyed. This procedure may take anywhere from a few minutes to several hours. Report any discomfort to the physician and/or nurse during the procedure. A cardioverter defibrillator may need to be implanted for some serious dysrhythmias. You will be taken to an operating room and will receive sedation and anesthesia prior to your procedure. Your heart rate, rhythm, breathing, and blood pressure will be monitored throughout the procedure. An incision will be made below your collarbone and the cardioverter defibrillator will be inserted under the skin.		

DIET AND FLUIDS

Before		During		After	
Goal	Activities	Goal	Activities	Goal	Activities
You will take food and fluids as tolerated. You will be on a heart healthy diet. You will take nothing by mouth for at least 6 hours before the electrophysiology study.	For dysrhythmias: You will be on clear liquids, a heart healthy diet, or a diabetic diet (if you are diabetic), depending on your rhythm disturbance. An IV will be started in your arm. You may or may not have IV fluids infusing through the IV line. Pain medication can be given by mouth or your IV line.	You will not take anything by mouth during any of the tests or procedures.	You will not take anything by mouth during any of the tests or procedures. An IV with or without fluids will be continued. Pain medication and medications to help you relax will be available to you through your IV line.	You will stay hydrated. You will continue a heart healthy diet.	You will take fluids to stay well hydrated. This is particularly important after the electrophysiology study. You should try to drink one glass of fluid every hour for several hours after the study. The nurse will let you know how much. Pain medication or sedation can be given by mouth or through your IV line.

You will eat a heart healthy or a diabetic diet (if you have diabetes):

- limit your fat intake to less than 30% of your total daily calories
- limit your saturated fat intake to less than 10% of your daily calories
- limit your cholesterol intake to less than 300 milligrams per day
- restrict calories if needed
- restrict salt if needed

For the electrophysiology study: You may take nothing by mouth for at least 6 hours before the procedure. Medications, especially the ones for dysrhythmias, may be withheld. A sedative will be given before and during the procedure to help you relax.

For the cardioverter defibrillator: You may take nothing by mouth for at least 6 hours before the procedure.

ACTIVITY

	Before		During		After
Goal	**Activities**	**Goal**	**Activities**	**Goal**	**Activities**
You will maintain an activity level as tolerated and as directed by tests.	You will need to stay on bed rest until your condition can be thoroughly assessed. Before an electrophysiology study and cardioverter defibrillator insertion, you will be placed on a stretcher and taken to a preparation area to get ready for your procedure.	You will maintain an activity level as tolerated and as directed by tests.	You can advance your activities as tolerated and as advised by your doctor and nurse. During a Holter monitor study, you will perform your usual activities. A diary will be given to you so you can document any symptoms, especially those similar to the ones that brought you into the hospital. You will wear this monitor for 24 hours. During an electrophysiology study, you will remain flat on your back on a hard table. If you have back discomfort, let the nurse know. Pain medication will be available. During a cardioverter defibrillator insertion, you will be kept under general anesthesia (asleep).	You will maintain an activity level as tolerated and as directed by tests. You will start an exercise program.	You can advance your activities as tolerated and as advised by your physician and nurse. After an electrophysiology study, you will remain flat in bed for several hours. A tight bandage will be applied to the catheter entry site (usually the groin). If you must cough or sneeze, place your hand over the bandage and apply pressure. You will be advised as to when you can get up. Do not get up the first time without help. Tell the nurse if you feel any dizziness, chest discomfort, or weakness with activity. After a cardioverter defibrillator is inserted, you will remain on bed rest until you are fully awake. The nurse will advise you as to when you can get up. Your response to activity will be monitored. Walking is usually well tolerated within 24 hours after the procedure. Your arm may be immobilized

Dysrhythmias Patient Education Outcome Pathway (continued)

ACTIVITY (continued)

Before		During		After	
Goal	Activities	Goal	Activities	Goal	Activities
					up to 24 hours. Avoid above the shoulder arm movements for four weeks. An ice bag may be applied over the incision. You may be referred to a cardiac rehabilitation program. When exercising at home, monitor your response to activity. Report any of the following to your doctor: • fast heart rate • irregular heart rate • palpitations • skipped beats • fainting • dizziness

MEDICATIONS

In the Emergency Room/At Time of Admission		During Your Hospital Stay		Before Discharge	
Goal	Activities	Goal	Activities	Goal	Activities
You will receive medications to treat your dysrhythmia.	You may receive the following types of medications: • oxygen • digoxin: This drug causes your heart to beat stronger and more efficiently. Because it also lowers your heart rate, your pulse will be monitored so the desired rate is achieved. Your potassium level will also be checked, since a low potassium level could cause the digoxin level to rise in your blood, potentially leading to dysrhythmias. Digoxin is	You will receive medications during your hospital stay to treat your dysrhythmia.	You may receive the following medications while you are in the hospital: • oxygen • digoxin • beta-blockers • calcium channel blockers • antidysrhythmics • sedatives	You will be able to state the name of your medications and why you need them during your hospitalization. You will be able to state the name of your medications upon discharge, how much to take, major side effects, and drug interactions.	The nurse and physician will provide education regarding your medications. You will be asked to repeat back information regarding your medications, including the name of your medications and why they were prescribed. In addition, you will be asked to state the major side effects and interactions of the medications you take on a routine basis and those on discharge.

frequently used for dysrhythmias with rapid heart rates and in certain kinds of congestive heart failure.

- Beta-blockers: These drugs reduce the amount of work on the heart and suppress dysrhythmias. They are commonly used for angina, high blood pressure, dysrhythmias, and after a heart attack.
- Calcium channel blockers: These drugs reduce how hard the heart pumps and they slow your heart rate. They also suppress dysrhythmias. They are used for high blood pressure, dysrhythmias, and certain types of angina.
- Antidysrhythmics: These drugs suppress abnormal rhythms.

Medications may be given either orally or through an IV.

DISCHARGE PLANNING

	Before		During		After	
	Goal	Activities	Goal	Activities	Goal	Activities
	You will begin planning your discharge with the hospital staff upon admission.	The nurse will ask you about your home life and plans for care after discharge. Let the nurse know early if you will need the social services department to help you coordinate your care after discharge.	Discharge planning will continue.	You will be discharged from the hospital when your heart rhythm and condition are stable.	You will understand the results of tests and procedures performed in the hospital. You will understand care and further tests needed after discharge.	Make an appointment with your physician for follow-up as instructed by your physician. Maintain a heart healthy diet as described earlier. Gradually increase your activity as advised by your physician. After an electrophysiology study, you will need to avoid lifting over 10 pounds for at least one week and take stairs slowly. The physician will let you know when you can return to work.

Dysrhythmias Patient Education Outcome Pathway (continued)

DISCHARGE PLANNING (continued)

Before		During		After	
Goal	Activities	Goal	Activities	Goal	Activities
					After a cardioverter defibrillator insertion, you will need to avoid lifting over 5 pounds for four weeks and to avoid above the shoulder arm movements for four weeks. You will also need to avoid driving. The physician will discuss the schedule with you.
					You may be referred to a cardiac rehabilitation program.
					Ask questions if you do not understand something.
					Keep a list of your medications, health problems, and any major procedures and surgeries in your wallet or purse.
					Ask your physician if you need to wear a Medic-Alert bracelet.
					Learn how to take your heart rate.
					Call your physician or go the emergency department if your dysrhythmia symptoms occur again.

Interventional Cardiology

Patient Education Outcome Pathway

During a percutaneous transluminal coronary angioplasty (PTCA) (balloon) procedure, a balloon-tipped catheter is placed into the area of blockage in one of the arteries of the heart. The balloon is inflated. This pushes the blockage up against the wall of the artery, thus creating a larger opening for blood flow.

An atherectomy (cutter) procedure uses a catheter with a small cutting device on the end. The cutter is placed into the area of blockage in one of the arteries of the heart. The cutter then slices away at the blockage, thus removing it entirely. With a few of the devices, the blockage is actually removed. With another device, the blockage is pulverized into small particles (smaller than a red blood cell) and released into the bloodstream.

A laser angioplasty procedure uses a catheter with lasing ability to create a larger passage through the blockage in one of the arteries of the heart.

A coronary stent is a small metal cage that is placed into an artery of the heart after it has been opened with one of the procedures just described. The stent is placed into the area to help it stay open.

PROCEDURE

Before		During		After	
Goal	Activities	Goal	Activities	Goal	Activities
You will understand what happens before the procedure.	The entry site for the catheter, usually the groin but may be the arm, will be washed with an antibacterial soap. The area may be shaved. One or two IV lines will be started in your arm. You will be given a sedative to help you relax, but you will still be awake.	You will understand what happens during the procedure.	The doctor will numb the area with a medication called xylocaine or lidocaine (similar to novacaine). This will burn until the area is numb. The doctor will make a small hole into the artery and will thread several catheters (hollow tubes) into your heart. You may be asked to cough, hold your breath, or turn your head to the left or right. For a balloon angioplasty: • A balloon-tipped catheter will be inserted into the artery. • Dye will be injected. • The balloon will be inflated several times from a few seconds to a few minutes to help push the area of plaque or blockage against the walls of the artery. • You may have some chest discomfort when the balloon is inflated. If you do, just let the nurse know. Pain medication will be available.	You will understand what happens after the cardiac procedure.	You will be returned to either the holding area or your room. You will stay flat in bed for 3–4 hours. You may raise the head of your bed 30 degrees after this time period. The nurse will let you know. You will have a tight bandage over the tubes in your leg. If you need to cough or sneeze, apply pressure with your hand over the bandage. If you feel a sensation of warmth or wetness, apply pressure with your hand over the bandage and call for the nurse. You must stay in bed while the sheaths (tubes) are in place and for several hours after they are removed. This will help prevent bleeding. You must keep your leg straight and still. Before the sheaths are removed, the nurse will give you some medication to help you relax. After they are removed, pres-

Interventional Cardiology Patient Education Outcome Pathway (continued)

PROCEDURE (continued)

Before		During		After
Goal	Activities	Goal	Activities	Activities
			For an atherectomy or cutter procedure:	sure will be applied by the nurse either manually or with a small machine. You must remain quiet. Pressure may be applied up to 1 hour to help prevent bleeding.
			• A balloon-tipped catheter with a small cutter on the end will be inserted into the artery.	A tight bandage will be applied once the tubes are removed.
			• Dye will be injected.	The nurse will check your heart rate, blood pressure, and the pulses in your legs frequently for several hours.
			• The cutter will be turned on several times and moved across the area of blockage. You will hear a sound similar to a dentist's drill. Several cuts are needed to remove the blockage.	You will be encouraged to drink lots of fluids, about one glass an hour for several hours.
			• You may have some chest discomfort when the cutter is on. If you do, just tell the nurse. Pain medication will be available.	Pain medication will be available.
				If you have any chest discomfort, let the nurse know immediately.
			• The blockage either will be removed or it may be crushed into small particles the size of red blood cells and released into the bloodstream.	You will be able to get out of bed a few hours after the sheaths are removed. Ask for help the first time you get up.
			For a laser angioplasty:	Most patients go home the next day.
			• A laser catheter will be inserted into the artery.	Avoid lifting over 10 pounds for one week.
			• You and the cath lab staff will wear special goggles to protect your eyes from the laser.	Take stairs slowly.
				The doctor will let you know when you can return to work.
			• Dye will be injected.	
			• The laser will be turned on and passed through the area of blockage several times to open the artery. You will hear a loud clicking sound.	
			• After the laser procedure is done, the doctor may decide	

to follow it with a balloon angioplasty. A small balloon-tipped catheter will be threaded into the area of blockage and inflated several times anywhere from a few seconds to a few minutes. This pushes the remaining blockage up against the walls of the artery.

- You may have some chest discomfort when the laser is on and/or with balloon inflations. Just tell the nurse if you do. Pain medication will be available.

For a stent:

- Sometimes after any of the procedures just described, a small stent or metal cage will be placed into the artery. The stent is placed to help prevent the artery from closing.
- The stent is placed on a balloon-tipped catheter. This catheter is then threaded into the area of blockage in the artery.
- The balloon is inflated, thus pushing the stent next to the walls of the artery. When the balloon is deflated, the stent remains in place.
- You may have some chest discomfort during the stent placement. If you do, just tell the nurse. Pain medication will be available.

Sometimes, one or more of the procedures just described may be performed depending on your condition.

When the doctor has the artery open, he or she will remove the catheters but will leave the tubes in your leg. They will stay in place for several hours.

Interventional Cardiology Patient Education Outcome Pathway (continued)

PROCEDURE (continued)

Before		During		After	
Goal	Activities	Goal	Activities	Goal	Activities
			A tight bandage will be placed on the tubes in your leg and you will be returned to either the holding area or your room. You may be given some pictures that show the area of blockage both before and after your procedure.		

TESTS

Before		During		After	
Goal	Activities	Goal	Activities	Goal	Activities
You and your family will understand the tests that will be done before your cardiac procedure.	Blood will be drawn to determine your complete blood cell count, clotting studies, electrolytes, and blood type. You may have a chest x-ray. An EKG will be done. You may be asked to provide a urine sample.	You will understand any tests that may be done during the cardiac procedure.	Your heart rate, rhythm, and blood pressure will be monitored throughout the entire procedure. Pressures inside your heart will be recorded during the procedure. The oxygen content in your blood will be monitored with a small sensor placed on one of your toes, fingers, or earlobes. The pulses in your feet will be checked frequently. Blood will be drawn through the sheaths (tubes) in your leg to monitor how well your blood is clotting. It is important to keep your blood thin during the procedure in an effort to prevent blood clots from forming.	You and your family will understand any tests that may be done after the cardiac procedure.	An EKG will be done after the procedure. Another may be repeated the morning after the procedure. Blood will be drawn to check your blood count, clotting studies, and cardiac enzymes two or three times after the procedure (usually every 6–8 hours for two times, but this routine varies from hospital to hospital and doctor to doctor). Your heart rate and rhythm will be monitored closely after the procedure.

DIET AND FLUIDS

Before		During		After	
Goal	Activities	Goal	Activities	Goal	Activities
You will take nothing by mouth for at least 6 hours before the procedure.	You may take nothing by mouth after midnight the night before your procedure. If your procedure is scheduled for later in the day, you may be able to have a clear liquid breakfast. Your doctor or nurse will let you know.

Your doctor or nurse will let you know if you can take your usual medications with a small sip of water the morning of the procedure. Most of the time, you will be allowed to take your heart medications.

One or two IV lines will be started in your arm and fluids given.

A sedative will be given before the procedure to help you relax. However, you will still be awake.

If you have not had an aspirin that day, one will be given to you before the procedure if you are able to take aspirin.

If stent placement is planned, you may be given other medications to help keep your blood from clotting before the procedure. | You will not take anything by mouth during the procedure. | You will still take nothing by mouth during the procedure. However, you may be given some medication to take with a small sip of water if needed. This usually includes a calcium channel blocker and some medications to help prevent blood clots from forming during the procedure. You may also be given some medication to dissolve under your tongue.

IV fluids will be continued.

Medications to help you relax will be given though the IV in your arm.

Pain medication will be available and can be given through your IV line. | You will begin taking fluids in order to stay well hydrated and to help flush the dye from your system.

You will progress to a heart healthy diet as tolerated. | You should drink at least 8 ounces of fluid per hour for 6–8 hours after the procedure unless your doctor or nurse tells you otherwise.

The IV will be removed once you are taking fluids well.

You should drink extra fluids for several days after the procedure unless your doctor or nurse tells you otherwise.

You will be able to eat after the procedure.

You should follow a heart healthy diet:
• limit your fat intake to less than 30% of your calories for the day
• limit your saturated fat intake to less than 10% of your calories for the day
• limit your cholesterol intake to less than 300 mg per day
• restrict calories if needed
• restrict salt if needed |

Interventional Cardiology Patient Education Outcome Pathway *(continued)*

ACTIVITY

Before		During		After	
Goal	Activities	Goal	Activities	Goal	Activities
You should maintain your current activity level before the procedure.	Maintain your current activity level before the procedure as advised by your doctor. You will be placed on a stretcher in the preparation area to start getting ready for your procedure.	You will remain flat during the procedure.	During the procedure, you will remain flat on your back on a hard table. If you have back discomfort, let the nurse know. Pain medication will be available.	You will remain flat and in bed for several hours after the procedure. You will return to your preprocedure activity level. You may be referred to a cardiac rehabilitation program.	You will remain flat for several hours after the procedure (according to hospital protocol) during the time the sheaths are in your leg and for several hours after they are removed to prevent bleeding. After 3 or 4 hours, you may be able to raise the head of the bed 30 degrees. A tight bandage will be applied to the entry site (usually the groin). When the sheaths are removed, pressure to help stop the bleeding may be applied by the nurse or with a small machine. You will be given medication to make you more comfortable during this time. If you must cough or sneeze, place your hand over the bandage and apply pressure. If you feel a sensation of wetness or warmth at the bandage, apply pressure and call for the nurse. You may have a 5 pound sandbag over the bandage for several hours. You will walk about 4–6 hours after the sheaths are removed. You will need assistance your first time up. Do not get up the first time without help. After you have walked the first time, you may have bathroom privileges. Tell the nurse if you feel any dizziness, chest discomfort, or weakness with activity. You may begin an exercise program upon the recommendation of your doctor. You may be referred to a cardiac rehabilitation program.

MEDICATIONS

	Before		During		After	
	Goal	Activities	Goal	Activities	Goal	Activities
	You should be able to state your medications to the doctor and the nurse before your procedure.	The nurse and doctor will ask you about your medications. Be sure to know the name and dosage of all your medications. You may want to bring them to the hospital with you. You should be able to take your medications the morning of the procedure with a small sip of water. Ask your doctor or nurse about this. One or two IV lines will be started in your arm. A sedative may be given either orally or through the IV to help you relax before the procedure. Other medications to help prevent blood cloting may also be given. If you have not had an aspirin the morning of your procedure, one will be given to you if you are able to take aspirin without problems.	You will be kept as comfortable as possible during the procedure.	If needed, a sedative or pain medication may be given through the IV lines during the procedure. The IV is also maintained in case medications must be given to you quickly. Blood thinners may also be given through the IV lines during the procedure. You may be given some medication during the procedure to swallow with a small sip of water. Other medications may be placed under your tongue to dissolve.	You will be able to state your medications before discharge.	The IVs will be removed when you start drinking fluids. You will receive teaching about the medications you will take at home. Most people will go home on a calcium channel blocker (to lessen the workload of the heart) and an aspirin a day. You will probably take one aspirin a day for the rest of your life. If you have had a stent placed, you will be on other medications to help keep your blood from clotting. These medications are usually taken for at least four weeks. Report any chest discomfort to the nurse or doctor. You may have a prescription for pain medication if needed.

DISCHARGE PLANNING

	Before		During		After	
	Goal	Activities	Goal	Activities	Goal	Activities
	You will begin planning your discharge as soon as you are admitted.	The nurse will ask you about your home life when you are admitted. Let the nurse know if someone will be with you when you are discharged.	Discharge planning will continue.	You may be discharged from the hospital the day after your procedure.	You will understand the results of the procedure. You will understand care needed after discharge.	Make an appointment with your doctor as instructed for follow-up. Maintain a heart healthy diet. Gradually increase your activity. You may be referred to a cardiac rehabilitation program. The doctor will discuss the results of the procedure with you and your family.

Interventional Cardiology Patient Education Outcome Pathway *(continued)*

DISCHARGE PLANNING (continued)

Before		During		After	
Goal	Activities	Goal	Activities	Goal	Activities
					The doctor will discuss future care with you and your family.
					Ask questions if you do not understand something.
					Ask for a phone number to call if you have questions after discharge.
					Plan to have someone stay with you the day you are going home.
					Report any chest discomfort after you are discharged to your doctor. There is a small chance that the artery may close again.
					It is very important for you to modify your risk factors for heart disease to help prevent further blockages from occurring:
					• follow a heart healthy diet
					• do not smoke
					• exercise regularly
					• take any medications for high blood pressure or diabetes
					• lose weight if applicable
					• learn to manage stress

Kidney Transplant

Patient Education Outcome Pathway

Kidney transplant surgery is a very important and emotional time for you and your family. It is your chance to return to a more normal life. Transplantation is not a cure. It is a form of treatment for kidney failure. You will no longer need dialysis or a strict diet, and you will have more energy. You will need to take antirejection medications for the entire time you have a functioning kidney transplant or you will reject your kidney. You will also have to be careful to prevent infections that your body may not be able to fight due to the antirejection drugs. Most important for you and your family is to take an active role in your health care so you will be prepared for your new life.

TESTS

Before		During		After	
Goal	Activities	Goal	Activities	Goal	Activities
You and your family will understand the tests that will be done to ensure you are physically and mentally ready for a kidney transplant.	A health history and physical examination will be done by the transplant team. Blood will be drawn as baseline information or to rule out pre-existing disease by the following: • complete blood cell count: measures your white and red blood cells and your platelets • clotting studies: PT, PTT, and Ivy bleeding time; measures your body's ability to stop bleeding • electrolytes: potassium, sodium, and chloride; calcium, magnesium, and phosphorous • kidney function test: blood urea nitrogen (BUN) and creatinine (Scr) • liver and parathyroid function tests Blood will also be drawn to evaluate for possible infection with the following: VDRL, HIV, hepatitis screening, and viral titers.	You will understand the tests being used to monitor the kidney transplant during hospitalization.	The day of the transplant you will be called to the hospital. Again, several different tests will need to be done to determine if you are physically ready for a transplant: • medical history • urine sample to check for infection • chest x-ray • EKG • a lot of blood tests including a final cross match with the donor kidney's blood to determine if the kidney is compatible to put in your body Every day after the transplant the following tests will be monitored: • REP or SMA-7, which includes creatinine, BUN, sodium, chloride, potassium, carbon dioxide, and blood sugar. The most important in watching the kidney functioning is creatinine and BUN. A normal creatinine level is around	You will understand the tests being used to monitor your kidney transplant after discharge.	The routine tests used to monitor your health and the functioning of the kidney are blood tests. Usually blood tests will be drawn twice weekly for the first three to six months. The tests drawn are an SMA-18 (which include the BUN and creatinine), CBC, and immunosuppression drug levels (either cyclosporine or Prograf). As the kidney function and drug levels stabilize, blood tests will be changed to weekly and then to monthly at about a year. If the blood tests show any decline in kidney function, the blood tests could be done more often and other diagnostic tests would be ordered.

Kidney Transplant Patient Education Outcome Pathway (continued)

TESTS (continued)

	Before		During		After
Goal	Activities	Goal	Activities	Goal	Activities
	Blood drawn for immunologic tests that determine whether your body will accept the new kidney with the help of immunosuppressive drugs are ABO typing, tissue typing, and antibody screening. These tests will be done on a regular basis until you receive a transplant.		1.0 and BUN level is 20–27. After the transplant these do not return to normal immediately but will decrease each day until they equalize out to a level that is normal for your transplanted kidney. For example, your creatinine may go to 1.6 at the lowest and this is your normal level.		
	EKG to check your heart rhythm.		• Immunosuppression drug levels (cyclosporine or Prograf) will be drawn to make sure your body is getting enough of the drug but not too much.		
	Chest x-ray to check your lungs for infection and fluid.				
	You may have a barium enema, upper GI, and/or gallbladder ultrasound.		A kidney ultrasound may be done the day after surgery and periodically thereafter. This evaluates the size and shape of the kidney and measures the flow of blood through the vessels that supply blood to the kidney.		
	You will be evaluated for different forms of infection by urine, sputum, and nose cultures. You will be checked for fungal skin tests; TB, mumps, and candida.				
	A voiding cystourethrogram is an x-ray test to check the connections from your bladder to your kidney and the ability of the bladder to empty completely.		A renal scan is usually done the day after surgery as a baseline study. This is a special x-ray study of the transplanted kidney. A dye is injected into a vein and pictures are taken of the kidney to see how well it is working.		
	A dental evaluation and possible dental x-rays will be done to find any possible source of infection in your mouth.		A chest x-ray will be done periodically.		
	A psychological evaluation will be performed by a professional with the transplant team to make sure you can handle the responsibility of a kidney transplant.		If the kidney doesn't start to work or work well enough according to the transplant doctor, a kidney biopsy may be performed. This procedure		
	Other tests may be done depending on your individual needs.				

DIET AND FLUIDS

Before		During		After	
Goal	Activities	Goal	Activities	Goal	Activities
You will be adequately nourished so your body is in the best condition possible to receive a kidney transplant.	Your need for a change in diet will depend on how much kidney function you still have and on what form of dialysis you choose: hemodialysis or peritoneal dialysis. With either choice a dietitian will set up an individualized plan for you. If you are on hemodialysis, the following are general guidelines: • Protein: 1 g/kg of body weight per day. The majority of this protein needs to come from high biological value protein: meat, poultry, fish, eggs, and milk. This form of protein is more efficiently used by the body and doesn't leave as much waste product. The waste products are measured in your blood by the BUN test. • Calories: You need 35 kcal/kg body weight per day. Due to the other restrictions in the diet, this can be done by eating more sugars and fats. • Sodium: Sodium is restricted by not eating foods high in salt and by not adding table salt to food. Salt can make	You will be adequately nourished and hydrated.	When you are notified that a kidney is available you will not eat or drink anything until after the surgery. After surgery, you will have clear liquids for a few days. Then, depending on how well the kidney is functioning, you will go either on the renal diet or transplant diet. The renal diet would again restrict the amounts of protein and salt. The transplant diet is as follows: • High in protein (especially high biological value protein) to help your muscles and skin tone. • Low sodium to prevent fluid retention in the tissues and high blood pressure. • Restricted in sugar and carbohydrates to prevent weight gain and high blood sugar. • Low in fat to prevent excessive weight gain. • High in phosphorus, magnesium, and calcium. Obtainable by eating two to three low fat dairy products per day and eating whole grain breads, nuts, dried beans, and peas.	You will be adequately nourished and hydrated.	With your kidney function in a normal range, drink a lot of fluids daily. Follow the transplant diet or the diet individually prescribed for you.

requires inserting a needle into the kidney with the help of an x-ray camera. Then a piece of the kidney tissue is examined under a microscope to determine the condition of the kidney.

Kidney Transplant Patient Education Outcome Pathway (continued)

DIET AND FLUIDS

Before		During		After	
Goal	Activities	Goal	Activities	Goal	Activities
	the body crave water as well as hold it in the tissue. Use spices and herbs instead for flavoring. • Fluids: You need to measure your urine output for a full 24 hours. Your fluid intake should be restricted to 500–800 mL, or 17–27 ounces plus your urine output per day. Weigh yourself every morning after you first void; you should gain 1 to 2 pounds per day. • Potassium: You are usually restricted to 40 to 50 mEq daily of potassium. Foods high in potassium are protein foods, citrus fruits, beans, potatoes, and nuts. Don't use salt substitutes, which are high in potassium. • Phosphorus: You will also have to restrict food high in phosphorus. Protein and dairy products have the highest levels. Since all cannot be eliminated you will be ordered by the kidney doctor to take a phosphate binder medication *with* meals. • Calcium supplements may be necessary. • Vitamins will be prescribed for you by the kidney doctor to replace the water soluble vitamins that are washed away with each hemodialysis treatment.		Calories are only restricted if you have excessive weight gain over your ideal body weight. Again, a dietitian should develop an individualized plan and discuss it with you.		

- Iron and folate supplements may be necessary if you are anemic.

If you are on peritoneal dialysis the dietary restrictions are more liberal:

- Protein: 1.2 to 1.5 g/kg per day, majority of high biological value protein.
- Calories: 35 to 40 kcal/kg body weight per day.
- Sodium and fluid: Same as with a hemodialysis patient.
- Potassium: No restrictions, unless, after time, lab work shows an increase in the potassium level. Then a restriction is indicated by doctor and dietitian.
- Phosphorous and vitamin supplementation: Same as with a hemodialysis patient.

The most important aspect for you is to talk with a dietitian at the dialysis center and obtain an individualized plan that you understand and can follow.

This is an area of your care where you are in control. If you follow the diet and fluid restrictions, you will tolerate dialysis better and your body will be in good shape for your transplant.

ACTIVITY

Before		During		After	
Goal	Activities	Goal	Activities	Goal	Activities
You will be in the best physical condition possible before your transplant.	Discuss with your kidney doctor about starting an exercise program. After the doctor states you can start exercising, determine what kind of program you will do at least three times a week.	You will obtain optimal mobility by discharge.	Your first day postsurgery you will be on bed rest but will be turned every 2 hours. Usually by the second day you will be getting up in a chair with assistance.	You will obtain optimal physical condition over weeks and months post-transplant.	Follow the walking program provided by the transplant program. After three to four weeks at home you may resume driving.

Kidney Transplant Patient Education Outcome Pathway (continued)

ACTIVITY (continued)

	Before		During		After
Goal	Activities	Goal	Activities	Goal	Activities
	You can start a stretching and walking program at home. If you experience chest pain or shortness of breath while walking, stop, sit down, and rest. Notify your doctor as soon as possible. If you need a more structured program to give you incentive to continue, you can check with the local hospital about Phase III Cardiac Rehabilitation. These programs have treadmills and exercise bicycles. There are nurses available if you have any problems. You could also check into a health club program.		You will increase activity each day and be walking in the hall at least 100 feet several times without assistance before you are discharged from the hospital.		When your doctor approves, you can work back into your pre-transplant exercise program and probably improve upon it with time. An exercise program is very important post-transplant for physical and psychological benefits. Many of the drugs you will be taking will cause increased body weight and a change in where your fat is deposited. A lot is placed in your face and can give you an entirely different look. With weight control and exercise, this can be minimized over time.

MEDICATIONS

	Before		During		After
Goal	Activities	Goal	Activities	Goal	Activities
You should be able to state your medications to the doctor and nurse before your surgery.	The nurse and doctor will ask you about all your medications. Bring an exact list with name and dosage or bring all your medications to the hospital with you. You won't be eating or drinking at this time. The doctor will order the medications he or she wants you to take with a small amount of water until surgery. At least one IV line will be started in your arm.	You will be asleep and your body will be kept stable during surgery.	An anesthesiologist will put you to sleep and monitor your blood pressure, heart rate, oxygen level, and level of sedation throughout the surgery. Medications will be given during surgery to keep all of the above stable.	You and/or your family will be able to follow a medication chart correctly before discharge and will understand the dosage and purpose of all medications.	Usually transplant programs will give you a medication administration record to assist you in keeping track of your medications and when to take them. Once you start feeling better, a few days after surgery, start asking what medication you are receiving and why. Antirejection or immunosuppressive drugs are the most important medications you will be taking to help your body

---

accept your new kidney. The body thinks of the new kidney as foreign tissue. These drugs help your body accept the new kidney by decreasing your body's natural response to attack foreign tissue. *You must take these every day exactly as you are taught or you will reject your new kidney.* The next section lists antirejection drugs with their most common side effects.

Prednisone

Dose Adjusted according to your weight, length of time after transplant, how well your transplant is doing, and the other antirejection drugs used in combination.

Side Effects
- increased appetite with weight gain and fat deposits that can cause a round face and puffy cheeks
- emotional changes
- stomach pain or burning
- swelling from salt and water retention
- acne
- increased chance of infection

Imuran

Dose Adjusted according to your white blood cell count and weight.

Side Effects
- decrease in white blood cells and platelets, which lowers resistance to infections
- increased risk of viral diseases such as mouth ulcers or shingles

Just before going to surgery several IV medications will be given to prepare your body for surgery. They may consist of the following:
- Imuran and Solu-Medrol: both immunosuppressive or antirejection drugs
- Zantac or Tagamet: to prevent ulcers
- an antibiotic: to prevent infection

Kidney Transplant Patient Education Outcome Pathway (continued)

MEDICATIONS (continued)

	Before		During		After
Goal	Activities	Goal	Activities	Goal	Activities

Cyclosporine

Dose Prescribed in 25 mg and 100 mg capsules. Amount is ordered according to blood levels.

When to take
- a.m. dose: in the morning with breakfast
- p.m. dose: 12 hours after the morning dose
- food appears to increase absorption, so cyclosporine needs to be taken with food

Measuring blood levels
- Do not take your cyclosporine dose until after you have your blood drawn
- Dosage amounts vary with each patient and your dose will be adjusted on the level of drug in your blood

Side Effects
- fine hand tremors, which need to be reported to the transplant team
- swollen gums
- excessive hair growth
- high blood pressure
- kidney damage
- increase in potassium

You may be put on Calan SR in conjunction with cyclosporine because it has been shown that by taking both drugs the amount of cyclosporine needed can be lowered.

A combination of prednisone, Imuran, and cyclosporine will most commonly be used as your antirejection medications.

Prograf (FK506)

Dose Prescribed in 1 mg or 5 mg capsules. Amount is ordered according to blood levels.

Relatively new drug that was developed to be used with liver transplants and has started to be used with kidney transplants.

Side Effects

- tremors
- headache
- insomnia
- diarrhea
- hypertension
- nausea
- kidney damage

When Prograf is used, you will not be on cyclosporine. The antirejection drug combination will be prednisone, Imuran, and Prograf.

All side effects need to be reported to the transplant team so they can monitor how the drug regimen is affecting you.

The following medications are given post-transplant to prevent different infections that the antirejection medications make you more prone to catch.

Mycostatin (nystatin)

Purpose To prevent a fungal or yeast infection in your mouth commonly known as thrush.

Dose 5 mL or one teaspoon four times a day. Taken for the first six months after a transplant.

When to take After meals and at bedtime. Swish and hold in your mouth 5 minutes and then swallow.

Side Effects

- constipation, diarrhea, and nausea

Kidney Transplant Patient Education Outcome Pathway (continued)

MEDICATIONS (continued)

Before		During		After	
Goal	Activities	Goal	Activities	Goal	Activities
					Bactrim SS (trimethoprim sulfur)
					Purpose Prevents lung and urinary tract infections.
					Dose Usually one a day for the first six months after transplant.
					Side Effects
					• nausea, vomiting, and diarrhea
					• increased sensitivity to the sun
					• lowered white blood cell count
					Zovirax (acyclovir)
					Purpose To prevent viral infections.
					Dose 800 mg four times per day for the first three months or as ordered by your doctor. The dosage may be lowered if kidney function is not within normal limits for a transplanted kidney.
					Side Effects
					• nausea, vomiting, and diarrhea
					Other medications usually given are as follows:
					Zantac
					Purpose To prevent ulcers.
					Dose 150 mg two times a day.
					Multivitamin supplement twice a day.
					Then other medications may be given, depending on your particular needs.

The easiest way to keep track of your medication and when to take it is to follow the medication administration record. Then set up pill boxes by the time of day each medication is taken.

Remember: if you have any questions, call the transplant nurse who is available 24 hours a day.

PROCEDURE/HOSPITALIZATION

Before		During		After	
Goal	Activities	Goal	Activities	Goal	Activities
You will understand what happens before the transplant.	You will be called any time of the day or night when a kidney becomes available and asked to come to the hospital where the transplant is to be performed. Tests will be performed to determine if you are physically ready for the transplant. Blood tests will be done to determine if the kidney is compatible with your body. You may receive dialysis. If you are on peritoneal dialysis, bring in supplies for two or three exchanges so you may continue dialysis until surgery. You will not be allowed anything to eat or drink until it is decided if you will have the transplant. An IV will be started and just before surgery you will receive medication to make you sleepy.	You will understand what will happen during your surgery.	You will be given medication to put you to sleep for your surgery. Usually the surgery takes 3 or 4 hours. An incision is made on either the right or left side of your lower abdomen. This area is selected because it offers a good blood supply and because the kidney is somewhat protected by the large pelvis bone. Often the kidney begins to make urine immediately, but it is not unusual for it to take some time before it begins to work.	You will understand what happens after the surgery.	After you wake up you will be in the recovery room or the intensive care unit. You will be in the intensive care unit for one or two days. During the first one or two days, vital signs (blood pressure, pulse, respirations, and temperature), blood tests, fluid input, and urine output will be monitored frequently. You will have a special IV called a central line in place near your shoulder where the nurses will measure readings in your heart to determine if you need fluid or if you need fluid removed. The central line will be monitored with your other vital signs. A catheter in your bladder will keep an accurate record of how much urine you are making. Your urine will be pink in color and there may be clots. You will probably have a continuous bladder irrigation connected to the catheter to remove the blood and clots so that the clots do not stop up

Kidney Transplant Patient Education Outcome Pathway (continued)

PROCEDURE/HOSPITALIZATION (continued)

Before		During		After	
Goal	Activities	Goal	Activities	Goal	Activities
					the catheter. You may feel some bladder spasms as long as the catheter is in place. Medication will be available to relieve discomfort from the spasms. The catheter is usually removed five to seven days after the surgery.
					You will be on oxygen either by face mask or nasal cannula, which will be tapered off as you improve after surgery.
					You will be expected to begin coughing and deep breathing and using the incentive spirometer while in the recovery room to prevent pneumonia. The incentive spirometer measures how much air you can inhale. You will be taught to take a deep breath, hold your breath for 5 seconds, then exhale very slowly. This will cause some discomfort, but you will have pain medication available to you. You can reduce the discomfort by holding a pillow over the incision area while attempting to deep breathe or cough.
					You will be started on the medications as previously discussed in the medication section.
					After you move out of the ICU, you will be moved to a regular hospital room. A semiprivate room is fine as long as your roommate does not have an infectious disease and your

white blood cell count is not low.

Everything done in ICU will continue to be done but less often, and by the end of the hospital stay you will be responsible for monitoring intake and output (I & O) and vital signs (blood pressure, temperature, and heart rate), since you will need to do it at home.

When stomach and bowel function return, you will start on a clear liquid diet and advance up to a renal transplant diet as described under Diet and Fluids.

You will be weighed daily before breakfast. It is important to weigh in the morning after voiding with the same clothes. Weight gain can be one of the signs of rejection of your new kidney.

Periodically you will be asked to collect a clean catch urine specimen to watch for infection. To obtain a clean catch urine specimen, clean yourself with an antiseptic pad, urinate a small amount in the toilet, then collect the rest of your urine in a specimen container that will be sent to the lab.

A 24 hour urine collection may be done at some time before going home to test kidney function along with the daily blood test.

You may also have an ultrasound and renal scan of the transplanted kidney done before discharge.

You will be monitored for signs and symptoms of "acute" rejection, since you are at highest risk for this to occur in the first three months. The signs of acute rejection are as follows:

Kidney Transplant Patient Education Outcome Pathway (continued)

PROCEDURE/HOSPITALIZATION (continued)

Before		During		After	
Goal	Activities	Goal	Activities	Goal	Activities
					• tenderness or pain over your kidney
					• a flu-like "ache" feeling
					• swelling in hands and legs
					• fever over 100°F
					• sudden increase in weight
					• blood pressure goes up
					• urine output goes down
					• blood creatinine goes up
					Some of the signs can still be related to your surgery, but if you have any doubt ask the transplant nurse or doctor.
					You will also be closely monitored the entire hospitalization for signs and symptoms of infection. The antirejection medications weaken the immune system to prevent rejection but also make you more prone to infection. The transplant team will monitor you for the following signs of infection:
					• fever over 100°F
					• flulike symptoms
					• cough or shortness of breath
					• sore throat
					• nausea, vomiting, and/or diarrhea
					• pain over transplant site
					• urgency, frequency, or burning with urination
					• redness, swelling, or drainage at the incision site
					Visitors at the hospital and in your home the first month

should be limited to your immediate family. For the first three to six months, try as much as possible to avoid crowds and avoid people with infectious conditions.

DISCHARGE PLANNING

Before		During		After	
Goal	Activities	Goal	Activities	Goal	Activities
You will begin planning your discharge as soon as you are admitted.	The nurse will ask about several different aspects of your home life on admission. You need to have someone with you for the first three to four weeks after discharge because you cannot drive for this period of time. You may need help caring for yourself.	Discharge planning will continue.	You will usually be in the hospital at least seven days, but the length of stay is different for each patient. Your length of stay depends on how soon the kidney works and how your body responds to the kidney and your new medications. You will become more responsible each day for keeping your own intake and output, recognizing correct medication and dosage, and learning to take your own vital signs.	You will understand all the care needed after discharge and what situations require notifying your transplant team.	You will keep records of your weight and vital signs as recommended by the transplant team. Make appointments with the transplant doctor and your kidney doctor as ordered. Keep your appointments for lab tests as ordered. You will call the transplant team with any signs or symptoms of rejection or infection. You will stay away from people with colds or infectious diseases. Take your medication exactly as prescribed and if you forget a dose, do not double up the dose. Call the transplant nurse. You will follow the prescribed diet. See a dentist for dental care every six months. Before going, tell your kidney doctor so antibiotics can be started to prevent an infection. You or your children must never receive immunizations for smallpox, measles, rubella, or any vaccine containing a *live* virus. This would cause you to have the disease instead of preventing it. See your kidney doctor for immuniza-

Kidney Transplant Patient Education Outcome Pathway (continued)

DISCHARGE PLANNING

Before		During		After	
Goal	Activities	Goal	Activities	Goal	Activities
					tions. Your children need to be vaccinated with *dead* virus immunizations, and you need to make their pediatrician aware that you are a transplant patient.
					You should not smoke because you are at higher risk for lung infections and cancer.
					If you drink alcohol you may drink up to two glasses of wine or beer per day. But be careful because alcohol is irritating to the stomach and can cause liver damage.
					Before taking over the counter medication for any reason, check with the transplant nurse or your kidney doctor. You can take acetaminophen for occasional aches and pains. *Never* take aspirin or nonsteroidal anti-inflammatory drugs (ibuprofen). Nonsteroidal anti-inflammatory drugs may cause kidney damage.
					You may resume sexual activity four weeks after transplant. If a female you need to discuss an appropriate birth control method before becoming sexually active.
					If you get home and have any questions at all, call the transplant nurse at the number given at discharge.
					Plan to have someone stay with you for up to three to four weeks until you are fully capable of caring for yourself.

Pacemakers

Patient Education Outcome Pathway

A cardiac pacemaker is a device implanted in the body that electrically establishes and maintains a rhythmic heartbeat. It is actually a two-part system: the pulse generator commonly called the pacemaker, and the pacing lead(s). The pulse generator contains the battery and electronic circuitry. It produces a pacing pulse that stimulates the heart to beat and acts as the "brain" for the pacing system. The lead(s) are insulated wires that carry the impulses to the heart and signals from the heart back to the pacemaker. Another way to visualize a pacemaker is as a battery-operated "mini-computer" that is implanted in the body to help regulate the heartbeat.

All pacemakers manufactured today are programmable, meaning the doctor or nurse can use a special computer to communicate with the pacemaker before and after it is placed inside your body. A form of *radio frequency* is used to "talk" to the pacemaker through the skin, allowing the pacemaker to have its settings customized for your needs. This painless procedure ensures the best performance from the pacemaker and actually helps the battery last longer.

Most pacemakers typically are small in size, about 1.5 inches long and about 0.25 inches thick. They usually weigh an ounce or less. The pulse generator is usually implanted in the upper chest (on either side) just below the collarbone. The insulated wires are passed through a vein in the chest area and placed directly inside the heart. This approach is called an *endocardial* system. Sometimes, the pacing leads are placed directly on the outside of the heart and the pulse generator is placed in a pocket in the abdominal area. This approach, known as the *epicardial* approach, is used in instances when the patient is already having some other type of open chest surgery.

A pacing system may be implanted using one or two lead wires connecting the pulse generator to your heart. Your doctor will determine which type of system is best for you based on the reason for the pacemaker and any other health issues related to your care. In general, pacemakers are placed as a treatment for a slow heart rate. The two most common reasons for pacemaker implantation are *sick sinus syndrome* and *atrio-ventricular block*. In the first situation, the heart's natural pacemaker beats too slowly at times *(bradycardia)* or may alternately speed up and then slow down *(tachy-brady syndrome)*, resulting in an irregular heart rate and rhythm. In instances of atrio-ventricular block, the heart's own electrical wiring system fails to conduct the signal generated by the natural heart pacemaker, the *sinus node*. Sometimes, an artificial pacemaker is needed to help regulate the heart rate. Medication may still be needed. Certain medications help maintain a normal heart rhythm, but have the added side effect of abnormally slowing down the heart rate. *Rate-modulated pacemakers* have an artificial sensor added to the circuitry to help the heart rate speed up in proportion to everyday activities.

Regardless of the cause, the result is a heart rate that fails to meet the body's need for blood and oxygen. Symptoms often associated with an abnormally slow heart rate include weakness, fatigue, dizziness, blackout spells, and shortness of breath. The slow rate may compound problems associated with weak or ineffective pump function of the heart *(congestive heart failure)* resulting in increased swelling of the extremities and difficulty breathing. The artificial pacemaker helps you feel better by monitoring your own heart's electrical function and providing a tiny electric impulse similar to that produced by a healthy heart when your natural pacemaker fails. Present pacemaker technology is designed to reproduce and maintain a rate and rhythm similar to a healthy heart's electrical function.

PROCEDURE

Before		During		After	
Goal	Activities	Goal	Activities	Goal	Activities
You and your family will understand what happens during the procedure.	The area of the incision, usually the right or left side of your chest, will be washed with a special antibacterial soap to prevent infection. Any hair in the area must be shaved.	You will understand what to expect during the procedure.	Special sheets called sterile drapes will be placed around the site for the incision. These sheets will extend upward below your neck to prevent you from breathing on the site once it has been prepped.	You and your family will understand aspects of your care after the procedure.	You will be returned to either the recovery room or your own room after your surgery. The nurses will monitor your blood pressure, pulse, respiration, and temperature as well as your heart monitor. In gen-

Pacemakers Patient Education Outcome Pathway (continued)

PROCEDURE (continued)

Before		During		After	
Goal	Activities	Goal	Activities	Goal	Activities
	You will be connected to the heart monitor and blood pressure machine.		These sheets will block your vision of the surgical site, but will not be over your face. A nurse usually sits at the head of your bed to monitor your condition and provide verbal reassurance during the procedure.		eral, most patients remain on the heart monitor 24 hours or longer after lead wire(s) insertion to ensure that dislodgment does not occur or is detected before hospital discharge. Should this occur, your doctor will advise you if a repeat operation will be needed to correct the problem.
	Some patients require a temporary pacemaker placed either externally or on the opposite side of the chest from the permanent pacemaker.		The doctor will numb the area with a medication similar to that used in dental procedures. Again, should you feel any pain during the procedure, tell the doctor so more medication may be given.		An ice pack is sometimes placed on the incision site to decrease swelling and discomfort.
	Oxygen may be given through a small tube in your nose during the procedure.		A small incision about 1–2 inches long is made under your collarbone. The doctor will then locate and isolate one or two blood vessels in this area called veins. Generally, a guiding sheath called an introducer is placed within the vessel and serves as a passageway for the lead wire(s) through the vein and into the heart. Once the leads are inside the heart, these introducers are removed and thrown away.		Pain medication may be given orally as needed.
	Let your doctor know if you have a dominant hand preference and whether or not you shoot a rifle or shotgun. Your doctor will probably try to place your pacemaker on the opposite side to prevent future friction or pressure on the site.				You will resume your normal activities, diet, and medication as ordered by your doctor. Remember to request assistance the first time you get out of bed as you may be weak or dizzy following your period of inactivity.
	An IV will be started or your existing IV site checked to ensure normal function.				Your IV will be removed once you are taking liquids.
	A mild sedative will be given to help you relax, but you will remain awake during the procedure.		The doctor will manipulate the lead wire(s) into position using special x-ray equipment to see the approximate location. The lead wire(s) are then connected to the external pacing system analyzer and a series of electrical measurements are recorded. These measurements determine if		Your doctor may order a daily 12 lead EKG until discharge to document normal pacemaker function.
					Blood work may be drawn to ensure your body has the appropriate level of medication and chemistry before hospital discharge.

the physician will leave the lead wire(s) in that location or try to reposition the lead(s) to a different place. You may be asked to breathe deeply or cough to ensure the lead wire(s) are in a secure location.

Once the doctor is satisfied with the lead wire(s) placement, a few stitches will be placed around the area where the leads enter the vein. This helps hold the lead(s) in a stable position while the system heals. The pulse generator is then connected to the lead wire(s).

A pocket is then gently formed under the skin and the pacemaker is placed into this pocket. Usually the incision is closed with self-absorbing suture material, meaning the internal stitches will self-dissolve as healing occurs. The outside skin layer will then be covered with thin bandages called steri-strips, which will gradually loosen over one to two weeks and can then be removed.

The doctor will observe the heart monitor to ensure your new pacing system is functioning normally. He or she may order specific changes to customize the settings during or after the implantation procedure. Any fine tuning of the device settings is usually done in the doctor's office or pacemaker clinic as an outpatient. Generally, a chest x-ray will be taken prior to leaving the procedure room.

Pacemakers Patient Education Outcome Pathway (*continued*)

TESTS

Before		During		After	
Goal	Activities	Goal	Activities	Goal	Activities
You and your family will understand the tests that will be done before your pacemaker is implanted.	A 12 lead EKG will be done. If you are an inpatient, you will probably be on a portable heart monitor that sends the picture of your EKG to the nurses' station. As an outpatient, you may have an event recorder or 24-hour Holter monitor. The purpose of each of these is to record the electrical activity of your heart to help your doctor in deciding which type of pacemaker is best for your body.

Blood work including a chemistry profile, clotting studies, and medication levels will be taken.

A chest x-ray may be done.

You may be asked to provide a urine sample to screen for infection.

Occasionally, additional cardiac studies are performed, which may include an electrophysiology study, cardiac catheterization, echocardiogram, or a tilt-table study. When indicated, these studies assist your doctor in determining the extent of your heart problem so the safest, most efficient treatment plan may be developed. | You will understand any tests that may be done during the procedure. | Your heart rate, rhythm, and blood pressure will be monitored by an external finger probe called a pulse oximeter.

Once the doctor has placed the lead wire(s) into your heart, proper position will be verified by taking electrical readings from an instrument called a **pacing system analyzer.**

Portable moving x-ray equipment will be used during the procedure to allow the doctor to see the path of the lead wire(s) during the insertion procedure.

You may be asked to take a deep breath or cough once the lead wire(s) are secured to ensure they will not become dislodged once you are moved from the table.

You will hear the doctor and nurses talking during the procedure. Once the doctor has placed the lead wire(s) in your heart, you will begin to hear the staff talk about numbers. This is when the staff helps the doctor decide if the lead wire(s) are in the best location. The numbers are actually the electrical measurements taken from the lead wire(s) that identify successful placement of the lead wire(s). | You and your family will understand any tests that may be performed after your pacemaker implantation. | A chest x-ray will be taken to confirm the exact location of the lead wire(s) and will serve as a reference guide for future comparison.

A 12 lead EKG with and without a magnet placed over the pulse generator will be done. Placing a magnet over a permanent pacemaker forces the device to "turn on" versus its typical function of only when needed. Each device has its individual characteristic response to magnet application that your doctor or nurse can interpret to confirm normal device function.

You will probably remain on the heart monitor for up to 24 hours and sometimes longer following insertion of new lead wire(s) to confirm there has been no lead wire dislodgment.

Follow-up blood work may be ordered to help your doctor regulate your medicines before you are sent home. |

DIET AND FLUIDS

Before		During		After	
Goal	Activities	Goal	Activities	Goal	Activities
You will take nothing by mouth for at least 6 hours before the procedure.	Generally, your doctor will tell you to take nothing by mouth after midnight the night before your surgery. This will decrease the risk of nausea and vomiting during the procedure. If your surgery is scheduled for late in the day, you may be allowed a clear liquid breakfast. Your doctor or nurse will inform you. An intravenous (IV) line will be started before the procedure. This will be used to give fluids if the doctor decides it is necessary. Also, a mild sedative will be given through the IV site to help you relax during the surgery. You will be calm but awake and able to talk with your doctor and nurses during the procedure. You will usually be allowed to take your medications with a small sip of water the day of surgery. Your doctor or nurse will advise you.	You will take nothing by mouth during the procedure.	You will take nothing by mouth during the procedure. IV fluids may be given. Medications to help you stay relaxed may be given through your IV line. Pain medicine will be available and can be given through your IV line.	You will begin to take fluids by mouth to prevent dehydration. You will progress to your normal diet as ordered by your doctor within a few hours of your procedure.	You will begin with clear liquids and progress to full liquids and finally your regular diet within a few hours after surgery. The IV will be removed once you are taking oral fluids well. You may see a dietitian before hospital discharge. Having a permanent pacemaker does not directly affect your diet. However, you should follow the principles of good nutrition, eating a balanced diet or a heart healthy diet with limited fat intake. Consult with your physician regarding the best diet for you. You should follow a heart healthy diet: • limit your fat intake to less than 30% of your calories per day • limit your saturated fat intake to less than 10% of your calories per day • limit your cholesterol intake to less than 300 mg per day • restrict calories if needed • restrict salt if needed

ACTIVITY

Before		During		After	
Goal	Activities	Goal	Activities	Goal	Activities
You should maintain your normal activity prior to surgery.	If you have been an inpatient, be aware you may be slightly weaker than normal due to bed rest and changes in your	You will be positioned either flat or with a towel roll between your	During the procedure it is important that you lie still to assist the doctor with lead wire(s) placement.	You will return to your previous activity level. Many people report a dra-	You may move about in bed as tolerated following your pacemaker implantation. Should you need help to reposition

Pacemakers Patient Education Outcome Pathway (continued)

ACTIVITY (continued)

Before		During		After	
Goal	Activities	Goal	Activities	Goal	Activities
	heart rhythm and rate. Ask for help when getting out of bed to prevent falls. You will be transferred to a stretcher for transportation to the surgery suite or cardiac catheterization laboratory where the procedure will be performed.	shoulder blades during the procedure.	Occasionally, the doctor may request a nurse to pull down on one of your arms to reposition the location of your collarbone and first rib. Special straps may be placed over your arms and legs to protect you while positioned on the procedure table and to prevent accidental movement during the procedure. If you experience back discomfort, tell the nurse. Pain medication or a slight change in your position may be used to relieve the discomfort.	matic improvement in their activity level after pacemaker implantation. You may be referred to a cardiac rehabilitation program.	yourself in bed, the hospital staff should use a "lift sheet" rather than pulling you up from your armpits. This technique will prevent unnecessary tension and possible dislodgment of your lead wire(s). Let the hospital staff help you the first time you get out of bed after your procedure. Once you have walked without difficulty, you may have independent bathroom privileges. Generally, you will be allowed to shower after a few days, but most doctors prefer you do not take a tub bath until the incision is completely healed. You may perform your own personal hygiene such as shampooing your hair in the shower. Avoid unnecessary lifting of the arm on the side of your pacemaker implant above your shoulder for the first week. Try to avoid activities requiring exaggerated arm extension for several weeks following your pacemaker implant to decrease the risk of lead wire dislodgment. Examples include golf, swimming, tennis, and lifting objects weighing more than 10 pounds. Check with your doctor for any specific instructions regarding your activity level, driving an automobile, or returning to work.

Be sure to notify the nurse of any pain, dizziness, weakness, or chest discomfort with activity.

Most doctors will allow an ice bag to be placed over the incision for the first day or two after surgery to reduce any local discomfort.

Depending on your overall cardiac status, your doctor may advise you to enter a cardiac rehabilitation program so your activity tolerance can be monitored and gradually advanced to your optimal level.

MEDICATIONS

Before		During		After	
Goal	Activities	Goal	Activities	Goal	Activities
You should know the name, dosage, and frequency of all your medications before you are admitted to the hospital.	Keep a written list of all your medications or bring the actual medication bottles with you to the hospital. Depending on your circumstances, your doctor may add or change your heart medications before your pacemaker placement. Check with your doctor or nurse for instructions regarding which medications you should take the morning of your procedure.	Medication may be given during the procedure to prevent discomfort or to help stabilize your heart rhythm during the procedure.	An IV line will be started in case medication must be given to you quickly. A mild sedative or pain medication may be given to decrease any anxiety or discomfort you may feel during the procedure. A local skin anesthetic such as novacaine is used to numb the area before making the skin incision. It is normal to feel some pushing and pulling at the site during the procedure, but not sharp pain. Be sure to tell the doctor or nurse if you experience any actual pain so more numbing medicine can be injected into the area.	You should be able to describe your medications by name, dosage, frequency, and appearance before going home.	A mild analgesic (pain medication) is usually ordered as needed after your surgery. Some tenderness and minor discomfort at the site is normal and generally responds to acetaminophen or ibuprofen. Do not take aspirin unless approved by your doctor because aspirin has a tendency to thin the blood and could make bruising worse at the implant site. Again, the use of an ice bag may help reduce swelling and discomfort. Your IV will be removed once you are taking oral fluids normally. It is important to remember that your pacemaker works in combination with the overall treatment prescribed by your physician. Most patients require some heart medications for the rest of their lives. *Do not change the dose or stop any of your medication without consulting your doctor.*

Pacemakers Patient Education Outcome Pathway (continued)

MEDICATIONS (continued)

Before		During		After	
Goal	Activities	Goal	Activities	Goal	Activities
					Remember, the pacemaker will treat your slow heart rate, but cannot change the force of your heart's contraction. For many patients, medication helps maintain the normal rhythm and the pacemaker maintains a normal heart rate.

DISCHARGE PLANNING

Before		During		After	
Goal	Activities	Goal	Activities	Goal	Activities
Your discharge planning will begin before admission to the hospital.	Most patients are discharged a few hours or in one to two days after pacemaker implantation. Your doctor will keep you advised depending on your overall physical condition and any complicating factors related to your care. Your doctor and nurses will probably ask you about your usual activity level and tolerance prior to hospital admission. This information is useful in prescribing the best type of pacemaker for you. Let the nurse know if someone will be with you when you are discharged.	The doctor and nurses may offer helpful information regarding your care during the procedure. Planning for your return to your usual activities will continue.	Any pertinent instructions/information discussed during your hospital stay should be given to you in writing. If anything is unclear, speak up and ask the doctor or nurse to clarify the information. Many patients ask their family to be present during instruction for the added confidence in having someone assist them once discharged from the hospital.	You will understand the reason for your pacemaker and how the device will help you. You will understand the care needed after hospital discharge.	Prior to your discharge, you should be enrolled into a pacemaker follow-up program. Most doctors use a combination approach with telephone checks alternated with in-office evaluations. Trans-telephonic monitoring (TTM, or telephone transmissions) allows you to send a tracing of your heart's EKG over the telephone directly into your doctor's office or pacemaker clinic. A typical transmission takes only a few minutes every one to two months as prescribed by your doctor or follow-up staff. Usually, patients are given a pacemaker telephone transmitter and taught how to use it before hospital discharge. A

nonmagnet EKG allows the staff to see the interaction of the pacemaker and your heart's own electrical system. A magnet EKG allows the staff to confirm device operation and battery stability.

During in-office checks, a special computer programmer is used to talk with your pacemaker and allow evaluation of the pulse generator and lead wire(s). During these visits, the device settings may be adjusted to provide optimal benefit, safety, and battery life.

You will probably need to schedule your first in-office checkup in seven to ten days after surgery to allow the doctor/nurses to inspect the incision area for healing, evaluate your device function, and answer any questions you may have about your care. Your doctor or nurses will let you know when to return to see the doctor.

Tell your doctor or nurse of any symptoms of infection: increasing redness/swelling, drainage from the incision area, excessive tenderness, feeling heat at the insertion site, or separation of the incision edges. Also, should you develop a fever without obvious signs of a cold or flu, call your doctor's office immediately. *Do not wait until your next scheduled appointment* because infection of a pacing system is a rare, but serious medical emergency.

You will notice bruising around the incision site and may be aware of the pacemaker's presence for the first few days.

Pacemakers Patient Education Outcome Pathway (continued)

DISCHARGE PLANNING (continued)

Before		During		After	
Goal	Activities	Goal	Activities	Goal	Activities
					Once the incision begins to heal, the bruising and tenderness will gradually subside. Your doctor or nurse will advise you about returning to your daily routine. Generally, a shower is allowed after 24–48 hours. The incision may be gently cleansed with an antibacterial soap and rinsed under running water. Soaking in the bathtub is not recommended until the incision is completely healed.
					Most doctors advise their patients to wait until their first postoperative visit to return to work, drive an automobile, or operate machinery. If in doubt, ask your doctor or follow-up staff.
					As stated earlier, take your medications exactly as prescribed by your doctor. Many complications can be prevented by simply following your doctor's advice.
					Modern technology has resulted in vast improvements in cardiac pacemaker design, function, and reliability. Very few things encountered in your normal home environment can interfere with your pacemaker function. Microwave ovens, electrical appliances, power tools, and office electronic equipment are all safe to use. Power stations, arc welders, ham radios, certain

medical equipment, and some types of cellular telephones produce strong electromagnetic (EMI) fields that may alter the function of your pacemaker. In general, it is best to avoid these situations because you may experience symptoms similar to those you had before your pacemaker was implanted. EMI interference may produce symptoms such as dizziness or feeling faint. These symptoms usually disappear by moving away from the equipment producing the interference. Sometimes, patients may be unaware of this interference, which is why your doctor and nurses give you these precautions. Again, your doctor or nurse should be able to answer any questions you may have regarding potential sources of interference.

Always tell your doctor, hospital staff, and dentist that you have a cardiac pacemaker. They are knowledgeable about sources of interference and what precautions to take to protect you and your pacemaker. For example, pacemaker patients may not receive an MRI (magnetic resonance imaging) test. Deep heat treatment (diathermy), transcutaneous electronic nerve stimulator (TENS) units, and radiation therapy all require special precaution. Also, certain medical and dental procedures may require you to be premedicated with an antibiotic to prevent infection in your bloodstream from settling in your heart. This condition, known as bacterial

Pacemakers Patient Education Outcome Pathway (continued)

DISCHARGE PLANNING (continued)

Before		During		After	
Goal	Activities	Goal	Activities	Goal	Activities
					endocarditis, is very serious, and its best treatment is prevention.
					The manufacturer of your pacemaker should supply you with an identification card that lists the specific model and serial number of your pacemaker and lead wire(s), the date of implantation, and follow-up information about your doctor. You should be given a temporary card prior to discharge from the hospital and the manufacturer will mail you a permanent card in six to eight weeks. *Always carry your pacemaker identification card with you.* Many doctors also give their patients a copy of the computer printout listing the most current device settings. In an emergency situation, this information will greatly assist the medical staff in your treatment. The ID card is about the size of a driver's license.
					Many patients also obtain a Medic-Alert bracelet or necklace. This is especially helpful if they have more than one chronic illness, medication allergy, or certain conditions such as diabetes, take blood thinners, or are at high risk for loss

of consciousness. Emergency medical technicians are trained to look for these alert tags, and such information may save valuable time in an emergency. Be aware that some airport and courthouse security checkpoints may react to the metal in your pacemaker. Most patients simply notify the security personnel they have a pacemaker and produce their wallet identification card. Generally, a hand spot-check is conducted rather than having the person pass through the security gate. The security gate may temporarily alter your pacemaker's function due to the powerful magnetic field, but simply stepping away from the magnetic source will restore normal function of your pacemaker.

Finally, pacemakers are safe, reliable, and extremely "smart" in their function. Most patients feel much better following the placement of their pacemaker. Many are able to resume activities that had become too physically burdensome prior to the pacemaker implant. While a pacemaker will not artificially prolong your life, it will greatly improve your quality of life and often help prevent some disease-related complications. Consult your doctor or follow-up nurse for any questions related to your pacemaker or your health.

Pneumonia

Patient Education Outcome Pathway

Pneumonia is an infection that occurs in the lungs. When the tiny air sacs (called alveoli) of the lungs are filled with infection, they are unable to accept oxygen. Pneumonia may occur by itself or as a complication of another disease. Most pneumonias are caused by bacteria. The incidence of bacterial pneumonia has increased due to the widespread use of antibiotics. Many people have become resistant to some of the most commonly used antibiotics. Resistant germs may reside in your nose or throat and can cause an infection if your immune system becomes weak or stressed.

TESTS

Before		During		After	
Goal	Activities	Goal	Activities	Goal	Activities
You and your family will understand the tests that will be completed.	You will be asked to cough up a sputum specimen, which will be sent to the lab to be cultured, tested, and analyzed to determine the best treatment for you. Blood and urine samples will also be collected and tested to detect any signs of infection in your blood or kidneys. An arterial blood gas (ABG) will be drawn to check your oxygen and carbon dioxide levels to see how well your lungs are working. A chest x-ray will be done to see where the areas of infection are occurring in your lungs.	You and your family will understand any tests that need to be completed.	Your temperature, blood pressure, heart rate, and breathing rate will be monitored by the nurses. A chest x-ray may be done to see how the pneumonia is improving. Your oxygen level may be monitored with a pulse oximeter, a device placed on your finger, toe, or earlobe.	You and your family will understand any tests that need to be completed.	You may need to have a follow-up chest x-ray or ABG once discharged.

DIET AND FLUIDS

Before		During		After	
Goal	Activities	Goal	Activities	Goal	Activities
You will take lots of fluids to stay well hydrated. You will eat a well-balanced diet.	You will need to drink at least 6–8 glasses of water per day to stay well hydrated. This makes it easier to cough up phlegm and lung secretions. If you are unable to drink enough fluids, IV fluids will be given to you.	You will take lots of fluids to stay well hydrated. You will eat a well-balanced diet.	You will continue to take in 6–8 glasses of water a day and a heart healthy diet. The nurses will keep track of how much fluid you are taking in and how much fluid you are putting out.	You will take lots of fluids to stay well hydrated. You will eat a well-balanced diet.	Continue to drink 6–8 glasses of water a day once home. This should not include caffeinated, carbonated, or alcoholic beverages. You should follow a heart healthy diet:

- limit your fat intake to less than 30% of your calories for the day
- limit your saturated fat intake to less than 10% of your calories for the day
- limit your cholesterol intake to less than 300 mg per day
- restrict calories/learn weight-gaining techniques if needed
- restrict salt if needed

The nurses will check your weight each day.

Once able to eat, you will be started on a heart healthy diet.

ACTIVITY

Before		During		After	
Goal	Activities	Goal	Activities	Goal	Activities
You should rest until your body recovers from the pneumonia.	You will be on bed rest until you feel stronger and your energy level improves.	You should progress your activity slowly until your energy returns.	The staff will help you get up to the bathroom until your energy level improves and you can safely get up and down without assistance. You will continue to progress your activity level as tolerated. The staff will plan frequent periods for you to rest between activities. You may need oxygen therapy to improve your activity level. Your oxygen level may be monitored with a pulse oximeter during activity.	You should be able to return to the activity level you had prior to getting pneumonia.	You will continue to advance your activity level once home. Begin a progressive exercise program once your energy returns. The nurse/respiratory therapist/physical therapist will help you get started. Plan rest periods once home. It may be helpful to take a nap during the day until your normal energy level returns. Remember that it takes at least a few months to recuperate from pneumonia, and bodily defenses may still be low. You may be very susceptible to further lung/upper respiratory tract infections. You may be referred to a pulmonary rehabilitation program.

Pneumonia Patient Education Outcome Pathway (continued)

MEDICATIONS

	Before		During		After
Goal		**Goal**		**Goal**	
	Activities		**Activities**		**Activities**
You should be able to state any medications you are on and why you take them.	Tell the doctor or nurses about any medications you are on and why you take them.	You should know any medications you are taking and why you are taking them. If you are on inhalers, you should know the proper way to take these medications.	You will be given antibiotics through an IV line to fight the pneumonia. You may be given medications through an IV, orally, or via inhalers to help open your airways further and make it easier to breath. You may be given breathing treatments to help improve your lung function and to make it easier to cough up phlegm and secretions. If you are on inhalers, the nurse or respiratory therapist will review how to take these. It may be recommended to use a spacer device with inhalers. The inhaler is attached to the spacer and then the spacer is placed in your mouth. Compress the inhaler medication and slowly inhale. Try to hold your breath for 5 seconds. You may need acetaminophen (e.g., Tylenol) if you have a fever.	You should know any medications you are taking and why you are taking them.	If you are given a prescription for an antibiotic to continue at home, be sure to take all of the medication exactly as prescribed. You will receive teaching about any medications you will be taking at home. If you will be using an inhaler at home, demonstrate the proper technique with or without a spacer device.

TREATMENTS

	Before		During		After
Goal		**Goal**		**Goal**	
	Activities		**Activities**		**Activities**
Your lungs will work as well as possible.	The doctors, nurses, and therapists will listen to your lung sounds frequently. You may be on oxygen therapy until your lungs improve. Do not remove the oxygen device unless the nurses/doctors say it is all right to take it off.	Your lungs will work as well as possible.	The nurses and respiratory therapists will teach you breathing exercises if needed to help conserve your energy. The nurses and respiratory therapists will teach you different cough techniques that will make it easier for you to cough up phlegm such as:	Your lungs will work as well as possible.	Continue breathing exercises, relaxation exercises, or energy conservation exercises as needed at home. Coordinate your breathing exercises with your activities. Continue to use the cough techniques as needed to help cough up phlegm.

- huff cough (forcing your air out as hard and fast as you can)
- cascade cough (coughing through one entire exhalation of your breathing cycle)

The nurses will show you relaxation techniques to keep your chest and lungs relaxed so that you can breathe as efficiently as possible.

DISCHARGE PLANNING

Before		During		After	
Goal	Activities	Goal	Activities	Goal	Activities
We will begin planning your discharge as soon as you are admitted.	The nurse will ask you about your home life when you are admitted. Let the nurse know if someone will be with you when you are discharged.	Discharge planning will continue.	Once your temperature is down to normal, you are feeling better, and your chest x-ray/ABGs are improved, you will be discharged from the hospital. You will be evaluated for potential risk factors that may contribute to developing pneumonia such as being over 65 years old, having other diseases such as cancer, AIDs, other lung problems (emphysema, asthma, chronic bronchitis), or whether you are bedridden. If you smoke, you will be *strongly encouraged to stop smoking.* Plans will be made to arrange any equipment that you may need at home such as oxygen therapy or home nebulizers (breathing treatments). If you need a visiting nurse at home, this will be arranged.	You will understand care needed after discharge.	Make an appointment with your primary doctor or lung doctor as instructed for follow-up. Know what medications you should be taking and the proper way to take them. Call the doctor if you notice: • increased breathing difficulties • fever • change in color, amount, or thickness of phlegm or lung secretions Ask for a number to call if you have questions. To avoid further occurrences of pneumonia, you will be encouraged to: • avoid crowds during peak flu seasons • get an annual flu shot • get a pneumonia shot every five years • avoid sudden changes in climate • continue adequate water intake (6–8 glasses per day) If you smoke, you will be given information on smoking cessation. You may be referred to an outpatient smoking cessation program.

Thoracic Surgery

Patient Education Outcome Pathway

Chest or thoracic surgery may be performed for a variety of conditions such as emphysema, cancer, infection, or injury. Sometimes the purpose of the surgery is to try to determine the problem or diagnosis. The preparation for the procedure and the follow-up care will vary based on the primary cause of your illness or injury.

The procedure usually involves a large incision in the chest, affecting major muscle groups. When possible a muscle-sparing procedure is done to reduce pain and improve recovery. In some patients a small incision is used and a scope inserted into the chest to help visualize the structures. This is called a *thoracoscopy*.

TESTS

Goal	Before		After	
	Activities		**Activities**	
You and your family will understand the tests that will be done to prepare you for the surgery.	Blood will be drawn to determine your blood cell count, electrolytes, and blood type. Your doctor will likely want to have blood products available for you during your surgery in case they are needed. Many tests can be performed on the blood sample to help determine your general state of health. You will have a chest x-ray and EKG. You may have pulmonary function tests and a bronchoscopy. Pulmonary function tests give us much information about how your lungs are working. A bronchoscopy involves placing a tube through your throat and into your lungs. If these are ordered you will be given information about these tests.		Blood will be drawn to determine your oxygen and carbon dioxide levels, your blood count, and electrolytes. Your heart rate and rhythm will likely be monitored continuously for one or more days. Follow-up chest x-rays will be done. Your oxygen saturation will be checked frequently for the next one to two days. This usually involves placing a sensor on one of your fingers or on your earlobe to tell the nurses the oxygen content in your blood.	

Goal				
You and your family will understand any tests that may be done after the surgery.				

DIET AND FLUIDS

Goal	Before		After	
	Activities		**Activities**	
Your stomach will be empty during the surgery.	You should not eat or drink anything after midnight the night before your surgery. Check with your nurse or doctor about any routine medications that you normally take. These drugs may need to be given by another route or you may be told to take them with a few sips of water before surgery. Two IV lines will be started in your arm and fluids given. A sedative will be given before your surgery to help you relax.		As soon as you are fully awake and recovered from the anesthesia, you will be able to start drinking fluids. This will usually be the next morning after surgery. You will gradually progress to solid foods as soon as your bowel sounds are normal. The IVs will be removed when they are no longer needed for medications and you are taking fluids well. You should follow a heart healthy diet: • limit your fat intake to less than 30% of your calories for the day	

Goal				
You will maintain or restore your fluid balance and nutrition. You will progress to a heart healthy diet as tolerated.				

- limit your saturated fat intake to less than 10% of your calories for the day
- limit your cholesterol intake to less than 300 mg per day
- restrict calories if needed
- restrict salt if needed

PHYSICAL ACTIVITY

Before		After	
Goal	Activities	Goal	Activities
You will maintain body strength and conditioning. You will continue your usual activity level before surgery.	You should maintain your current activity level before the procedure if at all possible. Some patients participate in a pulmonary rehabilitation program before their surgery. You should discuss this with your doctor.	As you recover from surgery, you will gradually resume activity to prevent complications such as pneumonia and blood clots. You will return to or improve your presurgery activity level.	You will remain in bed until you are fully awake and your blood pressure is normal. As soon as you are stable, your nurse will assist you to dangle on the side of the bed and then get up and sit in a chair. You will have one or more tubes in your chest to drain blood and air from the operation. It is very important to move after surgery. The chest tubes will usually be removed in two to three days and it will be easier for you to walk. You may also have special stockings on your legs to reduce the likelihood of blood clots. You may have an epidural catheter in your back for pain medication. An oxygen cannula will be in your nose to increase your oxygen level. Your level will be monitored by pulse oximetry. A small sensor will be placed on your toe, finger, or earlobe. Getting out of bed may seem very complicated, but your nurse will assist you to gradually increase your activity level. For example, you might walk 50 feet the first time and 100 feet the second time. Depending on your disease and type of operation, an aggressive pulmonary rehabilitation program may be initiated shortly after your operation. This will probably be started in the hospital and may be continued after surgery. You will be given an exercise program to do at home.

Thoracic Surgery Patient Education Outcome Pathway (*continued*)

MEDICATIONS

Before		After	
Goal	Activities	Goal	Activities
You should be able to tell the doctor/nurse which medications you are taking at home.	Make a list of the medicines and dosages you are taking or bring them to the hospital when you come for your surgery. Include the medicines you buy over the counter such as antacids, vitamins, and so on. Be sure to know the name and dosage of all your medications, including over-the-counter medicines.	You will understand the medications you are receiving while in the hospital. You will be able to state the medicine, purpose, and several common side effects of the medicines you will be taking when you go home.	You will be receiving medication for pain and it is important to take it as needed so that you will be able to deep breathe, cough, and walk in the hall. The pain medication may be given through the IV in your arm or by mouth as you can tolerate. You may have pain medication given through a patient-controlled analgesia (PCA) device. The nurse will show you how to work it. You will likely receive antibiotics to reduce the risk of infection. Additional medications will be based on other conditions you may have such as heart disease, emphysema, or diabetes. You will likely receive a prescription for pain medication when you go home.

PROCEDURE

Before		During		After	
Goal	Activities	Goal	Activities	Goal	Activities
You will understand what will happen to you before the procedure.	Some patients will be admitted the evening before surgery if testing still needs to be completed. Many people can come in the morning of surgery. It will be very important that your skin is as clean as possible before you go to surgery. You may be given a special soap to reduce the bacteria on your skin. Your chest and any other areas involved will be cleaned and shaved prior to your surgery either in your hospital room or in the operating room. At least one IV line will be placed before surgery.	You will understand what will happen during your procedure.	The procedure will be based on your disease but most often a segment or lobe of diseased lung is removed. The length of time in the operating room will depend on the procedure. An additional IV line is placed as well as an arterial line to monitor your blood pressure and oxygen levels. This line is usually placed in an artery in your wrist. A breathing tube (endotracheal tube) will be placed in your trachea and connected to a ventilator after you are asleep. This tube may be removed before you wake up in the	You will understand what happens after your surgery.	After your operation you will spend 2 or more hours in the recovery room. Depending on your procedure you may go to an intensive care unit (ICU) or a monitored area for one to two days to continue your recovery. Your blood pressure, pulse, respirations, breath sounds, and chest tubes will be checked frequently by the nurse. It will be important for you to ask for pain medication so that you can assist with increasing activity, deep breathing, and coughing.

You may receive a sedative to help you relax before the surgery.

An anesthesiologist will see you before surgery.

You may be given an antibiotic through your IV line before surgery.

recovery room. If not, it will be removed as soon as you are able to breathe on your own after surgery. While this tube in place, you will be unable to speak.

One or more tubes will be placed in your chest to drain excess fluids. You will have a large bandage over your incision and chest tube sites.

A catheter may be placed in your back to provide continuous pain medication or a pump may be connected to one of your IV lines to provide pain medication that you can control. This is called a PCA pump (patient-controlled analgesia). Let the doctor or nurse know if you are allergic to any pain medications.

You will have a bandage on your chest that the nurse will check often.

If you have any discomfort, let the nurse know immediately.

You will be able to dangle on the side of the bed and possibly get out of bed the day after your surgery. Most patients go home within one week. You will need help at home.

Your doctor will let you know when you can return to work and resume your normal activities at home.

Watch for signs of infection and call your doctor should they occur:

- fever
- cough
- green/yellow mucus
- wheezing
- shortness of breath
- fatigue
- weight gain/loss of 5 pounds or more within a week
- swelling of ankles

DISCHARGE PLANNING

Before		After	
Goal	Activities	Goal	Activities
You and your health care professionals will begin planning your discharge as soon as you come to the hospital and, in some cases, even before admission to the hospital.	Tell the nurse of any potential problems that may complicate your returning home such as stairs, need for home health. Let the nurse know if someone will be with you when you are discharged.	You will understand the results of your surgery and any follow-up care needed.	Your doctor will discuss the results of the procedure and any follow-up care. Ask questions if you do not understand something. Ask for a phone number to call if you have questions or problems. Your nurse and/or discharge planner will consider any possible home care needs such as home oxygen and assist you in obtaining them. You may be referred to a pulmonary rehabilitation program. Maintain a heart healthy diet: • limit your fat intake to less than 30% of your calories for the day

Thoracic Surgery Patient Education Outcome Pathway (*continued*)

DISCHARGE PLANNING (continued)

	Before		During
Goal		Goal	
	Activities		Activities
			• limit your saturated fat intake to less than 10% of your calories for the day
			• limit your cholesterol intake to less than 300 mg per day
			• restrict calories if needed
			• restrict salt if needed
			Gradually increase your activity.
			Plan to have someone stay with you awhile after surgery.
			Smoking cessation is critical. There are various ways to assist you such as medication and support groups. The American Lung Association and American Cancer Society can help. It is never too late to quit!

Valve Replacement

Patient Education Outcome Pathway

The heart is an organ that contains four chambers. The top two chambers are called the atria, and the bottom two chambers are the ventricles. Four heart valves separate the chambers from each other and the main blood vessels.

The pulmonic valve separates the right atrium from the right ventricle. The tricuspid valve separates the right ventricle from the pulmonary artery, which is the vessel that carries blood from the right side of the heart to the lungs. The mitral valve separates the left atrium from the left ventricle. The aortic valve separates the left ventricle (the main pumping chamber of the heart) from the aorta, which is the largest artery in the body. Any of these valves can become damaged or diseased and need to be replaced.

Valve replacement occurs when one or more of the heart valves must be replaced due to damage or disease. The valves may be porcine (pig), bovine (cow), or mechanical (artificial). The procedure to replace the valves, regardless what they are made from, is similar. Valve replacement usually requires open chest surgery. Some repairs can be done without open chest surgery. Also, some hospitals are now doing minimally invasive valve replacement, which requires just one or two small incisions into the chest wall. All of the procedures are discussed here.

PROCEDURE

Before		During		After	
Goal	Activities	Goal	Activities	Goal	Activities
You will understand what happens before the procedure.	You will meet with a nurse who will explain what will happen over the next few days. The nurse will explain the surgery and care afterward in the recovery room and open heart area. You will probably receive some booklets to read. The nurse will explain the various tubes you will have after surgery and what the intensive care unit (ICU) is like. You may have the chance to visit the ICU before your surgery. You may take nothing by mouth after midnight the night before your surgery. Tell your family to arrive approximately 90 minutes before your surgery is scheduled. You may be taken to an area for preparation for surgery before the actual time of your surgery.	You will understand what happens during the procedure.	For valve replacement using an open chest approach: • a large incision will be made down the center of your chest along the breastbone or sternum • the ribs are spread so the surgeon can reach your heart • you will be placed on a heart/lung bypass machine • the surgeon then replaces the valve • the sternum is wired together • the heart/lung machine is stopped • your chest is then closed For valve replacement using a minimally invasive approach: • the surgeon will make a small incision (about 4 inches) either across the top of the breastbone or sternum or along the side of the sternum	You will understand what happens after the surgery.	You will wake up either in the recovery room or in the open heart unit. When you first wake up, you will notice you have a lot of tubes in place: • You may still be on a respirator (ventilator). If so, there will be a large tube in your windpipe that goes through your throat and is connected to a machine to help you breathe. Once you are able to breathe on your own, this tube will be removed. Usually the tube is removed within a few hours after surgery or by the next morning. As long as this tube is in place, you will not be able to talk. The nurses will help you communicate (hand signals, nods, eye blinks, or magic slates).

Valve Replacement Patient Education Outcome Pathway (continued)

PROCEDURE (continued)

Before		During		After	
Goal	Activities	Goal	Activities	Goal	Activities
	Your chest will be washed with an antibacterial soap. Your chest may be shaved (done in some hospitals).		• you will be placed on a heart/lung bypass machine		• You will have at least two chest tubes in to help drain blood and air from your chest. These will go to a suction machine at the bedside. You may hear a bubbling noise.
	You will meet with an anesthesiologist who will tell you how he or she will put you to sleep during the surgery. If you have had any problems with anesthesia before, tell the anesthesiologist.		• the surgeon will then replace the valve		• Once you are taken off the respirator, oxygen will be given to you through a small tube (cannula) in your nose.
	One or two IV lines will be started in your arm.		• the heart/lung machine is stopped		• You may also have a tube in your nose that goes into your stomach to help keep your stomach empty and prevent nausea. This is usually removed one or two days after surgery.
	You will be given a sedative to help you relax before surgery.		• the incision is closed		• You will have a catheter in your bladder.
					• You may have a warming blanket on to help raise your body temperature after surgery. The body temperature is usually lowered during surgery.
					• You will have several IV lines.
					• You will have a small tube in your radial artery (in the wrist), which will help the nurses watch your blood pressure at all times.
					• There may a line directly into your heart to monitor pressures inside your heart at all times.
					• You may have a temporary pacing wire for a few days.

All of these lines and tubes should be removed within a few days.

You should be able to see your family within one to two hours after surgery.

You will stay in bed at least overnight. As soon as you are able, your activity will be increased. Here is an example of how your activity will be increased:

- dangle at the bedside
- sit in a chair several times a day
- walk 200 to 300 feet three or four times a day
- climb a flight of stairs before you go home

After you go home, you will either start a home exercise program or be referred to an outpatient cardiac rehabilitation program. The doctor or nurse will let you know.

You will have a bandage on your chest. The nurse will check it frequently.

Your blood pressure and pulse will be monitored continuously while you are in the ICU. After you are transferred to another unit, you may still stay on a heart monitor for several days. Once you are transferred, your activity level will be increased.

Pain medication will be available. Do not hesitate to ask for it. Once you are fully awake, you may be placed on a device called patient-controlled analgesia (PCA pump). This device allows you to control when and how much pain medication you receive. You will be taught how to use the pump. You will start receiving

Valve Replacement Patient Education Outcome Pathway (continued)

PROCEDURE (continued)

Before		During		After	
Goal	Activities	Goal	Activities	Goal	Activities
					morphine or a similar medication immediately after surgery. As you progress, this medicine will be changed to less strong pain relievers, such as the nonsteroidal anti-inflammatory agents. Be sure to let the nurses know when you have any discomfort.
					Let the nurses know if you have any:
					• chest discomfort
					• shortness of breath
					• bleeding
					• dizziness
					• nausea and vomiting
					• indigestion
					You will have several lab tests done for a few days after your surgery.
					You will be weighed daily.
					The nurses will keep a record of how much you drink and how much you urinate.
					You must cough and deep breathe several times a day to prevent pneumonia. You will use a pillow to help splint your chest. The nurse will show you how to use the pillow properly.
					Call your doctor if any of the following occur:
					• chest discomfort
					• redness or drainage at the site of the incision
					• shortness of breath
					• bleeding

- dizziness
- swelling
- weight gain over 2–3 pounds
- fever over 100°F

You will be started on blood thinners a few days after your surgery.

TESTS

Before		During		After	
Goal	Activities	Goal	Activities	Goal	Activities
You and your family will understand the tests that will be done before your valve replacement.	Blood will be drawn to determine your complete blood cell count, clotting studies to show how well your blood clots, electrolytes (potassium, sodium, chloride), and blood type. You may have a chest x-ray. A 12 lead EKG will be done.	You will understand any tests that may be done during the valve replacement	Your heart rate, rhythm, and blood pressure will be monitored throughout the entire procedure.	You and your family will understand any tests that may be done after the valve replacement.	Blood will be drawn to check your blood count and clotting studies several times during your hospitalization. If you have a porcine or bovine valve, you will remain on blood thinners at least six weeks. If you have a mechanical valve, you will take blood thinners the rest of your life. You will need to have clotting studies done frequently while you are taking a blood thinner. The doctor or nurse will let you know. Your heart rate, rhythm, and blood pressure will be monitored closely after the procedure.

DIET AND FLUIDS

Before		During		After	
Goal	Activities	Goal	Activities	Goal	Activities
You will take nothing by mouth after midnight the night before your surgery.	You may take nothing by mouth after midnight the night before your surgery. One or two IV lines will be started in your arm and fluids given before and during surgery.	You will not take anything by mouth during the procedure.	IV fluids will be continued throughout the surgery. Medications to help you relax before the surgery will be given through the IV.	You will begin taking fluids orally after you are off the ventilator (respirator).	While you are on the ventilator, a large tube will be in your mouth. You will not be able to speak or eat while this tube is in place.

Valve Replacement Patient Education Outcome Pathway (continued)

DIET AND FLUIDS (continued)

Before		During		After	
Goal	Activities	Goal	Activities	Goal	Activities
	A sedative will be given before your surgery to help you relax.				You will begin taking fluids as soon as you are able. You will be given a clear liquid diet. As you proceed in your recovery, your diet will be advanced to a heart healthy diet, which you should remain on after discharge: • limit your fat intake to less than 30% of your calories for the day • limit your saturated fat intake to less than 10% of your calories for the day • limit your cholesterol intake to less than 300 mg per day • limit your salt intake to less than 2,000 mg per day (about ½ teaspoon of salt); watch for salt in other foods (canned goods, baked goods, chips, processed meats) • limit your calorie intake if you need to lose weight You will meet with a dietitian before discharge.

ACTIVITY

Before		During		After	
Goal	Activities	Goal	Activities	Goal	Activities
You should maintain your current activity level before the surgery.	Maintain your current activity level before the surgery. You will be placed on a stretcher in the preparation area to start getting ready for your surgery.	You will remain asleep and motionless during the surgery.	During the surgery, you will be under anesthesia and kept motionless. When you wake up in the recovery room, you will be on a stretcher or in a bed.	You will remain in bed for several hours after the surgery. You will gradually increase your activ-	You will remain in bed for several hours after the surgery. The head of the bed may be elevated for comfort. The nurse will let you know.

	Before		During		After	
	Goal	Activities	Goal	Activities	Goal	Activities
(ACTIVITY, continued)					ity level after surgery. You will return and ideally progress past your presurgery activity level. You may be referred to an outpatient cardiac rehabilitation program.	The nurse or physical therapist will help you with some arm and leg exercises, which you should do several times a day. You will get up in a chair at the bedside on the first or second day after the surgery. You will begin walking on the second or third day after the surgery. You will gradually increase your walking to 200 to 300 feet three or four times a day. You will climb up and down a flight of stairs before you go home. You may be referred to an outpatient cardiac rehabilitation program after discharge. If not, you will be given an exercise program to do at home. You should not do any heavy lifting or pulling (over 10–15 pounds) for two to three months.

MEDICATIONS

Before		During		After	
Goal	Activities	Goal	Activities	Goal	Activities
You should be able to state your medications to the doctor and the nurse before your surgery.	The nurse and doctor will ask you about your medications. Be sure to know the name and dosage of all your medications. You may want to bring them to the hospital with you. One or two IV lines will be started in your arm. A sedative may be given through the IV line to help you relax before the surgery.	You will receive medications through the IV line during the surgery.	Various medications may be used during the procedure such as: • medications to help you relax • medications to induce or cause anesthesia • medications to regulate your heart rhythm • medications to control blood clotting	You will be able to state your medications before discharge. You will know how to take your medications properly, especially the blood thinners.	The IVs will be removed a few days after surgery. Once you are able to take fluids, most of the medications may be given orally. However, some medications, such as antibiotics, may still be given through the IV. You will receive teaching about the medications you will take at home. All patients will go home on a blood thinner. If you have a porcine (pig) or bovine (cow) valve, you will take blood thinners for at least six weeks after surgery. If you

Valve Replacement Patient Education Outcome Pathway (continued)

MEDICATIONS (continued)

Before		During		After	
Goal	Activities	Goal	Activities	Goal	Activities
					have a mechanical heart valve, you will be on a blood thinner for the rest of your life.

Precautions with blood thinners:

- Be sure to have your clotting levels checked frequently. The doctor or nurse will let you know how often.
- Avoid contact sports.
- Avoid activities that increase your odds of getting hurt.
- Always wear your seatbelt.
- Always wear shoes.
- If you notice bleeding (gums, urine, bowel movements), call your doctor right away.
- If you injure yourself and are bleeding, apply pressure for 10–15 minutes until the bleeding stops. If this is not effective, go to the nearest emergency room.
- If you have a large injury, go immediately to an emergency room.
- Drink the same amount of coffee, tea, or colas as you did in the hospital.
- Avoid foods that may interfere with clotting. You will receive a list of these before you leave the hospital.

You will have a prescription for pain medication. Take it as prescribed.

DISCHARGE PLANNING

	Before		During		After	
Goal	Activities	Goal	Activities	Goal	Activities	
You will begin planning your discharge as soon as you are admitted.	The nurse will ask you about your home life when you are admitted. Let the nurse know if you are planning to return home or stay with someone else after surgery. You should have someone with you the first week at home.	Discharge planning will continue.	You may be discharged from the hospital approximately five to seven days after surgery.	You will understand the results of the procedure. You will understand care needed after discharge.	Make an appointment with your doctor for follow-up. Maintain a heart healthy diet. Start your exercise program when you are able and increase as tolerated. You may be referred to a cardiac rehabilitation program. The doctor will let you know when you can return to work. Avoid lifting or pulling objects over 10–15 pounds for two to three months. The doctor will discuss the results of the procedure with you and your family. The doctor will discuss future care with you and your family. Ask questions if you do not understand something. Ask for a phone number to call if you have questions. You may be referred to an open heart support group. You may be followed by a home health agency for a few weeks after discharge. Call your doctor should any of the following occur: • chest discomfort • redness or drainage at the incision site • shortness of breath • bleeding • dizziness • swelling of the ankles • weight gain over 2–3 pounds • fever over 100°F Your doctor may want you to take antibiotics before any surgical or dental procedure. Ask about this.	

References

Introduction

Gottschlich, M.M., Matarese, L.E., Shronts, E.P. (1993). *Nutrition support dietetics core curriculum* (2nd ed.). Silver Springs, Md.: Aspen.

Hillegass, E.A., Sadowsky, S. (1994). *Essentials of cardiopulmonary physical therapy.* Philadelphia: W.B. Saunders.

Page, C.P., Hardin, T.C., Melnik, G. (1994). *Nutritional assessment and support: a primer* (2nd ed.). Baltimore: Williams and Wilkins.

Pedretti, L. (1990). *Occupational therapy: practice skills for physical dysfunction.* St. Louis: C.V. Mosby.

Chapter 1

Abdominal Aortic Aneurysm

Dalsing, M.C., Sawchuk, A.P. (1994). Surgery of the aorta. In V.A. Fahey (Ed.), *Vascular Nursing* (2nd ed., pp. 251–290). Philadelphia: W.B. Saunders.

Lessig, M.L., Lessig, P.M. (1991). Cardiovascular system. In J.G. Alspach (Ed.), *Core curriculum for critical care nursing* (4th ed., pp. 132–314). Philadelphia: W.B. Saunders.

Painter, L.M. (1995). Abdominal aortic aneurysm pathway: outcome analysis. *Journal of Vascular Nursing, 13*(4), 101–103.

Parthum, J. (1996). Vascular emergencies. In J.M. Clochesy, C. Breu, S. Cardin, A.A. Whittaker, E.B. Rudy (Eds.), *Critical care nursing* (2nd ed., pp. 535–557). Philadelphia: W.B. Saunders.

Carotid Endarterectomy

Christensen, C.R. (1997). Carotid endarterectomy clinical pathway: a nursing perspective. *Journal of Vascular Nursing, 15*(1), 1–6.

Fahey, V.A. (1994). *Vascular nursing* (2nd ed., pp. 325–345). Philadelphia: W.B. Saunders.

O'Brien, M.S. (1994). Postoperative treatment of patients undergoing carotid endarterectomy. *Journal of Vascular Nursing, 12* (1), 1–5.

Rogers, P.G., Henne-Mauk, S., Basham, K., Wicke, J., Miller, D., Polston, A. (1996). Carotid endarterectomy critical care outcome pathway. Louisville, Ky.: Baptist Hospital East.

Congestive Heart Failure

Moser, D.K., Cardin, S. (1996). Heart failure. In J.M. Clochesy, C. Breu, S. Cardin, A.A. Whittaker, E.B. Rudy (Eds.), *Critical care nursing* (2nd ed., pp. 380–406). Philadelphia: W.B. Saunders.

Newkirk, T., Leeper, B. (1996). Congestive heart failure: mapping the way to quality outcomes. *American Journal of Nursing, 96*(5), Supplement, 25–27.

Coronary Artery Bypass Surgery

Cronin, S.N., Logsdon, C., Miracle, V. (1997). Psychosocial and functional outcomes in women after coronary artery bypass surgery. *Critical Care Nurse, 17*(2), 19–24.

De Angelis, R. (1991). The cardiovascular system. In J.G. Alspach (Ed.), *Core curriculum for critical care nursing* (4th ed., pp. 132–314). Philadelphia: W.B. Saunders.

Gross, S., Coleman, B., Flavell, C., Salamandra, J. (1996). Patients undergoing cardiothoracic surgery and transplants. In J.M. Clochesy, C. Breu, S. Cardin, A.A. Whittaker, E.B. Rudy (Eds), *Critical care nursing* (2nd ed., pp. 458–512). Philadelphia: W.B. Saunders.

Lombness, P.M. (1994). Difference in length of stay with care managed by clinical nurse specialists or physician assistants. *Clinical Nurse Specialist, 8*(5), 255–260.

Pozehl, B., Barnason, S., Zimmerman, L., Nieveen, J., Crutchfield, J. (1995). Pain in the postoperative coronary artery bypass graft patient. *Clinical Nursing Research, 4*(2), 208–222.

Dysrhythmias

American Heart Association. (1994). *Advanced cardiac life support.* Dallas, Tex.: AHA.

DeAngelis, R. (1991). The cardiovascular system. In J.G. Alspach (Ed.), *Core curriculum for critical care nursing* (4th ed., pp. 200–205). Philadelphia: W.B.Saunders.

Guaglianone, D., Tyndall, A. (1995). Comfort issues in patients undergoing radiofrequency catheter ablation. *Critical Care Nurse, 2,* 47–50.

Medtronic, Inc. (1995). *Restoring the rhythms of life. Living with your cardioverter-defibrillator.* Minneapolis: Medtronic.

Menzel, L.K., White, J.M. (1996). Electrocardiogram interpretation. In J.M. Clochesy, C. Breu, S. Cardin, A.A. Whitaker, E.B. Rudy (Eds.), *Critical care nursing* (2nd ed., pp. 127–166). Philadelphia: W.B. Saunders.

Heart Transplantation

Gross, S., Coleman, B., Flavell, C., Salamandra, J. (1996). Patients undergoing cardiothoracic surgery and transplants. In J.M. Clochesy, C. Breu, S. Cardin, A.A. Whittaker, E.B. Rudy (Eds.), *Critical care nursing* (2nd ed., pp. 458–512). Philadelphia: W.B. Saunders.

Moroney, D.A., Reedy, J.E. (1994). Understanding ventricular assist devices: a self study guide. *Journal of Cardiovascular Nursing, 8*(2), 1–15.

Skinn, A.E., Joseph, D. (1994). Concepts of intraaortic balloon counterpulsation. *Journal of Cardiovascular Nursing, 8*(2), 45–60.

Vaska, P.L. (1993). Common infections in heart transplant patients. *American Journal of Critical Care, 2*(2), 145–154.

Interventional Cardiology

DeAngelis, R. (1991). The cardiovascular system. In J.G. Alspach (Ed.), *Core curriculum for critical care nursing* (4th ed., pp. 132–314). Philadelphia: W.B. Saunders.

Fowlow, B., Price, P., Fung T. (1995). Ambulation after sheath removal: a comparison of 6 and 8 hours of bed rest after sheath removal in patients following a PTCA procedure. *Heart and Lung, 24*(1), 28–37.

Goodkind, J., Coombs, V., Golobic, R.A. (1993).

Excimer laser angioplasty. *Heart and Lung, 22*(1), 26–35.

Gulanick, M., Naito, A. (1994). Patients' reactions to angioplasty: realistic or not? *American Journal of Critical Care, 3*(5), 368–373.

Miracle, V.A. (1992). Coronary atherectomy. *Critical Care Nurse, 12*(3), 41–48.

Shickel, S., Cronin, S.N., Mize, A., Voelker, C. (1996). Removal of femoral sheaths by registered nurses: issues and outcomes. *Critical Care Nurse, 16*(2), 32–36.

Topol, E.J., Leya, F., Pinkerton, C.A., Whitlow, P.L., Hofling, B., Simontin, C.A., et al. (1993). A comparison of directional atherectomy with coronary angioplasty in patients with coronary artery disease. *New England Journal of Medicine, 329*(4), 221–227.

Minimally Invasive Cardiac Surgery

Gross, S., Coleman, B., Flavell, C., Salamandra, J. (1996). Patients undergoing cardiothoracic surgery and transplants. In J.M. Clochesy, C. Breu, S. Cardin, A.A. Whittaker, E.B. Rudy (Eds.), *Critical care nursing* (2nd ed., pp. 458–512). Philadelphia: W.B. Saunders.

Mathias, J.M. (1996). New technique takes pain out of saphenous vein harvesting. *OR Manager, 12*(7), 16–17.

Mizell, J.L., Maglish, B., Matheny, R. (1997). Minimally invasive direct coronary artery bypass graft surgery. *Critical Care Nurse, 17*(3).

Myocardial Infarction

De Angelis, R. (1991). The cardiovascular system. In J.G. Alspach (Ed.), *Core curriculum for critical care nursing* (4th ed., pp. 132–314). Philadelphia: W.B. Saunders.

Reinhart, S.I. (1995). Uncomplicated acute myocardial infarction: a critical path. *Cardiovascular Nursing, 31*(1), 1–7.

Wilson, R.F. (1992). *Critical care manual: applied physiology and principles of therapy* (2nd ed.). Philadelphia: F.A. Davis.

Peripheral Vascular Disease

De Angelis, R. (1991). The cardiovascular system. In J.G. Alspach (Ed.), *Core curriculum for critical care nursing* (4th ed., pp. 132–314). Philadelphia: W.B. Saunders.

Hanssen, C.S. (1992). Assessing the extremities. *Nursing 92, 22*(8), 32C–32F.

Henderson, L.J., Kirkland, J.S. (1995). Angioplasty with stent placement in peripheral arterial occlusive disease. *AORN Journal, 61*(4), 671–685.

Parthum, J. (1996). Vascular emergencies. In J.M. Clochesy, C. Breu, S. Cardin, A.A. Whittaker, E.B. Rudy (Eds.), *Critical care nursing* (2nd ed., pp. 535–551). Philadelphia: W.B. Saunders.

Thrombolytic Therapy

Donnell, L. (1996). Complications of MI beyond the acute stage. *American Journal of Nursing,* September, pp. 25–31.

Magee, M. (1989). Nursing care of the patient receiving thrombolytic therapy. *Supplement to Journal of Emergency Nursing,* March/April, pp. 165–173. St. Louis: C.V. Mosby.

NIH. (1993). Emergency department: rapid identification and treatment of patients with acute myocardial infarction. Washington, D.C.: U.S. Department of Health and Human Services. National Heart, Lung, and Blood Institute. Pub. no. 93-3278.

Ondrusek, R. (1996). Spotting an MI before it's an MI. *RN,* April, pp. 26–29.

Ramsden, C. (1988). *Management of the acute myocardial infarction patient.* N.J.: Gardiner-Caldewell Synermed.

Valve Replacement

De Angelis, R. (1991). The cardiovascular system. In J.G. Alspach (Ed.), *Core curriculum for critical care nursing* (4th ed., pp. 132–314). Philadelphia: W.B. Saunders.

Goran, S.F. (1996). From counterpulsation to paralysis: a case presentation. *Critical Care Nurse, 16*(2), 54–57.

Gross, S., Coleman, B., Flavell, C., Salamandra, J. (1996). Patients undergoing cardiothoracic surgery and transplants. In J.M. Clochesy, C. Breu, S. Cardin, A.A. Whittaker, E.B. Rudy (Eds.), *Critical care nursing* (2nd ed., pp. 458–512). Philadelphia: W.B. Saunders.

Sanford, M.M. (1997). Rewarming cardiac surgery patients: warm water vs warm air. *American Journal of Critical Care, 6*(1), 39–45.

Schakenbach, L.H. (1996). Patients with valvular disease. In J.M. Clochesy, C. Breu, S. Cardin, A.A. Whittaker, E.B. Rudy (Eds.), *Critical care nursing* (2nd ed., pp. 428–457). Philadelphia: W.B. Saunders.

Thomson, S.C., Well, S., Maxwell, M. (1997). Chest tube removal after cardiac surgery. *Critical Care Nurse, 17*(1), 34–38.

Vascular Emergencies

Bruni, K.R., Hoosier-Paty, D.M., Hoffman, G.T. (1996). The quality of life of the limb threatened patient after lower extremity revascularization. *Journal of Vascular Nursing, 14*(4), 99–103.

DeAngellis, R. (1991). The cardiovascular system. In J.G. Alspach (Ed.), *Core curriculum for critical care nursing* (4th ed., pp. 132–314). Philadelphia: W.B. Saunders.

Edwards, R., Abullarade, C., Turnbull, N. (1996). Nursing management and follow-up of the postoperative vascular patient in a clinic setting. *Journal of Vascular Nursing, 14*(3), 62–67.

Fahey, V.A. (1995). Heparin-induced thrombocytopenia. *Journal of Vascular Nursing, 13*(4), 112–116.

Painter, L.M., Dudjak, L.A., Breiner, K., Langford, A. (1995). Abdominal aortic aneurysm pathway: outcome analysis. *Journal of Vascular Nursing, 13*(4), 101–105.

Parthum, J. (1996). Vascular emergenices. In J.M. Clochesy, C. Breu, S. Cardin, A.A. Whittaker, and E.B. Rudy (Eds.), *Critical care nursing* (2nd ed., pp. 535–552). Philadelphia: W.B. Saunders.

Chapter 2

Acute Respiratory Failure

Henneman, E.A. (1996). Patients with acute respiratory failure. In J.M. Clochesy, C. Breu, S. Cardin, A.A. Whittaker, E.B. Rudy (Eds.), *Critical care nursing* (2nd ed., pp. 630–648). Philadelphia: W.B. Saunders.

Adult Respiratory Distress Syndrome

Burns, S.M., Burns, J.E., Truwit, J.D. (1994). Comparison of five clinical weaning indices. *American Journal of Critical Care, 3,* 342–352.

Enger, E.L. (1996). Patients with adult respiratory distress syndrome. In J.M. Clochesy, C. Breu, S. Cardin, A.A. Whittaker, E.B. Rudy (Eds.), *Critical care nursing* (2nd ed., pp. 656–681). Philadelphia: W.B. Saunders.

Asthma

Janson-Bjerklie, S., Ferketech, S., Benner, P., Becker, G. (1992). Clinical markers of asthma severity and risk: importance of subjective as well as objective factors. *Heart and Lung, 21*(3), 265–272.

Miracle, V.A. (1994). Treating asthma in adults. *Perspectives in Respiratory Nursing, 5*(4), 1, 3–5.

National Asthma Education Program. (1991). *Executive summary: guidelines for the diagnosis and management of asthma.* Bethesda, Md.: U.S. Department of Health and Human Services.

Samuelson, W.M., Kapita, J.M. (1995). Management of the difficult asthmatic: gastroesophageal reflux, sinusitis, and pregnancy. *Respiratory Care Clinics of North America, 1*(2), 287–299.

Tasota, F.J. (1996). Patients with chronic obstructive pulmonary disease. In J.M. Clochesy, C. Breu, S. Cardin, A.A. Whittaker, E.B. Rudy (Eds.), *Critical care nursing* (2nd ed., pp. 601–619). Philadelphia: W.B. Saunders.

Wilmoth, D.F., Carpenter, R.M. (1996). Preventing complications of mechanical ventilation: permissive hypercapnia. *AACN Clinical Issues, 7*(4), 473–481.

Chronic Obstructive Pulmonary Disease

Dossey, B., Guzzetta, C., Kenner, C. (1992). Acute respiratory failure: the patient with chronic obstructive lung disease. C*ritical care nursing body-mind-spirit* (3rd ed., pp. 332–339). Philadelphia: J.B. Lippincott.

Tasota, F. (1996). Patients with chronic obstructive pulmonary disease. In J.M. Clochesy, C. Breu, S. Cardin, A.A. Whittaker, E.B. Rudy (Eds.), Critical care nursing (2nd ed., pp. 601–619). Philadelphia: W.B. Saunders.

Wimbush, F.B., Wright, J.E. (1993). Acute respiratory infection. In J.E. Wright and B.K. Shelton (Eds.), *Critical care nursing* (pp. 136–146). Boston: Jones and Bartlett.

Chronic Ventilator-Dependent Patients

Burns, S.M., Burns, J.E., Truwit, J.D. (1994). Comparison of five clinical weaning indices.

American Journal of Critical Care, 3, 342–352.

Wilson, D.J. (1996). Chronic ventilator dependent patients. In J.M. Clochesy, C. Breu, S. Cardin, A.A. Whittaker, E.B. Rudy (Eds.), *Critical care nursing* (2nd ed., pp. 689–705). Philadelphia: W.B. Saunders.

Lung Cancer

Acute Pain Management Guidelines Panel. (1992). *Acute pain management: operative or medical procedures and trauma.* Rockville, Md.: U.S. Department of Health and Human Services, Public Health Service, Agency for Health Care Policy and Research. AHCPR Pub. No. 92-0032.

American Pain Society. (1992). Principles of analgesia use in the treatment of acute pain and cancer pain. Skokie, Ill.

Brenner, Z.R., Addona, C. (1995). Caring for the pneumonectomy patient: challenges and changes. *Critical Care Nurse, 15*(5), 65–72.

Clark, J.C., McGee, R.F. (1988). *Core curriculum for oncology nursing.* Philadelphia: W.B. Saunders.

Howland, W.S., Graziano, C.C. (1985). *Critical care of the cancer patient.* Chicago: Year Book Medical.

Hudzinski, D.M. (1995). An algorithmic approach to cancer pain management. In D.J. Wilke (Ed.), *Nursing Clinics of North America, 30*(4), 711–723.

Jacox, A., Carr, D.B., Payne, R., et al. (1994). *Clinical practice guideline: management of cancer pain.* Rockville, Md.: U.S. Department of Health and Human Services, Public Health Service, Agency for Health Care Policy and Research. AHCPR Pub. No. 94-0592.

Neagley, S.R. (1991). The pulmonary system. In J.G. Alspach (Ed.), *Core curriculum for critical care nursing* (4th ed., pp. 1–131). Philadelphia: W.B. Saunders.

Niles, R. (1995). Pharmacologic management of cancer pain. In D.J. Wilke (Ed.), *Nursing Clinics of North America, 30*(4), 745–763.

Roth, J.A., Ruckdeschel, J.C., Weisenburger, T.H. (1989). *Thoracic oncology.* Philadelphia: W.B. Saunders.

Sebiston, D.C., Spencer, F.C. (1990). *Surgery of the chest* (Vol. 1, 3rd ed.). Philadelphia: W.B. Saunders.

Sloman, R. (1995). Relaxation and the relief of cancer pain. In D.J. Wilke (Ed.), *Nursing Clinics of North America, 30*(4), 679–709.

Lung Volume Reduction Surgery

American Thoracic Society (Medical Section of the American Lung Association). (1995). Standards for the diagnosis and care of patients with chronic obstructive pulmonary disease. *American Journal of Respiratory and Critical Care Medicine, 152*(5), S78–S121.

Casabari, R. (1993). *Principles and practice of pulmonary rehabilitation.* Philadelphia: W.B. Saunders.

Cooper, J.D., Patterson, G.A. (1996). Lung volume reduction surgery for severe emphysema. *Seminars in Thoracic and Cardiovascular Surgery, 8,* 52–60.

Emery, C.F., Leatherman, N.E., Burker, E.J.,

MacIntyre, N.R. (1991). Psychological outcomes of a pulmonary rehabilitation program. *Chest, 100*(3), 613–617.

Hodgelan, J. (1993). *Pulmonary rehabilitation.* Philadelphia: J.B. Lippincott.

Kersten, L. (1989). *Comprehensive respiratory care.* Philadelphia: W.B. Saunders.

Malen, J.F. (1992). Pulmonary rehabilitation of thoracic surgery patients. *Perspectives in Respiratory Nursing, 3*(4).

McGraw, L. (1997). Lung volume reduction surgery: an overview. *Heart and Lung, 26*(2), 131–138.

Miller, D. (1996). Personal communication.

Reis, A. (1995). Effects of pulmonary rehabilitation on physiologic and psychosocial outcomes on patients with COPD. *Annals of Internal Medicine, 122*(11), 823–832.

Szeleky, L. et al. (1997). Preoperative predictors of operative morbidity and mortality in COPD patients undergoing bilateral lung volume reduction surgery. *Chest, 111*(3), 550–558.

Pneumonia

Ryan, C.J. (1996). Pulmonary infections. In J.M. Clochesy, C. Breu, S. Cardin, A.A. Whittaker, E.B. Rudy (Eds.), *Critical care nursing* (2nd ed., pp. 620–629). Philadelphia: W.B. Saunders.

Wimbush, F.B., Wright, J.E. (1993). Acute respiratory infection. In J.E. Wright and B.K. Shelton (Eds.), *Critical care nursing* (pp. 136–146). Boston: Jones and Bartlett.

Pulmonary Embolism

Dossey, B., Guzzetta, C., Kenner, C. (1992). Acute respiratory failure: the patient with chronic obstructive lung disease. In *Critical care nursing body-mind-spirit* (3rd ed., pp. 367–385). Philadelphia: J.B. Lippincott.

Wimbush, F.B., Wright, J.E. (1993). Acute pulmonary embolism. In J.E. Wright and B.K. Shelton (Eds.), *Critical care nursing* (pp. 164–181). Boston: Jones and Bartlett.

Thoracic Surgery

Brooks-Brunn, J. (1997). Predictors of postoperative pulmonary complications following abdominal surgery. *Chest, 111*(3), 564-571.

Byes, J., Smyth, K. (1997). Effect of a music intervention on noise annoyance, heart rate, and blood pressure in cardiac surgery patients. *American Journal of Critical Care, 6*(3), 183-191.

Davidson, J. (1997). Thoracoscopy: nursing implications for optimal patient outcomes. *Dimensions of Critical Care Nursing, 16*(1), 20-28.

Finkelmeier, B. (1995). *Cardiothoracic surgical nursing.* Philadelphia: J.B. Lippincott.

Shields, T.W. (1994). *General thoracic surgery* (4th ed.). Baltimore: Williams & Wilkins.

Stannard, D., et al. (1996). Clinical judgement and management of postoperative pain in critical care patients. *American Journal of Critical Care, 5*(6), 433-441.

Vaca, K., Osterlock, J., Daake, C., Noedel, N. (1996). Nursing care of the thoracoscopic lung volume patient. *American Journal of Critical Care, 5,* 412–419.

Wilson, S.F., Thompson, J.M. (1990). *Respiratory disorders.* St. Louis: Mosby Year Book.

Chapter 3

Cirrhosis and Portal Hypertension

Briones, T.L. (1991). The gastrointestinal system. In J.G. Alspach (Ed.), *Core curriculum for critical care nursing* (4th ed., pp. 970–1007). Philadelphia: W.B. Saunders.

Kelso, L.A. (1994). Alcohol-related end-stage liver disease and transplantation: The debate continues. *AACN Clinical Issues in Critical Care Nursing, 5*(4), 501–506.

Siconolfi, L.A. (1995). Clarifying the complexity of liver function tests. *Nursing 95, 25*(5), 39–44.

Smith, S.L. (1996). Patients with liver dysfunction. In J.M. Clochesy, C. Breu, S. Cardin, A.A. Whittaker, E.B. Rudy (Eds.), *Critical care nursing* (2nd ed., pp. 1048–1085). Philadelphia: W.B. Saunders.

Gastrointestinal Bleeding

Ruppert, S.D., Englert, D.M. (1996). Patients with gastrointestinal bleeding. In J.M. Clochesy, C. Breu, S. Cardin, A.A. Whittaker, and E.B. Rudy (Eds.), *Critical care nursing* (2nd ed., pp. 1022–1047). Philadelphia: W.B. Saunders.

Pancreatitis

Briones, T.L. (1997). Caring for people with hepatic, biliary, and pancreatic disorders. In J. Luckmann (Ed.), *Saunders manual of nursing care* (pp. 1301–1348). Philadelphia: W.B. Saunders.

Hennessy, K. (1996). Patients with acute pancreatitis. In J.M. Clochesy, C. Breu, S. Cardin, A.A. Whittaker, E.B. Rudy (Eds.), *Critical care nursing* (2nd ed., pp. 1091–1104). Philadelphia: W.B. Saunders.

Kohn, C.L., Bronzenec, S., Foster, P.F. (1993). Nutritional support for the patient with pancreatobiliary disease. *Critical Care Nursing Clinics of North America, 5,* 37.

Krumberger, J.M. (1993). Acute pancreatitis. *Critical Care Nursing Clinics of North America, 5,* 185.

Chapter 4

Acute Head Injury

Acorn, S. (1995). Assisting families of head-injury survivors through a family support program. *Journal of Advanced Nursing, 21,* 872–877.

Kerr, M.E., Lovasik, D., Darby, J. (1995). Evaluating cerebral oxygenation using jugular venous oximetry in head injuries. *AACN Clinical Issues, 6*(1), 11–20.

Nikas, D.L. (1991). The neurologic system. In J.G. Alspach (Ed.), *Core curriculum for critical care nursing* (4th ed., pp. 315–471). Philadelphia: W.B. Saunders.

Zwimpfer, T.J., Moulton, R.J. (1993). Neurologic trauma concerns. *Critical Care Clinics, 9*(4), 727–739.

Acute Ischemic Stroke

Albers, G.W. (1996). Medical treatment for acute ischemic stroke. Unpublished manuscript. Stanford University Medical Center Stroke Center, Palo Alto, Calif.

Caplan, L.R. (1986). *Stroke: a clinical approach.* Stoneham, Mass.: Butterworth.

Clochesy, J.M. (1996). Patients with cerebral vascular disorders. In J.M. Clochesy, C. Breu, S. Cardin, A. Whittaker, E.B. Rudy (Eds.), *Critical care nursing* (2nd ed., pp. 781–802). Philadelphia: W.B. Saunders.

Frankel, M.R. (1996). The use of intravenous tissue plasminogen activator for acute ischemic stroke: questions and answers on the NINDS tPA Stroke Study. *The Neurologist, 2*(5), 254–262.

Gallo, B.M., Hudak, C.M. (1994). *Critical care nursing: a holistic approach.* Philadelphia: J.B. Lippincott.

Gillyatt, P., Husten, L. (1996). *Stroke: A Harvard Health Letter special report,* pp. 8–33. Boston: Harvard Medical School Health Publications Group.

Harvey, R., Green, D. (1996). Deep vein thrombosis and pulmonary embolism in stroke. *Topics in Stroke Rehabilitation, 3*(1), 54–70.

National Institute of Neurological Disorders and Stroke rt-PA Study Group. (1995). Tissue plasminogen activator for acute ischemic stroke. *New England Journal of Medicine, 333*(24), 1581–1587.

Guillain-Barré Syndrome

Nikas, D.L. (1991). The neurologic system. In J.G. Alspach (Ed.), *Core curriculum for critical care nursing* (4th ed., pp. 315–471). Philadelphia: W.B. Saunders.

Thompson, K.S. (1996). Patients with Guillain-Barré syndrome. In J.M. Clochesy, C. Breu, S. Cardin, A.A. Whittaker, E.B. Rudy (Eds.), *Critical care nursing* (2nd ed., pp. 831–845). Philadelphia: W.B. Saunders.

Villaire, M. (1995). ICU: from the patient's point of view. *Critical Care Nurse, 15*(1), 80–87.

Subarachnoid Hemorrhage

Campbell, V. (1991). Effects of controlled hyperoxygenation and endotracheal suctioning on intracranial pressure in head injured adults. *Applied Nursing Research, 4*(3), 138–140.

Carpenito, L. (1993). *Nursing diagnosis application to clinical practice.* Washington, D.C.: American Psychological Association.

Fuller, J., Schaller-Ayers, J. (1994). *Health assessment: a nursing approach.* Philadelphia: J.B. Lippincott.

Marshall, S., Marshall, L., Voss, H., Chesnut, R. (1990). Intracranial pressure monitoring. *Neuroscience critical care pathophysiology and patient management.* Philadelphia: W.B. Saunders.

Rusy, K. (1996). Rebleeding and vasospasm after subarachnoid hemorrhage: a critical care challenge. *Critical Care Nurse, 16*(1), 41–47.

Clochesy, J.M. (1996). Patients with cerebral vascular disorders. In J.M. Clochesy, C. Breu, S. Cardin, A.A. Whittaker, E.B. Rudy (Eds.), *Critical care nursing* (2nd ed., pp. 781–802). Philadelphia: W.B. Saunders.

Winkelman, C. (1994). Advances in managing increased intracranial pressure: a decade of selected research. *AACN Clinical Issues in Critical Care Nursing, 5*(1), 9–14.

Chapter 5

Acute Renal Failure

Whittaker, A.A. (1996). Patients with acute renal failure. In J.M. Clochesy, C. Breu, S. Cardin, A.A. Whittaker, E.B. Rudy (Eds.), *Critical care nursing* (2nd ed., pp. 926–941). Philadelphia: W.B. Saunders.

End-Stage Renal Disease/Kidney Transplantation

Albee, B., Beckman, N.J., Schell, H.M. (1996). Patients with end-stage renal disease. In J.M. Clochesy, C. Breu, S. Cardin, A.A. Whittaker, E.B. Rudy (Eds.), *Critical care nursing* (2nd ed., pp. 949–968). Philadelphia: W.B. Saunders.

Stark, J.L. (1991). The renal system. In J.G. Alspach (Ed.), *Core curriculum for critical care nursing* (4th ed., pp. 472–608). Philadelphia: W.B. Saunders.

Chapter 6

Adrenal Crisis

Brown, D. (1996). Patients with disorders of the neurohypophysis, thyroid, and adrenals. In J.M. Clochesy, C. Breu, S. Cardin, A.A. Whittaker, E.B. Rudy (Eds), *Critical care nursing* (2nd ed., pp. 1122–1130). Philadelphia: W.B. Saunders.

Gotch, P.M. (1991). The endocrine system. In J.G. Alspach (Ed.), *Core curriculum for critical care nursing* (4th ed., pp. 609–674). Philadelphia: W.B. Saunders.

Diabetic Ketoacidosis

Gotch, P.M. (1991). The endocrine system. In J.G. Alspach (Ed.), *Core curriculum for critical care nursing* (4th ed., pp. 609–674). Philadelphia: W.B. Saunders.

Guthrie, D.W. (1996). Patients with disorders of glucose metabolism. In J.M. Clochesy, C. Breu, S. Cardin, A.A. Whittaker, E.B. Rudy (Eds.), *Critical care nursing* (2nd ed., pp. 1107–1115). Philadelphia: W.B. Saunders.

Jones, T.L. (1994). From DKA to hyperglycemic hyperosmolar nonketotic syndrome: the spectrum of uncontrolled hyperglycemia in diabetes mellitus. *Critical Care Nursing Clinics of North America, 6*(4), 703–720.

VanBuskirk, M.C., Vanderbilt, D. (1995). Evaluating patient care by the use of a DKA CareMap in an intensive care unit setting. *Journal of Nursing Care Quarterly, 9*(3), 59–68.

Chapter 7

Acute Pain Management

Acute Pain Management Guidelines Panel. (1992). *Acute pain management: operative or medical procedures and trauma*. Rockville, Md.: U.S. Department of Health and Human Services, Public Health Service, Agency for Health Care Policy and Research. AHCPR Pub. No. 92-0032.

American Pain Society. (1992). *Principles of analgesic use in the treatment of acute pain and cancer pain*. Skokie, Ill.

Ferrell, B.R. (1995). The impact of pain on quality of life. In D.J. Wilke (Ed.), *Nursing Clinics of North America, 30*(4), 609–624.

Grant, M., Ferrell, B.R., Rivera, L.M., Lee, J. (1995). Unscheduled readmissions for uncontrolled symptoms. In D.J. Wilke (Ed.), *Nursing Clinics of North America, 30*(4), 673–682.

Meehan, D.A., McRae, M.E., Rourke, D.A., Eisenring, C., Inperial, F.A. (1995). Analgesic administration, pain intensity, and patient satisfaction in cardiac surgical patients. *American Journal of Critical Care, 4*(6), 435–442.

Reede, S. (1996). Patients with pain. In J.M. Clochesy, C. Breu, S. Cardin, A.A. Whitaker, E.B. Rudy (Eds.), *Critical care nursing* (2nd ed., pp. 1381–1412). Philadelphia: W.B. Saunders.

Chronic Pain Management

Ferrell, B.R. (1995). The impact of pain on quality of life. In D.J. Wilke (Ed.), *Nursing Clinics of North America, 30*(4), 609–624.

Grant, M., Ferrell, B.R., Rivera, L.M., Lee, J. (1995). Unscheduled readmissions for uncontrolled symptoms. In D.J. Wilke (Ed.), *Nursing Clinics of North America, 30*(4), 673–682.

Hudzinski, D.M. (1995). An algorithmic approach to cancer pain management. In D.J. Wilke (Ed.), *Nursing Clinics of North America, 30*(4), 711–723.

Jacox, A., Carr, D.B., Payne, R., et al. (1994). *Clinical practice guideline: management of cancer pain*. Rockville, Md.: U.S. Department of Health and Human Services, Public Health Service, Agency for Health Care Policy and Research. AHCPR Pub. No. 94-0592.

Niles, R. (1995). Pharmacologic management of cancer pain. In D.J. Wilke (Ed.), *Nursing Clinics of North America, 30*(4), 745–763.

Reede, S. (1996). Patients with pain. In J.M. Clochesy, C. Breu, S. Cardin, A.A. Whitaker, E.B. Rudy (Eds.), *Critical care nursing* (2nd ed., pp. 1381–1412). Philadelphia: W.B. Saunders.

Sloman, R. (1995). Relaxation and the relief of cancer pain. In D.J. Wilke (Ed.), *Nursing Clinics of North America, 30*(4), 679–709.

Burns

Bolinger, B. (1995). Burn care in the home. *Journal of WOCN, 22*(3), 122–127.

Caine, R.M. (1996). Patients with burns. In J.M. Clochesy, C. Breu, S. Cardin, A.A. Whittaker, E.B. Rudy (Eds.), *Critical care nursing* (2nd ed., pp. 1279–1303). Philadelphia: W.B. Saunders.

Richard, R.L., Staley, M.J. (1994). *Burn care and rehabilitation: principles and practice*. Philadelphia: F.A. Davis.

Disseminated Intravascular Coagulation

Dressler, D.K. (1996). Patients with coagulopathies. In J.M. Clochesy, C. Breu, S. Cardin, A.A. Whittaker, E.B. Rudy (Eds.), *Critical care nursing* (2nd ed., pp. 1147–1161). Philadelphia: W.B. Saunders.

Jennings, B.M. (1991). The hematologic system. In J.G. Alspach (Ed.), *Core curriculum for critical care nursing* (4th ed., pp. 675–748). Philadelphia: W.B. Saunders.

HIV

Centers for Disease Control. (1987). Public Health Service Guidelines for counseling and antibody testing to prevent HIV infection and AIDS. In *Mortality and Morbidity Weekly Report, 36*, 509–515.

Centers for Disease Control and Prevention. (1993). Recommendations for HIV testing services for inpatients and outpatients in acute care settings and technical guidance on HIV. In *Mortality and morbidity Weekly Report, 42*(RR-2), 1–17.

Minkoff, H.L., DeHovitz, J.A. (1991). Care of women infected with the Human Immunodeficiency virus. *Journal of American Medical Association, 266*(16), 2253–2258.

Muma, R., Lyons, B.A., Borucki, M.J., Pollard, R. (1994). *HIV manual for health care professionals.* Norwalk: Conn.: Appleton & Lange.

Obstetric Crises

Goff, K., Hull, B. (1996). Patients with obstetric crises. In J.M. Clochesy, C. Breu, S. Cardin, A.A. Whittaker, E.B. Rudy (Eds.), *Critical care nursing* (2nd ed., pp. 1458–1469). Philadelphia: W.B. Saunders.

Morgan, J. (1994). Nutrition and pregnancy: problems and solutions. *Nursing Times, 90*(46), 31–33.

Shuster, E.A. (1994). Seizures in pregnancy. *Emergency Medical Clinics of North America, 12*(4), 1013–1025.

Sepsis/Systemic Inflammatory Response Syndrome

Clochesy, J.M. (1996). Patients with systemic inflammatory response syndrome. In J.M. Clochesy, C. Breu, S. Cardin, A.A. Whittaker, E.B. Rudy (Eds.), *Critical care nursing* (2nd ed., pp. 1359–1370). Philadelphia: W.B. Saunders.

Hazinski, M.F. (1994). Mediator-specific therapies for the systemic inflammatory response syndrome, sepsis, severe sepsis, and septic shock. Present and future approaches. *Critical Care Nursing Clinics of North America, 6*(2), 309–319.

Secor, V.H. (1994). The inflammatory/immune response in critical illness. Role of the systemic inflammatory response syndrome. *Critical Care Nursing Clinics of North America, 6*(2), 251–264.

Shelton, B.K. (1994). Disorders of hemostasis in sepsis. *Critical Care Nursing Clinics of North America, 6*(2), 373–387.

Trauma

Bayley, E.W., Turcke, S.A. (1991). *A comprehensive curriculum for trauma nursing.* Boston: Jones and Bartlett.

Cardona, V.D., Hurn, P.D., Mason, P.B., Scanlon-Schilpp, A.M., Veise-Berry, S.W. (1988). *Trauma nursing: from resuscitation through rehabilitation.* Philadelphia: W.B. Saunders.

Klein, D.G. (1996). Patients with trauma. In J.M. Clochesy, C. Breu, S. Cardin, A.A. Whitaker, E.B. Rudy (Eds.), *Critical care nursing* (2nd ed., pp. 1335–1358). Philadelphia: W.B. Saunders.

Lanros, N.E. (1988). *Assessment & intervention in emergency nursing* (3rd ed.). Norwalk, Conn.: Appleton & Lange.

Mowad, L., Ruhle, D.C. (1988). *Handbook of emergency nursing: the nursing process approach.* Norwalk, Conn.: Appleton & Lange.

Rea, R., Bourg, P., Parker, J.G., Rushing, D. (1987). *Emergency nursing core curriculum* (3rd ed.). Philadelphia: W.B. Saunders.

Wirtz, K.M., La Favor, K.M., Ang, R. (1996). Managing chronic spinal cord injury: issues in critical care. *Critical Care Nurse, 16*(4), 24–35.

Normal Hemodynamic Values

Cardiac output	4–8 L/min
Cardiac index	2.5–4.0 L/min/m^2
Stroke volume	60–130 mL/beat
Stroke volume index	40–50 mL/beat/m^2
Mean arterial pressure	70–100 mmHg
Pulmonary artery (PA) pressure	15–25 mmHg systolic/8–15 mmHg diastolic
Mean PA pressure	10–15 mmHg
Pulmonary capillary wedge pressure (PCWP)	6–12 mmHg
Right atrial pressure (RAP) or central venous pressure (CVP)	2–8 mmHg
Right ventricular pressure	15–25 mmHg systolic/2–8 mmHg diastolic
Systemic vascular resistance (SVR)	800–1,300 dynes-sec/cm^5
Systemic vascular resistance index (SVRI)	1,970–2,390 dynes-sec/cm^5
Pulmonary vascular resistance (PVR)	150–250 dynes-sec/cm^5
Pulmonary vascular resistance index (PVRI)	160–280 dynes-sec/cm^5
Left ventricular stroke work	60–80 g/beat
Left ventricular stroke work index (LVSWI)	45–65 g/beat/m^2
Right ventricular stroke work	10–15 g/beat
Right ventricular stroke work index (RVSWI)	5–10 g/beat/m^2

Oxygenation Parameters

SaO_2	90–100%
SpO_2	92–100%
SvO_2	60–80%
a-A ratio	> 60%: normal
	25–60%: significant degree of intrapulmonary shunting
	< 25%: severe degree of intrapulmonary shunting
Hemoglobin	12–16 g/dL
Arterial oxygen content (CaO_2)	16–20 mL/dL
Oxygen transport	800–1,200 cc/min
Lactic acid	1–2 mEq/L

Arterial Blood Gases

pH	7.35–7.45
PCO_2	35–45 mmHg
PaO_2	80–100 mmHg (assuming sea level)
HCO_3^-	22–26 mEq/L
Base excess	−3– +3.0

Respiratory Parameters

Tidal volume (Vt)	2–5 cc/kg
Vital capacity (VC)	10–15 cc/kg
Minute ventilation (Ve)	6–10 L/min
Negative inspiratory force	> -20
Respiratory rate	< 30/min

Laboratory Values

Serum Chemistry (SMA-6, 7, 12, 18)

Sodium $(Na)^+$	135–145 mEq/L
Chloride $(Cl)^-$	98–106 mEq/L
Potassium $(K)^+$	3.5–5.0 mEq/L
Blood urea nitrogen (BUN)	12–25 mg/dL
Creatinine	0.5–1.2
Glucose	60–110 mg/dL
Serum osmolality	280–295 mOsm/kg
Calcium $(Ca)^{++}$	8.5–10.5 mg/dL (4.5–5.5 mEq/dL)
Phosphate $(PO_4)^{+++}$	3.0–4.5 mg/dL
Magnesium $(Mg)^{++}$	1.5–2.0 mEq/L
Albumin	3.5–4.0 g/dL
	2.8–3.5 g/dL: mild depletion
	2.9–2.7 g/dL: moderate depletion
	< 2.1 g/dL: severe depletion
Prealbumin	> 15 mg/dL
	10–15 mg/dL: mild depletion
	5–10 mg/dL: moderate depletion
	< 5 mg/dL: severe depletion
Bilirubin	0.2–0.9 mg/dL
Aspartate aminotransferase (AST)	40 units

Alanine aminotransferase (ALT)   45 units
Ammonia   11–35 Umol/L
Total cholesterol   120–200 mg/dl
Low density lipoprotein cholesterol (LDL)   < 130 mg/dL
High density lipoprotein cholesterol (HDL)   > 45 mg/dL

Urine chemistry

24 hour creatinine clearance   115–125 mL/min
Urine osmolality   50–1,200 mOsm/L
Urine electrolytes Na^+: 40–80 mEq/L
          K^+: 20–40 mEq/L
Urine specific gravity   1.010–1.030
Urine pH   4.6–6.0

Complete Blood Count

Hemoglobin   12–16 g/dl
Hematocrit   38–50%
Platelet count   150,000–450,000
White blood cell count   5,000–10,000
Differential:
          Segmented neutrophils   56% (1,800–7,800 mcg)
          Band neutrophils   3% (0–700 mcg)
          Eosinophils   2.7% (0–450 mcg)
          Basophils   0.3% (0–200 mcg)
          Lymphocytes   34% (1,000–4,800 mcg)
          Monocytes   4% (0–800 mcg)

Index